DILEMMAS IN THE MANAGEME
NEUROLOGICAL PATIENT

DILEMMAS IN THE MANAGEMENT OF THE NEUROLOGICAL PATIENT

Edited by

Charles Warlow BA, MB BChir, MD, FRCP
Clinical Reader in Neurology, University Department of Clinical Neurology, Radcliffe Infirmary, Oxford, UK

John Garfield MChir, FRCS, FRCP
Consultant Neurosurgeon, Wessex Neurological Centre, Southampton, UK

CHURCHILL LIVINGSTONE
EDINBURGH LONDON MELBOURNE AND NEW YORK 1984

CHURCHILL LIVINGSTONE
Medical Division of Longman Group Limited

Distributed in the United States of America by
Churchill Livingstone Inc., 1560 Broadway, New
York, N.Y. 10036, and by associated companies,
branches and representatives throughout the world.

First published 1984
  Reprinted 1985

ISBN 0-443-03551-2

British Library Cataloguing in Publication Data
Dilemmas in the management of the neurological
    patient.
    1. Nervous system —— diseases   2. Therapeutics
    I. Warlow, Charles   II. Garfield, John
    616.8′046   RC346

Library of Congress Cataloging in Publication Data
Dilemmas in the management of the neurological
patient.
    1. Nervous system —— Diseases —— Treatment
—— Addresses, essays, lectures. I. Warlow, Charles
P., 1942–   II. Garfield, John (John
Samuel) [DNLM: 1. Nervous system diseases ——
Therapy ——Congresses. WL 100 D576 1982]
RC349.8.D54 1983   616.8′046   83–7513

Printed in Great Britain by
Butler & Tanner Ltd, Frome and London

Contributors

John R. Bartlett MB BChir, FRCS
Consultant Neurosurgeon, Brook General Hospital, London, UK

L. D. Blumhardt MB ChB, FRACP
Senior Lecturer in Neurology, University of Liverpool, UK

Michael Briggs MB BS, FRCS
Consultant Neurosurgeon, Radcliffe Infirmary, Oxford, UK

David Chadwick MA, BM BCh, MRCP
Consultant Neurologist, Department of Neurology, Walton Hospital,
Liverpool, UK

David de Bono MD FRCP(Ed)
Consultant Cardiologist, Department of Cardiology, The Royal Infirmary,
Edinburgh, UK

J. B. Foster MB BS, FRCP
Consultant Neurologist, Newcastle General Hospital, Newcastle upon Tyne,
UK

John Garfield MChir, FRCS, FRCP
Consultant Neurosurgeon, Wessex Neurological Centre, Southampton, UK

Neil Gordon MB ChB, FRCP
Consultant Paediatric Neurologist, Booth Hall Children's Hospital,
Manchester, UK

Stephen J. Haines MD
Assistant Professor of Neurosurgery, University of Minnesota, Minneapolis,
Minnesota, USA

M. J. G. Harrison MA, BM BCh, FRCP
Consultant Neurologist, Department of Neurological Studies, Middlesex
Hospital, London, UK

D. Hilton-Jones MA, MB BChir, MRCP
Registrar in Neurology, Radcliffe Infirmary, Oxford, UK

Anthony Hopkins MD, FRCP
Physician in Charge, Department of Neurological Sciences, St Bartholomew's
Hospital, London, UK

Richard A. C. Hughes MD, FRCP
Consultant Neurologist, Guy's Hospital, London, UK

A. J. Lees MB BS, MRCP
Consultant Neurologist to the National Hospitals for Nervous Diseases,
University College Hospital and the Whittington Hospital, London, UK

Maurice Longson MB ChB
Professor of Virology, Consultant Virologist, North Manchester Regional
Virus Laboratory, Clinical Laboratories, Manchester Royal Infirmary,
Manchester, UK

A. P. Lonton
Department of Education, Manchester University, Manchester, UK

D. L. McLellan MA, MB, PhD, FRCP
Senior Lecturer in Neurology and Consultant Neurologist, University of
Southampton, UK

Klim McPherson
Lecturer in Medical Statistics, Department of Community Medicine and
General Practice, Radcliffe Infirmary, Oxford, UK

John Marshall MB ChB, FRCP
Professor of Neurology, National Hospitals for Nervous Diseases, London,
UK

W. B. Matthews DM, FRCP
Professor of Clinical Neurology, University of Oxford, Oxford, UK

J. Douglas Miller MD, PhD, FRCS(ed), FRCS(Glas), FACS, FRCP (Ed)
Professor of Surgical Neurology, University of Edinburgh, Edinburgh, UK

Pauline Monro MB BS, FRCP
Consultant Neurologist, St. George's Hospital and St James' Hospital,
London, UK

P. K. Newman MB ChB, MRCP
Consultant Neurologist, Regional Neurological Centre, Newcastle General
Hospital, Newcastle upon Tyne, UK

J. D. Pickard MB MChir, FRCS
Consultant Neurosurgeon, Wessex Neurological Centre, Southampton General
Hospital, Southampton, UK

Jonathan Punt FRCS
Senior Neurological Registrar, Wessex Neurological Centre, Southampton, UK

D. J. Read MA, DM, MRCP
Senior Medical Registrar, St James's University Hospital, Leeds, UK

Michael M. Sharr MB BS, MRCP, FRCS
Consultant Neurosurgeon, South East Thames Regional Neurosurgical Unit,
Brook General Hospital, London, UK

David Thrush MB BChir, MRCP
Consultant Neurologist, Department of Neurology, Freedom Fields Hospital,
Plymouth, UK

Contents

Introduction

There is no lack of dilemmas in patient management in medicine in general and, however much some neurologists and neurosurgeons pretend otherwise, medical and surgical neurology are not exceptional in this respect. The areas of controversy are usually quite easy to detect by noting the vaguer recommendations on treatment in undergraduate medical textbooks, the occasional flash of honestly admitted ignorance in review articles, conflicting data in original papers, and — most of all — by the informal comparison of methods of treatment used by different doctors for what appear to be the same conditions. Formal comparisons are, regrettably, rare.

Dilemmas owe their existence to inadequate data, or to the lack of methods to obtain or analyse data. Clinicians can usually do nothing about the latter, but we can improve on the former if, in the first place, we are prepared to admit our inadequacies. It is, of course, more comfortable to ignore controversial areas completely and merely use the 'recommended' treatment or procedure, a policy which unfortunately is nurtured in some teaching hospitals by the view that medical students should be told of the known, rather than of the unknown. We have, however, invited our contributors to take the more uncomfortable option, but the more interesting for those who question whether they are doing the best for their patients, and face some of the controversial areas of neurology and neurosurgery.

We have asked our contributors to review areas of controversy which trouble clinicians called on to manage patients, to try and identify why the controversies exist and what can be done to resolve them, and finally to define their current clinical practice. Not surprisingly, considering the individuality of neurologists and neurosurgeons, we have ended up with a variety of literary styles and scientific approaches which will not all appeal to all our readers. Nonetheless we hope that for every reader some chapters will be provocative and that clinicians will be encouraged to tackle some of the questions raised. Certainly the answer to some, or even most, of the problems are within our grasp if we are prepared to organize and to contribute to randomized controlled trials, to follow-up our patients and keep accurate records, to demand post-mortems, and to establish national registers of uncommon conditions. The causes of failure are not financial but a lack of motivation, and an inclination to 'muddle on'. To that is added the difficulty of persuading individuals to work together rather than against each other, and the lack of that most precious of all commodities to the hard-pressed clinician — time.

A note on how this book developed
Rather than simply ask our friends and colleagues to write a series of chapters on controversial issues, we thought we should try and educate ourselves and thus others by meeting together to discuss each topic in turn. This we did at Green College, Oxford, in May 1982, generously supported by Lipha Pharmaceuticals. Prior to the meeting each chapter author circulated an abstract of his views to all the other authors and ten minutes was allowed for the author to present his or her arguments verbally. A main discussant, who had previously been designated from one of the other chapter authors, then led the discussion that followed. In this way we hoped that the authors could introduce controversial ideas and provoke constructive criticism so they would then be able to write a better chapter. How effective this policy was cannot be answered without a randomized trial! However, the meeting was of considerable interest and we hope that the tone of informality and flavour of doubt has survived in print.

1. What does spinal cord stimulation offer the multiple sclerosis patient?

D. J. Read, W. B. Matthews

INTRODUCTION

'Each decade brings a new vogue in treatment and hopes of a cure are raised, only to be dashed when the new treatment is critically evaluated' was the editorial verdict on spinal cord stimulation in multiple sclerosis (MS) towards the end of its first decade of use (Anon, 1980a). The 'transistorised placebo' of the 1970s although novel, was not an original concept, and had in fact been preceded by much earlier attempts at electrical treatment of this chronic, incurable, neurological disease. In 1758 Brydone attempted, with apparently good results, the electrical cure of one Elizabeth Foster who, from the clinical description given, may well have had MS; and almost a century later La Beaume similarly electrified Sir Augustus D'Este, a grandson of George III and generally regarded as having kept the first diary of an MS sufferer (Firth, 1948), with rather less spectacular results:

> 'Electricity having been strongly recommended to me, on the 3rd of January and on the following two days it is administered to me by Mr La Beaume. If anything can be clear and apparent to a patient, it is clear and apparent to me that electricity is the most powerful agent to my injury instead of to my recovery'.

Based on the gate control therapy of pain of Melzack & Wall (1965), Shealy et al (1967) developed electrical stimulation of the spinal cord as a means of treating intractable pain, and in 1973 Cook and Weinstein published their observations on a patient who had both MS and intractable pain and who received spinal cord stimulation for the latter. She was not only relieved of the pain but was also, apparently, considerably improved neurologically, this purely chance observation leading to the subsequent development of spinal cord stimulation for the symptomatic treatment of patients with MS. It is unfortunate that in·the decade following this observation, the standard of most of the published work has done little to dispel the inheritance of over two centuries of medical disbelief in the therapeutic potential of judiciously applied electrical stimulation.

The application of 'the silent and invisible power of electricity' to the healing of bone fractures has also attracted some less than enthusiastic editorial comment

1

(Anonymous, 1980b) despite being able to draw on the world wide experience of more than 2000 orthopaedic surgeons and more than 3500 patients so treated (Bassett, 1980). The equivalent combined experience for MS involves probably no more than 600 patients of whom only 100 or so appear, from the published data, to have been carefully and objectively studied. This treatment is expensive, time consuming and exacting for both the physician and patient alike, and the potential user has to balance the enthusiastic and sweeping claims of some authors, based usually on large series of ill-defined cases documented poorly or not at all, against the much more cautious claims made by those authors whose publications show evidence of painstaking assessment, usually on relatively small numbers of patients. Guidance on what symptoms are likely to respond and in which patients is therefore difficult, based as it must be on such small numbers.

TECHNIQUE

The technique, which has been described in detail by Illis et al (1976), consists of the insertion, via hollow epidural needles, of two platinum tipped electrodes in the posterior thoracic epidural space, so that the tips lie one or two vertebral bodies apart and approximately in the mid-line. The final position of the electrodes is adjusted with the apparatus switched on in order to produce the stimulation sensation — pleasant warm paraesthesiae — in the trunk below the level of the electrodes and in one or both legs.

The procedure is carried out under local anaesthesia, as is the later subcutaneous implantation of the receiver. Continuous stimulation is applied to the spinal cord by means of an external pulse generator radio-coupled to the implanted receiver to which the distal ends of the electrodes are connected. There are no absolute electrical criteria for stimulation characteristics though a frequency of 33–50 Hz and a pulse width of 200–400 μs at the sensory threshold voltage (usually between 0.5 and 5 volts) is generally accepted. The pulses may or may not be of alternating polarity. There are a number of commercial systems available with similar and satisfactory electronic performance, the Achilles' heel of all systems being the electrodes.

In the early days, a fixed array of four to six electrodes was inserted at open laminectomy under general anaesthesia with all the risks and complications attending such a major procedure but with the advantage of a stable electrode position from which an appropriate combination could be chosen later by trial and error. The single long flexible electrodes now in use have exchanged this stability for the ease and lesser risks of percutaneous epidural insertion, but electrode slippage (and sometimes extrusion) with consequent loss of stimulator sensation and clinical effect remains the most troublesome and time consuming aspect of the procedure. Adjustment or re-insertion of new electrodes may have to be performed on more than one occasion before satisfactory function is obtained, though a multi-headed electrode currently under assessment may in future obviate this need, at least in part.

CLINICAL EXPERIENCE

Anecdotal evidence
The history of previous treatments for MS is such that the protagonists of any new therapy would do well to consider the experiences of Moxon (1875) who described the first clinical series of MS patients in this country over a century ago:

'The results of the treatment used in the forgoing cases will be seen from the reports to be most unsatisfactory; no approach to cure has been made. The patients, who, as a rule, are cheerful and thankful for what is done on their behalf, are apt to declare themselves generally rather better, so that the report of the clinical clerk putting down their answers may read like a statement of continual good progress towards recovery. But the general result has been that, after many months' stay in the hospital, the poor people are found to have grown steadily though slowly worse'.

The first MS patient treated with spinal cord stimulation (Cook & Weinstein, 1973) experienced what can only be described as a truly remarkable recovery which, unfortunately, has not proved to be repeatable in other hands. The patient was 55 years old at the time, had had MS for 35 years and could barely walk 3 or 4 yards with the aid of crutches. She was described as having a severe paraparesis, ataxia of all four limbs, dysarthria, dysphagia and sensory impairment of all four limbs. Spinal cord stimulation returned a full range of movement of nearly normal strength to the legs, abolished the ataxia, dysarthria and dysphagia and returned sensory function to near normal. It was stated that 'she could drive her car, walk, swim and even complete a tour of Europe that summer with dorsal column stimulation as her only aid'. At the time of publication the patient had been treated for a total of 21 months without relapse. The paper, which described four other patients, was anecdotal in style with little attempt at objective measurement, but the authors were sufficiently encouraged to conclude that 'chronic spinal cord stimulation produces a significant modification of abnormal neurologic signs and dysfunction in patients with MS'.

This enthusiastic conclusion continued to be supported wherever large numbers of patients were treated without attempts at detailed measurement of such objective neurological changes as can be quantified. Indeed, one paper (Dooley, 1977) stated that follow-up was in part conducted by telephone and postal questionnaire, from neither of which objective evidence could be expected. The majority of such papers emanate from the USA and most have appeared in the proceedings of two international symposia: the Sixth International Symposium on External Control of Human Extremities (1978), and the Third International Meeting on Spinal Cord Stimulation (1980). Overall, the second symposium added little to the first which has been reviewed elsewhere (Read et al, 1980). It is difficult to be certain of the precise number of patients treated as many of them probably appear in the published series more than once as part of a cumulative total in subsequent papers from the same centre, but a reasonable estimate would be about 500. Based on these patients, from whom conclusions unsupported by published objective data have been drawn, one might expect overall success rates varying from 60–100% with improvement in all areas of neurological dysfunction including visual disturbance, and one would be hard pressed to deny this revolutionary treatment to the large number of significantly disabled MS sufferers for whom depressingly little else can be done.

Objective evidence

There have been few centres where the effect of spinal cord stimulation on neurological disability appears to have been adequately assessed and the number of patients so studied totals no more than 100. With the exception of bladder dysfunction, which will be discussed separately, the picture which emerges is one of increasing pessimism paralleling increasing reliance on objective data rather than subjective impressions. It should be pointed out perhaps that any form of placebo controlled or cross-over trial is impossible. Stimulation sensation has to be introduced initially in order to place the electrodes accurately and thereafter it is difficult to convince the average patient that treatment is being given in the absence of the paraesthesiae so patiently striven for at electrode insertion. Moreover, ethical considerations forbid the insertion of deliberately non-functioning epidural foreign bodies. In addition to these difficulties, much that is claimed to improve is not susceptible to bias-free measurement, and the best that can be hoped for is 'blind' assessment, the difficulties of which are considerable, and so far this has been achieved, albeit partially, by only one author.

The first 'objective' papers appeared from the USA (Young & Goodman, 1979; Rosen & Barsoum, 1979), the 23 patients studied by the former authors being rather better assessed than the 9 of the latter. Neither found any objective improvement in motor, sensory or cerebellar function though 30% of each patient group claimed subjective improvement. Both sets of authors agreed in being unable to support the further use of spinal cord stimulation in the symptomatic treatment of MS, though neither of them studied bladder function. Ketelaer et al (1979) working in Belgium, reported 11 patients, assessed on two independent disability scoring scales. Functionally useful changes were seen in only 2 of the patients both of whom were only mildly disabled at the start, but who nevertheless provided support for the verdict of cautious approval. In this series subjective improvement was claimed by 6 of the 11 patients.

The Southampton group initially reported on 19 patients, assessing the response of motor function using the Kurtzke disability scale. They observed improvement in motor function in 5, sensory function in 5, and ataxia in 1, though only 2 patients improved by more than 1 grade (1 each in the motor and sensory group). In a later publication (Tallis et al, 1982) a quantitative estimation of the response of motor function to spinal cord stimulation was reported. The majority of the 23 patients referred to in this later study had been included in the earlier studies. Although 14 out of the 23 patients reported subjective improvement in some aspect of motor function, no significant improvement in walking speed, Tourtellotte (1965) tests or timed activities of daily living could be detected. They concluded that spinal cord stimulation did not have a major beneficial effect on the motor symptoms of multiple sclerosis. Hawkes et al (1980) used a formidable battery of tests on the 19 patients reported and were unable to convince themselves that the improvement in moblility and strength seen in 8 of the patients was due to anything other than motivation and practice. Using similar quantitative measurements this was also our conclusion (Read et al, al, 1980); in some patients 'blindly' assessed video tapes indicated a deleterious effect of spinal cord stimulation on walking. Of the 15 patients studied, however, 6 experienced a marked and sustained reduction in lower limb spasticity previously only described in traumatic paraplegic patients (Richardson et al, 1979). Twelve of these patients claimed significant improvement.

Although necessarily anecdotal, there are recorded a sufficient number of patients with 'central' pain who have experienced marked (usually complete) relief to warrant mention in this section. Also worthy of note is the high rate of subjective improvement in all the papers in which this is stated.

Bladder dysfunction
Only one beneficial therapeutic effect of spinal cord stimulation in MS is mentioned in practically every paper on this subject — that on the urinary bladder. Symptomatic relief, often marked, has been reported in urgency, hesitancy, frequency, poor stream, retention and even frank incontinence. There has, however, been little attempt at documenting these changes and six papers only need be considered. Abbate et al (1977) and Dooley et al (1978) performed limited tests and although the hard data is lacking from their publications it can be inferred that beneficial effects were produced in up to 75% of their 78 patients, supported by claims of changes towards the normal of some previously abnormal urodynamic variables.

The most complete published studies are those of Illis et al (1980), Hawkes et al (1980, 1981), and Read et al (1980) containing a total of 60 patients, to which has been added a further 9 in a forthcoming comprehensive review (Read et al, 1983). Symptomatic improvement occurred in 50-60% of patients treated, with some reduction in frequency, abolition of continuous or episodic incontinence in a small number (17) and significant improvement in urinary flow rates shown to be due to reduction in urethral closure pressure and relaxation of the urethral sphincter. Infrequent but definite reduction of bladder dyssynergia was seen in 5 patients as was reduction in detrusor instabilitiy in a larger number (13) which may explain the symptomatic improvement in urgency and frequency. These measured changes in bladder function provide the most compelling evidence that spinal cord stimulation produces a genuine therapeutic effect independent of any underlying placebo response.

CURRENT PRACTICE

Who should do it?
At present, spinal cord stimulation can only be regarded as being in a developmental stage with many problems to be overcome before it is offered as an established treatment other than on a purely research basis. Apart from the technical problems surrounding electrode design, yet to be fully explored are: different electrical parameters such as pulse width, polarity, frequency and duration of stimulation; optimal cord level; possible effect on progression of disease; and relation of effect to presence of plaques if known. On a broader

front the difficulties of disentangling failure of effect from natural progression of disease would have to be investigated with regard to the cost, time and hospital facilities that carefully studied large numbers implies, though it seems unlikely that this will ever be a practical proposition. All these factors argue in favour of keeping the expertise localised in a relatively small number of interested referral centres where experience can be concentrated and where the necessary equipment and skill required in assessing the response can be developed. There is no place for the sporadic amateur, 'let's give it a try' approach. One factor which should be considered however is the expense of the apparatus (at present a major obstacle in the way of more widespread use) which is unlikely to fall significantly unless the demand is sufficiently great — a troublesome dilemma.

For what and to whom should it be done?
Spinal cord stimulation is not a panacea for the ills of MS and with our present knowledge it seems reasonable to limit the majority of therapeutic efforts to disorders of bladder function as being the only system commonly affected in MS for which unequivocal evidence of stimulation associated benefit exists. There is at present no means of predicting patients likely to respond and no alternative to a period of trial stimulation before and during which full urodynamic assessment is mandatory. Only on rigorous objective criteria can the relatively few patients who will benefit, some markedly, be separated from the majority who will otherwise acquire an expensive electronic placebo. Two other symptoms are probably worth considering for a trial of treatment — the presence of 'central' pain for which excellent results, at least in the short term, have been reported from many centres including all three in the UK and secondly, severe lower limb spasticity or nocturnal flexor spasms in both of which good results have been claimed (Read et al, 1980). It is likely, given the common occurrence of symptoms (Miller et al, 1965) that both these categories of patients will also have bladder dysfunction thus providing documented justification for such a trial.

Although not an absolute bar to a trial of spinal cord stimulation, it is the experience of most workers in this field (see especially Illis et al, 1980) that disability sufficiently severe to confine the patient to a wheelchair is generally associated with little or no clinical response to spinal cord stimulation. One possible exception to this is that if the major cause of immobility is severe, lower limb spasticity then mobility (as well as bladder function) may improve (Read et al, 1980), though this has not been reproduced in other centres. Accordingly, attention should probably be directed mainly to the ambulant patient. The problem of what to do with the patient who claims significant subjective improvement in the absence of any objective evidence that this is so (and occasionally in the face of evidence of frank deterioration) is not one for which an easy solution exists. Individual cases have to be dealt with in whatever fashion seems appropriate, balancing the morale-depressing consequences of denying apparently effective treatment against the objective inability to justify the tying up of expensive apparatus better employed elsewhere. The decision is never easy and it is perhaps kinder to let the patient discover for himself that the treatment is not as wonderful as he first imagined, possibly after a second but delayed temporary trial before the receiver is subcutaneously implanted.

CONCLUSION

From this brief survey it can be seen that the initial all-embracing enthusiasm for the symptomatic effects of spinal cord stimulation in MS was based on insubstantial supporting evidence and that later and more critical examination has swung opinion in the other direction. Spinal cord stimulation does not offer much to the majority of MS patients, though it would be a mistake to dismiss it out of hand as an expensive electronic placebo without recognising its limited therapeutic potential especially with regard to the urinary bladder. Bladder problems in MS are the commonest cause of admission to long-term care institutions and consequent renal complications are the commonest cause of death in this group (Jameson, 1977). Any treatment which offers the possibility of reducing this morbidity should therefore be given a fair trial whatever the difficulties.

The anonymous leader writer quoted at the beginning of this chapter was merely re-stating the typical time course of all new treatments, especially electrical, expounded by H. L. Jones at the end of the last century:

'As each fresh important discovery in electrical science has been reached men's minds have been turned anew to the subject, and interest in its therapeutic properities have been stimulated. Then, after extravagant hopes and promises of cure, there have followed failures and disappointments, which have thrown the employment of this agent into disrepute, to be again after a time revived and brought into popular favour'.

(Jones, 1895)

It is to be hoped that spinal cord stimulation will eventually find its own level and become a useful adjunct in the management of at least one of the distressing symptoms of MS.

REFERENCES

Abbate A, Cook A W, Attallah M 1977 Effect of electrical stimulation of the thoracic spinal cord on the function of the bladder in multiple sclerosis. Journal of Urology 117: 285–288
Anonymous 1980a Dorsal column stimulation in multiple sclerosis. British Medical Journal i: 1287–1288
Anonymous 1980b Electricity and bones. British Medical Journal ii: 470–471
Bassett C A L 1980 Electricity and bones. British Medical Journal ii: 1428
Brydone P 1758 An instance of the electrical virtue in the cure of a palsy. Philosophical Transactions 50: 392–395
Cook A W, Weinstein S P 1973 Chronic dorsal column stimulation in multiple sclerosis. New York State Journal of Medicine 73: 2868–2872
Dooley D M 1977 Demyelinating degenerative and vascular disease. Neurosurgery 1: 214–225
Dooley D M, Sharkey J, Keller W, Kasprak M 1978 Treatment of demyelinating and degenerative diseases by electrostimulation of the spinal cord. In: Proceedings of the 6th International Symposium on External Control of Human Extremities, Belgrade: Yugoslav Committee for Electronics and Automation 529–544
Firth D 1948 The case of Augustus D'Este, Cambridge
Hawkes C H, Desmond A, Bultitude M I, Kanegaonakar G S 1980 Stimulation of dorsal column in multiple sclerosis. British Medical Journal i: 889–891
Hawkes C H, Fawcett D, Cooke E D, Emson P C, Paul E A, Bowcock S A 1981 Dorsal column stimulation in multiple sclerosis: effects on bladder, leg blood flow and peptides. Applied Neurophysiology 44: 62–70
Illis L S, Sedgwick E M, Oygar A E, Sabbahi Awaddalla M A 1976 Dorsal column stimulation in the rehabilitation of patients with multiple sclerosis. Lancet i: 1383–1386

Illis L S, Sedgwick E M, Oygar A E 1980 Spinal cord stimulation in multiple sclerosis: clinical results. Journal of Neurology, Neurosurgery and Psychiatry 43: 1–14

Jameson R M 1977 Multiple sclerosis and the urinary tract. Practitioner 218: 91–96

Jones H L 1895 Medical electricity, 2nd edn, London

Ketelaer P, Swartenbroekx P, Deltenre H, Carton H, Gybels J 1979 Perutaneous epidural dorsal cord stimulation in multiple sclerosis. Acta Neurochirugica 49: 95–101

Melzack R, Wall P D 1965 Pain mechanisms: a new theory. Science 150: 971–979

Miller H, Simpson C A, Yeates W K 1965 Bladder dysfunction in multiple sclerosis British Medical Journal: 1265–1269

Moxon W 1895 Eight cases of insular sclerosis of the brain and spinal cord. Guy's Hospital Reports 20: 437–478

Read D J, Matthews W B, Higson R H 1980 The effect of spinal cord stimulation on function in patients with multiple sclerosis. Brain 103: 803–833

Read D J, Tallis R C, Illis L S, Sedgewick E M 1983 Occasional review: spinal cord stimulation in the United Kingdom. Journal of Neurology, Neurosurgery and Psychiatry (in press)

Richardson R R, Cerullo L J, McLane D G, Gutierrex F A, Lewis V 1979 Percutaneous epidural neurostimulation in modulation of paraplegic spasticity. Acta Neurochirurgica 49: 235–243

Rosen J A and Barsoum A H 1979 Failure of chronic dorsal column stimulation in multiple sclerosis, Annals of Neurology 6: 66–67

Shealey C N, Mortimer J T, Reswick J B 1967 Electrical inhibition of pain by stimulation of the dorsal colums. Anaesthesia and Analgesia Current Research 46: 489–491

Sixth International Symposium on External Control of Human Extremities 1978 Yugoslav Committee for Electronics and Automation, Belgrade

Tallis R C, Illis L S, Sedgewick E M 1982 The quantitative assessment of the influence of spinal cord stimulation on motor function in patients with multiple sclerosis. International Rehabilitation Medicine (in press)

Third International Meeting on Spinal Cord Stimulation 1980 Proceedings published in Applied Neurophysiology 1981, 44

Tourtellotte W W, Haerer A F, Simpson J F 1965 Quantitative clinical neurological testing. Annals of the New York Academy of Sciences 122: 480–505

Young R F, Goodman S J 1979 Dorsal spinal cord stimulation in the treatment of multiple sclerosis 1979. Neurosurgery 5: 225–230

2. Does manipulation of the immune system help in multiple sclerosis?

Richard A. C. Hughes

INTRODUCTION

Some current therapeutic endeavours in multiple sclerosis (MS) are directed towards immunosuppression, others towards immunostimulation. Success has been claimed for each approach (Basten et al, 1980; Patzold & Pocklington, 1980). The paradox is explained by the opposing hypotheses that MS is due to abnormally increased immunity, probably to a myelin antigen, or to diminished immunity probably to a virus. Either hypothesis provides the prospect of controlling the inflammation which is at least partly responsible for the demyelination in MS.

Unfortunately not many therapeutic trials have used large enough numbers of patients or long enough periods of observation to have a reasonable chance of detecting even major changes in the clinical course of the disease (Brown et al, 1979). Many authors have compared the clinical course of individual patients before and after entry to a trial. This approach is always affected by the tendency for the relapse frequency to fall with passage of time regardless of treatment. Although reliance has often been placed on relapse frequency, a persistent increase in disability seems to me a more important criterion of the progress of MS. The number of patients required in order to detect a one grade difference in change on an 11 point disability scale (Kurtzke, 1965) at the end of 15 months are soberingly large. One hundred and fifty patients would be needed, half in the control and half in the treatment group, to have a 95% chance of detecting such a difference at the $P < 0.05$ significance level. Few of the trials to be reviewed approach this size.

EVIDENCE FOR AUTOIMMUNITY

The main evidence that MS is an autoimmune disease lies in its similarity to chronic relapsing experimental allergic encephalomyelitis (Wisniewski et al, 1982). The weakness of the autoimmune hypothesis has been the lack of satisfactory evidence for humoral or cell-mediated immune responses to myelin antigens in MS. In particular, conventional tests for antibody and cell-mediated immunity to myelin basic protein, the antigen responsible for the acute form of

9

EAE, have given results which were either negative or did not differ from those in patients with other neurological diseases (Hughes et al, 1982; Iivainen, 1981). According to unconfirmed reports antibodies to myelin basic protein can be detected in the cerebrospinal fluid (c.s.f.) and serum of patients with active MS with ultra-sensitive methods and also tests for antibody-dependent cell-mediated cytotoxicity (Frick & Stickl, 1982; Iivainen, 1981).

Most of the many reports of immune responses to myelin components other than myelin basic protein have also been disputed (Iivainen, 1981) and any responses which become established as real might be a secondary effect. A particularly important observation is that MS serum has a myelinotoxic effect on myelinated tissue cultures. The importance of this factor must now be doubted since the effect is not unique to MS serum. Furthermore, it is not due to immunoglobulin but to some other unidentified, and possibly non-specific, factor (Iqbal & Bornstein, 1980). The evidence that MS is an autoimmune disease has scanty clinical immunological support but the similarity to chronic relapsing EAE alone justifies trials of immunosuppression.

IMMUNOSUPPRESSION

ACTH and steroids

Acute relapses were the subject of a decade of conflicting anecdotal reports about the results of steroid treatment. Finally, in a small British controlled trial more of the 22 patients treated with ACTH were judged to have responded than of the 18 control patients (Miller et al, 1961). This conclusion was supported by a large American cooperative trial in which 103 patients were randomised to treatment with ACTH 80 units daily for a week, 40 units daily for 4 days and 20 units daily for 3 days and a similar number to placebo injections (Rose et al, 1970). The ACTH group fared slightly better during the month of observation. The major analysis compared the improvement of the patients on the Kurtzke (1965) scale. By the end of 4 weeks 65% of the ACTH treated patients had improved at least 1 point on this scale compared with only 48% of the control patients ($P < 0.05$). In acute retrobulbar neuritis an ACTH group recovered visual acuity more rapidly than the controls in one trial (Rawson & Liversedge, 1969) but not in another (Bowden et al, 1974).

Neurologists have been extraordinarily conservative in continuing to use ACTH in the management of MS while physicians in other branches of medicine have adopted oral steroids. This is unfortunate because there is no satisfactory evidence that ACTH exerts its immunological effects by any means other than stimulating the output of adrenal corticosteroids. The responses of different individuals to ACTH are variable. In one report the responses of MS patients were reduced compared with normal subjects (Maida & Summer, 1979). There have been no satisfactory controlled trials of oral steroids in the management of acute relapses. Anecdotal reports of benefit from medium and high dose steroid treatment are difficult to evaluate. There is an urgent need for a properly controlled comparison of ACTH with low and high dose prednisolone in the treatment of acute MS relapse. Two such trials are in progress in the United Kingdom.

10

Trials of chronic treatment with ACTH and/or steroids have failed to demonstrate any benefit. In an extremely well-conducted three-centre study Millar et al (1967) randomly allocated 181 patients to ACTH and 169 to non-steroid treatment. The dose of ACTH was adjusted between 15 and 25 units per 24 h to produce slight mooning of the face and so it could not be a blind study. Both groups deteriorated an average of 0·2 units on the Kurtzke disability scale by the end of 18 months and experienced about 0·74 relapses per patient year. Tourtellotte & Haerer (1965) randomised 38 patients to 8–12 mg methylprednisolone per 24 h and the same number to cyanocobalamin. Allegedly blind assessments revealed that after 18 months there was no significant difference between the groups in the relapse rate (0·39 per year on methylprednisolone, 0·51 on cyanocobalamin) or amount of deterioration on the Kurtzke disability scale. These controlled trials support the conclusion from large uncontrolled series that neither long-term ACTH nor steroids prevent the deterioration of patients with MS. The message to clinical neurologists is clear: there is no reason to add the disfiguring burden of iatrogenic Cushing's syndrome to MS.

The use of local, that is intrathecal steroids, might seem an attractive alternative but has been abandoned because of several reports of resultant arachnoiditis (Ellison & Myers, 1980).

Azathioprine
Azathioprine, an imidazole derivative of 6-mercaptopurine, is metabolised in the liver to 6-mercaptopurine itself and exerts its immunosuppressive effect by inhibiting the DNA synthesis of actively proliferating cells. It is not a particularly powerful agent but, in a chronic disease such as MS, has the advantage of being relatively non-toxic. Although usually well tolerated, azathioprine may cause gastrointestinal complaints, derangement of liver function and of course increased risk of infection. Teratogenicity and increased risk of cancer are theoretical risks which have to be considered in long-term treatment, although neoplasms have not proved a problem except in patients with renal transplants also being treated with steroids (Ellison & Myers, 1980).

Several uncontrolled trials of azathioprine in MS (reviewed by Ellison & Myers, 1978, 1980) have claimed reduction of the progression or relapse rate. The four available controlled trials, each with different merits and drawbacks, deserve individual mention. In the first controlled trial, an open study, 19 male patients were treated with azathioprine 2.5 mg/kg per 24 h and 24 with placebo for 2 years (Swinburn & Liversedge, 1973): no benefit was found but the study was too small to show anything other than a dramatic effect. Rosen (1979) performed a small controlled trial of azathioprine on women with the progressive stage of MS in his private practice. Assessments were not blind but the dose was more closely adjusted than in other trials to maintain the white cell count at about $3500/\mu l$ and continued for longer (at least 3 and average 4·5 years). Only 2 of 22 treated patients came to need a wheelchair in that time compared with 13 of 22 untreated patients. In a larger controlled but, again, unfortunately not 'blind' study 56 patients were treated with azathioprine 2 mg/kg per 24 h for an average of 2 years and 51 with control treatment which consisted of either levamisole or polyunsaturated fatty acids (Patzold & Pocklington, 1980). The neurological deficit of each patient was assessed every 4–8 weeks by one observer and each group of signs was combined into a single numerical scale. The rate of deterioration on this scale was less in the group treated with azathioprine than in the control group: this effect was attributable to slowing in the course of the disease of those who had been affected for less than 2 years. Patients who had been affected for longer did not benefit. These results have to be interpreted with caution since the randomisation process chanced not to provide evenly matched groups. At entry to the trial those treated with azathioprine had more severe disease and had been ill for longer than the controls. Since the azathioprine patients had more severe disease at entry they had less far to deteriorate which could have influenced the outcome of the trial in the direction observed.

Finally, in a small double-blind trial in London 43 patients were randomised to treatment with azathioprine 3 mg/kg and also antilymphocyte globulin and prednisolone for 1 month followed by azathioprine alone for 14 months, or to placebo (Mertin et al, 1982). There were no significant differences between the groups in the relapse rate or change in the Kurtzke disability score at the end of the period. Nevertheless there was a trend for the immunosuppressed patients to have less relapses and show less deterioration in their disability scores.

The evidence from the uncontrolled trials and these small controlled trials is that azathioprine does not prevent progression of MS but does not cause unacceptable side-effects. It may cause a moderate slowing of the course of the disease. Such slowing of the course should be detected by one of the large controlled trials in progress, one of steroids and azathioprine in Los Angeles and one of azathioprine alone in the United Kingdom.

Cyclophosphamide

Neurologists have been cautious about using immunosuppressive agents other than azathioprine. There are several reports of cyclophosphamide being used in short courses in small groups of patients with variable results (Ellison & Myers, 1978). It was the first immunosuppressive drug other than steroids to be used in MS (Aimard et al, 1966). It is an alkylating agent which cross-links complementary DNA strands and, unlike azathioprine, is active on both resting and dividing cells. It is a powerful and rapidly acting immunosuppressive agent, probably more effective on B than T lymphocytes. In some experimental situations it inhibits the action of suppressor T cells more than helper T cells and may therefore lead to an increase rather than decrease of some immune reactions. In clinical medicine it is used at doses which are cytotoxic to many bone marrow cells so that this paradoxical stimulation of immune reactions has not become a problem. In addition to gastrointestinal disturbances and bone marrow depression, cyclophosphamide produces some individual side-effects — alopecia, haemorrhagic cystitis, testicular atrophy and azoospermia.

In the largest trial (Gonsette et al, 1977) 110 patients were given a 2 week course of intravenous cyclophosphamide and followed for between 2 and 6 years. The dose was adjusted to maintain a leucopenia of $2000/\mu l$ and lymphopenia of $1000/\mu l$ for between 2 and 3 weeks. There was a reduction in the annual relapse rate: for instance 40 patients, who had had symptoms for between 4 and 6 years at entry, had an annual relapse rate of 0·80 before and 0·35 after treatment. Furthermore 67% of patients stabilised for 2 years following treatment. In another study a course of 8 g cyclophosphamide with prednisolone over about 4 weeks was considered to arrest the deterioration of 27 of 39 patients with chronic progressive MS (Hommes et al, 1980). On the other hand 21 patients treated with a similar short course of cyclophosphamide progressed at the same rate as 21 retrospectively matched patients not so treated (Theys et al, 1981). Some of the patients analysed by Theys et al (1981) had been included in the study of Gonsette et al (1977) who reached the opposite conclusion. This sort of controversy will remain unanswerable without resort to proper prospective randomised controlled trials. Whether a drug as toxic as cyclophosphamide is suitable for large scale controlled trials in a condition as chronic as MS is a legitimate subject for dispute.

Antilymphocyte serum
Antilymphocyte serum raised by immunising animals with human lymphocytes has been applied to many potentially immune-mediated diseases in the hope of suppressing the immune system without the harmful effects of cytotoxic immunosuppressive agents on irrelevant tissues. Antilymphocyte serum is effective in preventing and treating EAE. In MS several small trials with and without other immunosuppressive agents were conducted during the seventies. The largest controlled trial was the London trial of antilymphocyte globulin, prednisolone and azathioprine (Mertin et al, 1982) to which reference has already been made. During the first month of the 15 months of azathioprine treatment 15 infusions of antihuman lymphocyte globulin were given. This trial showed a non-significant reduction in relapse rate and slowing of disease progression in the treated group. If this effect was indeed due to treatment the antilymphocyte globulin may have contributed. In a small controlled trial of antilymphocyte globulin and ACTH 10 patients improved significantly more than 10 patients treated with ACTH alone. The improvement was maintained for a year but after 5 years there was no difference between the groups (Kastrukoff et al, 1978). The results from the available controlled trials and anecdotal reports are not particularly encouraging and the hazards of anaphylaxis with foreign protein treatment make continued use of antilymphocyte serum unlikely.

Plasma exchange
The addition of plasma exchange to other forms of immunosuppression has been claimed beneficial in several anecdotal reports. These are as difficult to evaluate as any other uncontrolled trial in MS. In the absence of controlled trials or any convincing evidence for circulating myelinotoxic factors specific for MS the use of plasma exchange will remain speculative (Van den Noort & Waksman, 1980).

Myelin basic protein
Since EAE can be prevented or treated by administering the causative antigen, myelin basic protein, in incomplete Freund's adjuvant (i.e. without killed Mycobacterium), this substance has been used to treat MS patients in three small trials. The results have been inconclusive. The treatment has great theoretical

interest but many practical difficulties including the hazard of developing acute EAE as happens with injections containing nervous tissue such as some rabies vaccines and brain tumour emulsions used in the immunotherapy of cerebral gliomas. There is also the problem of giving sufficient basic protein: Alvord et al (1979), who reviewed the relevant literature, calculated that the doses used in these trials were one thousand-fold too small by comparison with the amounts required to suppress EAE in guinea-pigs.

Prevention, and to some extent treatment of EAE, can be achieved by administering synthetic analogues of the encephalitogenic determinants of myelin basic protein which have been altered sufficiently from the native sequence that they are not themselves encephalitogenic. In pursuit of this idea a few individual patients with MS have been treated with a copolymer of alanine, glutamic acid, lysine and tyrosine, which has a molecular weight of 23 000 and the nickname Cop-1 (Bornstein et al, 1982). This material will suppress EAE in guinea-pigs and rabbits. It has not been found to suppress immune responses other than those to myelin basic protein. Cop-1 has obvious theoretical advantages over myelin basic protein and generalised immunosuppressant treatment and is being submitted to a randomised controlled trial in the United States.

EVIDENCE FOR IMMUNODEFICIENCY IN MS

Trials of immunostimulant treatment in MS are predicated on the hypothesis that the disease is due to a virus infection against which the immune response is deficient. The idea is attractive since several experimental models of chronic virus infection causing chronic CNS disease are known but much of the clinical evidence points in the opposite direction. There is no evidence of increased liability to infection in MS. Circulating and intrathecal humoral immune responses to measles and other viruses seem to be increased rather than decreased. On the other hand cell-mediated responses to measles, and possibly some other viruses, are decreased (Iivainen, 1981). The peripheral blood T cell subpopulation bearing the phenotype of suppressor cells is reduced at the time of relapses. While this reduction could be interpreted as a subtle form of immunodeficiency, its functional significance remains uncertain.

TREATMENT OF MULTIPLE SCLEROSIS WITH IMMUNOSTIMULANTS

Transfer factor

Transfer factor is a dialysable extract of leucocytes which is capable of transferring antigen-specific immunity to a naive recipient. The donor must be highly skin test positive to the relevant antigen. Unfortunately we do not know what the relevant antigen in MS is. Furthermore, transfer factor has not been characterised, may be a mixture of substances and cannot be standardised — factors which make experiments difficult to repeat. There is experimental support for the efficacy of transfer factor in correcting immunodeficiency in several

14

conditions including the Wiskott-Aldrich syndrome, coccidioidomycosis and chronic mucocutaneous candidiasis, and in preventing varicella-zoster infection in childhood leukaemia. Two uncontrolled and three controlled trials have failed to show any effect in MS but, in 1980, Basten et al published a prospective blind controlled study in which 29 treated patients deteriorated significantly less at 18 months than 29 placebo treated patients. By 24 months the transfer factor treated group had deteriorated $0 \cdot 79 \pm \cdot 2$ (mean $\pm$ s.d.) units on the Kurtzke disability scale, the control group $1 \cdot 86 \pm 1 \cdot 50$ ($P < 0 \cdot 005$). This result appears the most impressive of any controlled trial in this review. Of course one trial is insufficient to prove empirically that immunostimulant treatment is effective but it certainly justifies the further trials of transfer factor proposed in Australia.

Levamisole
Levamisole, originally marketed as an antihelminth, stimulates several immune functions including phagocytosis, chemotaxis and cutaneous delayed hypersensitivity. It has been beneficial in rheumatoid arthritis and recurrent aphthous ulceration. In MS the overall conclusion from three uncontrolled and three controlled trials is that it has no effect. In the largest trial on 54 patients the potential side-effects of serious granulocytopenia were not encountered (Gonsette et al, 1982).

Interferon
Interferons are glycoproteins released by cells infected by viruses and which induce antiviral activity in other cells. They are usually acid-stable. Chemically different, usually acid-labile, 'immune' interferons are produced by leucocytes in response to mitogens, endotoxins and both bacterial and viral infections. Interferons from human leucocytes and fibroblasts are now being produced on a large enough scale for limited clinical trials in viral infections and cancer. Only very preliminary observations have been made in MS. Leucocyte interferon production in vitro is probably reduced in MS, although there is some contradictory evidence and comparative information from other neurological diseases is not yet available. Interferon does not cross the blood-brain barrier so that intrathecal treatment is necessary if it is considered desirable to affect the immune responses occurring within the CNS. Despite this disadvantage a controlled trial of intrathecal human fibroblast interferon was pursued for 6 months and was claimed to show a reduction in relapse rate in 10 treated compared with 10 control patients during 18 months after entering the study (Jacobs et al, 1981). The authors considered that the treated but not the control patients showed a significant reduction in relapse rate compared with that before entry to the study. Unfortunately the small size of the treatment groups and 'open' study design prevent firm conclusions being drawn.

CONCLUSION

Immunopathological evidence, particularly the similarity with chronic relapsing EAE, favours an autoimmune aetiology for MS but is not conclusive. The controlled trials of azathiprine suggest that immunosuppression is effective but require confirmation. In one trial, however, immunostimulation with transfer factor (Basten et al, 1980) appeared to slow down progression of the disease. This paradox can be explained by modern immunological theory. The numbers of suppressor cells are depressed in the blood of patients at the time of acute relapses. Immunosuppression might work by halting a harmful immune response, immunostimulation by increasing the activity of the suppressor cells which normally control such harmful responses.

Even if these conclusions are not as clear as the reader may wish there is room for optimism. It does seem theoretically possible that the inflammation can be controlled by one of the immunological treatments discussed. It is encouraging that several current trials have large enough samples and long enough periods of observation to answer the question posed in the title of this chapter.

Acknowledgment
I am grateful to Fiona Woods, Pharmacy, Guy's Hospital for help with researching the bibliography.

REFERENCES

Aimard G, Girard P F, Raveau J 1966 Sclerose en plaques et processus d'autoimmunisation. Traitement par les antimitotiques. Lyon Medical 215: 345–352

Alvord E C, Shaw C M, Hruby S, Kies M W 1979 Has myelin basic protein received a fair trial in the treatment of MS? Annals of Neurology 6: 461–469

Basten A et al 1980 Transfer factor in treatment of MS. Lancet 2: 931–934

Bornstein M B, Miller A I, Teitelbaum D, Arnon R, Sela M 1982 Multiple sclerosis: trial of a synthetic polypeptide. Annals of Neurology 11: 317–319

Bowden A N, Bowden P M A, Friedmann A J, Perkin G D, Rose F C 1974 A trial of corticotrophin gelatin injection in acute optic neuritis. Journal of Neurology, Neurosurgery and Psychiatry 37: 869–873

Brown J R, Beebe G W, Kurtzke J F, Loewenson R B, Silberberg D H, Tourtellotte W W 1979 The design of clinical trials to assess therapeutic efficacy in MS. Neurology 29: suppl: 1–23

Ellison G W, Myers L W 1978 A review of systemic non-specific treatment of MS. Neurology 28: 132–139

Ellison G W, Myers L W 1980 Immunosuppressive drugs in multiple sclerosis: pro and con. Neurology 30: 28–32

Frick E, Stickl H 1982 Specificity of antibody-dependent lymphocyte cytotoxicity against cerebral tissue constituents in MS. Acta Neurologica Scandinavica 65: 30–37

Gonsette R E, Demonty L, Delmotte P 1977 Intensive immunosuppression with cyclophosphamide in multiple sclerosis. Follow up of 110 patients for 2-6 years. Journal of Neurology 214: 173–181

Gomsette R E, Demonty L, Delmotte P, Decree J, de Cock W, Verhaegen H, Symoens J 1982 Modulation of immunity in multiple sclerosis: a double-blind levamisole-placebo controlled study. Journal of Neurology (in press)

Hommes O R, Lamers K J B, Reekers P 1980 Effect of intensive immunosuppression on the course of chronic progressive multiple sclerosis. Journal of Neurology 223: 177–191

Hughes R A C, Gray I A, Gregson N A, Metcalfe R A 1982 Multiple sclerosis — lymphocyte transformation with multiple sclerosis and normal brain myelin basic protein and subcellular fractions. Acta Neurologica Scandinavica 65: 161–173

Iivainen M V 1981 The significance of abnormal immune responses in patients with multiple sclerosis (review). Journal of Neuroimmunology 1: 141–172

Iqbal I G, Bornstein M B 1980 Multiple sclerosis: serum gammaglobulin and demyelination in organ culture. Neurology 30: 749–754

Jacobs L, O'Malley J, Freeman A, Ekes R 1981 Intrathecal interferon reduces exacerbations of multiple sclerosis. Science 214: 1026–1028

Kastrukoff L K, McLean D R, McPherson T A 1978 Multiple sclerosis treated with antithymocyte globulin — a five year follow-up. Canadian Journal of Neurological Science 5: 175–178

Kurtzke J F 1965 Further notes on disability evaluation in MS with scale modifications. Neurology 15: 654–661

Maida E, Summer K 1979 Serum cortisol levels of multiple sclerosis patients during ACTH treatment. Journal of Neurology 220: 143–148

Mertin J, Rudge P, Kremer M, Healey M J R, Knight S C, Compston A 1982 Double-blind controlled trial of immunosuppression in the treatment of multiple sclerosis: final report. Lancet 2: 351–354

Millar J H D, Vas C J, Noronha M J, Liversedge L A, Rawson M D 1967 Long term treatment of multiple sclerosis with corticotrophin. Lancet 2: 429–431

Miller H J, Newell D J, Ridley A 1961 MS: treatment of acute exacerbations with ACTH. Lancet 2: 1120–1122

Patzold U, Pocklington P 1980 Azathioprine in MS — a three year controlled study of its effectiveness. Journal of Neurology 223: 97–119

Rawson M D, Liversedge L A 1969 Treatment of retrobulbar neuritis with corticotrophin. Lancet 2: 222

Rose A S, Kuzma J W, Kurtzke J F, Namerow N S, Sibley W A, Tourtellotte W W 1970 Cooperative study in the evaluation of therapy in multiple sclerosis: ACTH versus placebo. Neurology 20 suppl: 1–59

Rosen J A 1979 Prolonged azathioprine treatment of non-remitting multiple sclerosis. Journal of Neurology, Neurosurgery and Psychiatry 42: 338–344

Swinburn W R, Liversedge L A 1973 Azathioprine and multiple sclerosis. Journal of Neurology, Neurosurgery and Psychiatry 36: 124–126

Theys P, Gosseye-Lissoir F, Ketelaer P, Carton H 1981 Short-term intensive cyclophosphamide treatment in multiple sclerosis. Journal of Neurology 225: 119–135

Tourtellotte W W, Haerer A F 1965 Use of oral corticosteroids in the treatment of multiple sclerosis. A double-blind study. Archives of Neurology 12: 536–545

Van den Noort S, Waksman B H 1980 Plasma exchange: aid to therapy of multiple sclerosis. Neurology 30: 1111–1112

Wisniewski H M, Lassmann H, Brosnan C F, Mehta P D, Lidsky A A, Madrid R E 1982 Multiple sclerosis: immunological and experimental aspects. In: Matthews W B, Glaser G H (eds) Recent Advances in Clinical Neurology, 3. Churchill Livingstone, Edinburgh, p 96

3. Do evoked potentials contribute to the early diagnosis of multiple sclerosis?

L. D. Blumhardt

Over the last decade improved methods of recording evoked potentials (EP's) have resulted in their widespread adoption as routine clinical tests. A reputation as 'one of the most useful techniques in modern clinical neurophysiology' (Chiappa & Ropper, 1982) has been founded particularly on the high prevalence of abnormal visual, auditory and somatosensory EP's in patients with demyelinating disease. This evidence for the disseminated nature of the lesions has been hailed as 'one of the biggest advances in the diagnosis of multiple sclerosis' (Lancet, 1982). However, while the frequent occurrence of abnormal EP's in patients with unequivocal demyelination has been firmly established, the contribution of EP's to the investigation and management of patients with unexplained symptoms or signs that *may* be due to multiple sclerosis (MS), remains to be precisely defined.

To evaluate the role of a new, potentially diagnostic test, we need to know not only the proportion of patients with a positive result amongst those in whom the disease is established by a 'gold standard', but also in equivocal cases of the disease and in patients with other commonly confused conditions. What is the role of the new test in relation to established diagnostic techniques and what are its potential advantages and disadvantages? How reliable and reproducible are the results? How does the new test stand up against the 'gold standard'? As the prevalence of the disease in the population will clearly affect the 'abnormality rate', we need to know the methods of selection or preliminary screening of patients in the studies which evaluate the test. Finally, to determine the benefits for the patient, we need to know the positive and negative predictive abilities of EP's and the subsequent fate of the patients who had either normal or abnormal results.

In this chapter I intend to discuss these various aspects with particular emphasis on the pattern–reversal visual evoked potential (VEP), abnormalities of which usually make up the largest proportion of subclinical lesions demonstrated in multi-modality studies and provide the best evidence of anatomically-distinct lesions in patients with known spinal cord or brain stem disease.

18

EVOKED POTENTIAL ABNORMALITIES IN ESTABLISHED MULTIPLE SCLEROSIS

If the test is to be of potential diagnostic value it must be capable of demonstrating a high prevalence of abnormalities in proven cases of the disease in question. An abnormal EP in 'clinically-definite' multiple sclerosis is of course of no intrinsic value for diagnosis since this has been firmly established, by definition, on clinical grounds. Nevertheless, this initial requirement appears well-satisfied for the pattern VEP where abnormality rates in different series of 'clinically-definite' MS are between 75% and 97% (Table 3.1). However, in a disease where symptoms and signs relapse and remit and plaques of demyelination progressively accumulate in sensory pathways, these bald statistics provide little proof of the value of EP's for early diagnosis. Have the published series contained a reasonable cross-section of mild to severe and short to long duration cases? Is disease duration related to the abnormality rate of EP's in definite MS? To what extent do EP abnormalities remain static? Was the VEP

Table 3.1 Prevalence of abnormal VEP in 'clinically definite' MS with or without clinical evidence of optic nerve involvement. *Key*: ON, optic neuritis; a, acuity; r, refraction; c, colour vision; p, pupils; fi, fields; fu, fundoscopy; pr, intraocular pressure.

Reference	Overall abnormalities (%)	With history of ON	No history of ON	No history or signs of ON	Methods of excluding ON
Halliday et al (1973)	97	17/17 (100%)	16/17 (94%)	—	No systematic examination
Asselman et al (1975)	84	11/11 (100%)	15/20 (75%)	—	a,r,c,p,fi,fu.
Mastaglia et al (1976)	83	14/14[a] (100%)	—	5/9[a] (56%)	'No clinical evidence of optic neuropathy'
Mastaglia et al (1977)	80	27/27[a] (100%)	—	5/13[a] (38%)	a,c,p,fi,fu,r.
Hennerici et al (1977)	81	— (100%)	— (57%)	—	a,c,p,fi,fu,pr.
Zeese (1977)	92	9/10 (90%)	15/16 (94%)	7/8 (88%)	'No findings of optic neuritis'
Matthews et al (1977)	75	26/28 (93%)	9/13 (69%)	11/20 (55%)	fu,'pale discs'
Shahrokhi et al (1978)	82	37/41 (90%)	12/19 (63%)	—	Not described
Trojaborg & Petersen (1979)	96	17/18[b] (94%)	33/38[b] (85%)	—	Not described
Khoshbin & Hallett (1981)	76	—	—	6/15 (40%)	fu,fi,c
Purves et al (1981)	91	16/17 (94%)	—	14/16 (86%)	a,p,fi
Brooks & Chiappa (1982)	88	62/63 (99%)	—	16/26 (62%)	p,fi,fu,c
Walsh et al (1982)	84	—	—	21/42[b]	'No history or clinical evidence'

a Ratio assuming patients with normal VEP's had no signs and negative histories.
b Ratio of *eyes* recorded.

abnormality the only evidence of optic nerve damage and, if so, what were the clinical procedures against which the sensitivity of the VEP was measured? Few published studies provide satisfactory answers to these important questions.

Subclinical abnormalities of EP's in 'clinically-definite MS'

In most series the majority of patients in the 'clinically-definite' category have a positive history of optic neuritis. Not surprisingly, the highest VEP abnormality rates are found in these patients. The rates are almost invariably lower where a clear history of optic neuritis is lacking, (57–94%, Table 3.1). Although highly variable, these results have been interpreted as a surprising sensitivity of the VEP to 'subclinical' optic neuritis, a conclusion which does not allow for the visual signs in many of these cases, or for the observation that patients with MS not infrequently forget their previous, well-documented episodes of optic neuritis. The extent to which the VEP result has been correlated with *both* history and neuro-ophthalmological assessment of optic nerve damage, varies enormously in different studies (Tables 3.1 and 3.2). Where it is possible to extract such information it can be seen that 'abnormality detection rates' are often inflated by the inclusion of patients with positive clinical signs of optic neuritis (i.e. are merely confirmatory of optic nerve damage). Thus in one series, VEP abnormalities were detected in 69% of a group of patients who had a negative history for optic neuritis despite signs of optic atrophy and in only 55% of those with a negative history whose discs were judged normal on ophthalmoscopy (Matthews et al, 1977). A more detailed eye examination would be expected to lower still further the proportion of cases in whom evidence of optic nerve damage was provided solely by the VEP. In a few studies, where more rigorous criteria have both been applied and correlated with the VEP, the true 'hit-rates' are lower, although marked inter-study variability persists (Table 3.1). Apart from the rigor of the clinical eye examination, other factors such as differences in diagnostic criteria, definitions of 'normal' and VEP methodology, and variations in the patient sample, may contribute to this apparently variable sensitivity of the VEP to 'subclinical' optic nerve damage. Even wider interstudy variations are seen in patient populations in whom MS is suspected, but not established.

EVOKED POTENTIAL ABNORMALITIES IN EQUIVOCAL CASES OF DEMYELINATION

The proposed diagnostic role of the EP depends on its sensitivity to unsuspected plaques of demyelination in patients in whom the diagnosis is in doubt. Here we need to consider both the detection rate of subclinical lesions and the specificity of the recorded abnormalities. In most series the proportion of patients with abnormal EP's declines in parallel with the diagnostic certainty (Table 3.2). It should be noted here that although most authors use the McAlpine et al (1972) classification with or without minor modifications, few describe the preliminary screening tests carried out prior to classification of their patients. Inclusion in the 'possible' category, in this or similar schemata, requires that other causes have

Table 3.2 Prevalence of abnormal pattern VEP in patients suspected to have MS. *Key*: b, all ratios except *f* (below) are no. cases with abnormal VEP/total no. cases in group; +ON, positive history of optic neuritis; −ON, negative history of optic neuritis; −SS, no signs *or* symptoms (NB assumed in those studies where not clearly defined); epl: early possible or latent MS; sus, suspected MS. N.B. methods of excluding ON as for Table 3.1.

Reference	Overall probable MS	Overall possible MS	Probable MS +ON	Probable MS −ON	Probable MS −SS	Possible MS +ON	Possible MS −ON	Possible MS −SS	Methods of excluding ON
Halliday et al (1973)[b]	5/5	11/12 (92%)	1/1	4/4	—	6/6	5/6 (83%)	—	No systematic eye examination
Asselman et al (1975)[b]	5/6 (83%)	3/14 (21%)	4/4	1/2	—	—	3/14 (21%)	5/27[f] (19%)	a,r,c,p,fi,fu.
Lowitzsch et al (1976)[e]	25/42 (60%)	13/20 (65%)	26/42 (62%)	16/42 (38%)	5/42[g] (12%)	—	—	9/20[g] (45%)	a,c,fi,fu,sl,re.
Mastaglia et al (1976)[a]	3/9 (33%)	12/36 (33%)	—	—	2/9 (22%)	—	—	8/36 (22%)	Not described ('no evidence of optic neuropathy')
Mastaglia et al (1977)[c]	13/30[epl] (43%)	7/32[sus] (22%)	—	—	8/30 (27%)	—	—	7/32 (22%)	a,c,p,fi,fu,r. ('no signs of optic neuritis')
Matthews et al (1977)[b]	14/24 (58%)	10/28 (36%)	4/6	10/18 (56%)	7/13 (54%)	0/2	10/26 (38%)	8/24 (30%)	fu, 'pale discs'
Collins et al (1978)[c]	15/30[epl] (50%)	7/31[sus] (23%)	—	—	7/30 (23%)	—	—	5/31 (16%)	a,c,fi,fu,p ('no clinical involvement')
Nilsson (1978)[a]	8/9 (90%)	3/10 (30%)	—	—	—	—	—	—	—
Shahrokhi et al (1978)[b]	24/46 (52%)	12/43 (28%)	10/11 (91%)	—	14/35 (40%)	7/10 (70%)	—	5/33 (15%)	Not described ('no history or clinical evidence of optic neuritis')
Trojaborg and Petersen (1979)[a]	7/12 (58%)	2/10 (20%)	5/5	5/19 (26%)	—	—	2/20 (10%)	—	Not described
Kjaer (1980)[d]	3/3	11/19 (58%)	3/3	—	—	—	3/3	8/16 (50%)	Not described
Aminoff & Ochs (1981)[a]	—	21/96 (22%)	—	—	—	—	—	21/96 (22%)	Not described ('? subclinical optic nerve lesions')
Brooks & Chiappa (1982)[a]	43/61 (70%)	17/48 (35%)	—	—	16/32 (50%)	—	—	10/41 (24%)	p,fi,fu,c. (all patients did not have all tests)

a McAlpine et al (1972) classification of suspected MS.
b Modified McAlpine classification.
c McDonald & Halliday (1977) classification.
d Modified McDonald & Halliday classification.
e Bauer (1974) classification.
f Ratio represents 'hit-rate' in 'normal' *eyes* examined.
g Ratios based on cases 'reclassified'.

been eliminated by appropriate tests, including myelography in cases with progressive spinal cord disease. In patients with symptoms or signs typical of demyelination, in whom these qualifications have been rigorously applied, the risk of developing MS at some point in the future is clearly high whatever the EP result.

'Subclinical' abnormalities

As described above for 'definite MS', the potential usefulness of EP's tends to be overestimated in many reports by a failure to distinguish 'subclinical' from merely confirmatory abnormalities. The highest abnormality rates for the VEP therefore reflect the high proportion of patients with symptoms or signs (or both) of previous optic neuritis. The proportion of patients with 'subclinical' abnormalities (true 'hit-rates') lies between 12% and 54% for probable MS and 15% and 50% for 'possible' cases and is lowest when care has been taken to correlate neuro-ophthalmological findings (Table 3.2).

Disease duration is not considered in the majority of studies, although there are large differences between and within subcategories. In one series symptom duration ranged from 1 month to 30 years (Collins et al, 1978). Authors seldom separate suspected early cases of MS from patients with chronic progressive paraparesis, both of which fall within the McAlpine 'possible' category. In one of the few reports which mentions symptom duration, the mean values for 'definite', 'early probable or latent', and 'possible' groups, were 8·6 years, 4·4 years and 11·4 months, respectively (Mastaglia et al, 1977). However, even here no correlation was made with the EP results. If the increased abnormality rates merely reflect the progressive accumulation of plaques with time, we cannot expect EP's to predict in the early stages those who have MS and who will subsequently develop multiple lesions.

Only one study has attempted to assess the value of the VEP for detecting subclinical lesions in patients with a single, non-visual, neurological episode, highly suggestive of a first attack of demyelination and of less than 3 months duration (Matthews et al, 1977); only 2 of 39 cases (5%) had 'delayed' VEP's, although 6 were judged to have pale discs. In another study of 15 patients recorded within 3 months of an acute or subacute spinal cord lesion, in whom many alternative pathologies were excluded by appropriate blood tests and myelography, the VEP was delayed in only 2 of 15 cases (13%) (Blumhardt et al, 1982a). Similarly, although abnormalities of the sensory evoked potential (SEP) are common in unequivocal demyelination and there is a high risk of developing MS after optic neuritis, only 4 of 39 patients (10%) studied when they presented with acute optic neuritis, had abnormalities of cervical or cortical SEP's (Matthews, 1978). Thus either the majority of such patients do not have demyelinating disease, or the EP's cannot reliably predict the development of MS because they are insensitive to early, perhaps minor lesions or, more probably, because damage has not yet occurred at other sites in the c.n.s. The latter conclusion seems more likely both because, it is to be hoped, other diseases have been largely excluded by definition and because follow-up studies in similar groups of patients show that a majority of these patients eventually do develop MS (e.g. Marshall, 1955; Hutchinson, 1976).

EP's would be expected to be more helpful in patients with longer histories. In undiagnosed cases of spastic paraparesis there appears to be a three-fold increase in the proportion of VEP abnormalities when symptom duration exceeds 3 years, as compared with those with shorter histories (Blumhardt et al, 1982a). Longitudinal, serial EP studies of acutely-presenting patients with possible MS should provide interesting information on the evolution of subclinical abnormalities, although diagnosis on EP evidence will, of course, be delayed.

Recent efforts to improve the 'hit-rates' in suspected MS have been largely directed towards 'refinements' of the stimulus to increase the sensitivity of the VEP, or into multi-modality studies. Foveal stimulation (Hennerici et al, 1977), light-emitting diode arrays (Nilsson, 1978), lower stimulus luminance (Cant et al, 1978) and pattern-onset stimulation (Aminoff & Ochs, 1981), have all been claimed to increase the 'hit-rates' in possible MS. These slight 'improvements' remain to be substantiated. The increased sensitivity of foveal stimulation could not be confirmed in one recent study which found absent foveal responses in 37% of patients and 20% of healthy controls (Oepen et al, 1982).

Multi-modality studies have generally shown the VEP to be the most clinically useful test (e.g. Small et al, 1978; Deltenre et al 1982; Kjaer, 1980), although some studies have found the median SEP superior to the VEP (Mastaglia et al, 1976). Combined modality testing will clearly increase the proportion of abnormalities found but the positive brain stem auditory evoked potential (BAEP) and SEP results often merely confirm damage to the brain stem or spinal cord which cannot reliably be attributed to an anatomically separate lesion. Thus no patients could be reclassified on the SEP results in one study despite an abnormality rate of 55% (Kjaer, 1980). Surprisingly little work has been carried out to determine whether the patients with subclinical lesions detected in these combined studies, actually have MS.

ARE DELAYED EVOKED POTENTIALS DISEASE SPECIFIC?

From the earliest reports of the diagnostic value of EP's it has been stressed that abnormally-delayed responses are not specific for demyelinating disease (Halliday et al, 1973; Asselman et al, 1975). This warning has been amply emphasised by many subsequent studies. A wide variety of disorders affecting the visual pathways may be associated with prolongation of VEP latency (Table 3.3). Furthermore, while a consistently delayed VEP in a patient with spastic paraparesis provides good evidence of multiple lesions it cannot be regarded as diagnostic of MS without many qualifications and exclusions.

Delayed EPs in unrelated conditions
The delayed VEP may merely indicate an unrelated ocular condition incidental to the spinal cord lesion such as, for example, glaucoma. Delayed VEP's may occur in up to 74% of patients with this condition, including some with 'clinically silent' disease (Huber & Wagner, 1978). A similar false-positive result may also arise from lens opacities, drusen of the optic nerve head (Stevens & Newman, 1981) or amblyopia (Ikeda et al, 1978; Wanger & Nilsson, 1978). The VEP, therefore, is no substitute for a careful history and competent neuro-ophthalmological examination. It should also be mentioned here that spurious 'delays' may result from poor technique. EP's are notoriously variable and all apparently abnormal responses must be checked for consistency. Serious errors can arise through inadequate monitoring of fixation. For example, deliberate inattention or drooping of the eyelid with drowsiness or ptosis can result in marked delays (Carroll et al, 1982). Age, gender, pupil size and refractive error

Table 3.3 Examples of non-specificity of pattern VEP delays.

Pathology	Proportion of patients with delayed VEP	Reference
Amblyopia	2/10	Wanger & Nilsson (1978)
Glaucoma	15/21	Cappin & Nissim (1975)
	29/39	Huber & Wagner (1978)
Leber's optic atrophy	4/14	Carroll & Mastaglia (1979)
	2/2	Dorfman et al (1977)
Tropical amblyopia	1/1	Asselman et al (1975)
Ischaemic optic neuritis	3/3	Asselman et al (1975)
	3/10	Halliday et al (1977)
	5/5	Hennerici et al (1977)
	4/15	Wilson (1978)
Optic nerve/chiasmal compression	2/2	Asselman et al (1975)
	7/16	Halliday et al (1977)
'Spinocerebellar degeneration'	2/3	Asselman et al (1975)
	3/5	Halliday et al (1977)
Friedreich's ataxia	12/22	Carroll et al (1980)
	5/7	Pedersen & Trojaborg (1981)
Hereditary spastic paraplegia	3/13	Pedersen & Trojaborg (1981)
Hereditary cerebellar ataxia	4/11	Pedersen & Trojaborg (1981)
Peroneal muscular atrophy	5/9	Tackmann & Radu (1980)
Parkinson's disease	24/36	Bodis-Wollner & Yahr (1978)
Sarcoidosis	15/50	Streletz et al (1981)
B_{12} deficiency	5/6	Troncoso et al (1979)

may all affect the response latency and any alteration of the stimulus parameters requires the re-establishment of normal limits. Few authors describe methods for determining the reproducibility of their results and unrealistic definitions of the limits of normality tend to create non-disease (Meador, 1965). Authors using 2 s.d. criteria may classify 1 in 40 healthy responses as 'abnormal'.

The spinal cord disease and the abnormal VEP may be related but due to some condition other than MS. Here the delayed responses reported in pernicious anaemia, sarcoidosis, Arnold-Chiari malformation, posterior fossa tumours and the spinal and cerebellar degenerations are potentially serious causes of diagnostic confusion. Although the number of cases with these disorders that have been studied to date is small, and the laboratory conditions and criteria of abnormality often different to those used in MS studies, the proportions of patients with delayed responses are high (Table 3.3).

Similarly, abnormal short-latency BAEP or SEP responses may be found in a variety of different disorders. Delayed or attenuated BAEP's in patients with mixed pyramidal, cerebellar and cranial nerve syndromes may be associated with cerebello-pontine angle tumours (Selters & Brackman, 1977; Eggermont et al, 1980) or the Arnold-Chiari malformation (Robinson & Rudge, 1980) as well as demyelinating disease. Abnormal SEP's are similarly non-specific and may be recorded in system degenerations, cord tumours, B12 deficiency or cervical spondylosis, in addition to MS (Krumholz et al, 1981; Jones et al, 1980; Ganes, 1980).

The latency and waveform of the EP
While it must be accepted that abnormal EP's, including delayed VEP's, are non-specific for MS, there is a tendency in the recent literature to emphasise the

usefulness of 'typical' or 'characteristic' features of EP's in different conditions. While such generalisations are of considerable academic interest they are of little relevance to the *diagnosis* of individual cases, due to the large variety of EP abnormalities within and across disease boundaries. For example, the 'characteristically long delays' found in some patients with MS have been contrasted with the smaller average delays found in other conditions. However, in patients with possible MS where abnormal EP's have the greatest potential value, the delays reported in many studies are often of lesser degree than those found in patients with a more certain diagnosis (Nilsson, 1978). They are frequently marginal. Thus where the diagnosis is uncertain, slight adjustments of the definition of the 'normal upper limit' may result in large changes in the 'hit-rate' (see Matthews et al, 1977). Many hundreds of patients must have been 'reclassified' from 'possible' to 'probable' MS on the basis of delays which only exceeded 'normal' limits by a few milliseconds or less. The prognostic value of these slight delays, as compared with more markedly prolonged responses, has yet to be established (see below). At the other extreme, the very long 'delays' of perhaps 100 ms or even more, which have been reported in some studies, are invariably associated with distorted and attenuated potentials that are difficult to identify. Whether such responses contain a delayed P100 component is entirely speculative. In this type of recording some authors prefer to regard this wave as absent (Mauguière et al, 1982).

Whatever the explanation for these extreme examples it is clear that a wide range of delays is encountered in patients suspected to have MS. Furthermore, the delays reported in a variety of other diseases overlap with a large proportion of the mild to moderate delays found in patients with unequivocal demyelinating disease. For example, mean delays of 43 ms and a maximum delay of 48 ms have been reported in 30% of cases of hereditary spastic paraplegia, despite a conservative 3 s.d. criteria for the upper limit (Pedersen & Trojaborg, 1981). In patients with spinocerebellar degenerations mean delays varying between 12 ms and 30 ms have been reported (Carroll et al, 1980; Wenzel et al 1981; Pedersen & Trojaborg, 1981). In 24% of patients with sarcoidosis 'subclinical' delays ranged from 1–22 ms (Streletz et al, 1981) and maximum delays of the order of 26 ms have been encountered with spinal cord disease due to B12 deficiency (Troncoso et al, 1979; Fine & Hallet, 1980).

In other conditions where delayed EP's may be mistakenly attributed to a primary demyelinating lesion, such as ischaemic optic neuritis or chiasmal compression, some authors have emphasised the greater frequency of waveform alterations and amplitude changes. Again, however, there is a large variation in the effects of any particular disorder on the EP waveform which is more likely to be related to non-specific factors such as the premorbid waveform and the presence, severity and site of visual field defects, than the type of pathology (Blumhardt, 1982). Thus, while ischaemic optic neuritis may have a greater effect on response amplitude than latency, in contrast with the 'characteristic' effects of demyelination (Halliday et al, 1977), these features cannot distinguish one pathology from the other with any reliability. Thus grossly distorted or attenuated responses are found in some patients with unequivocal MS and delays have been reported in 26–100% of patients with ischaemic optic nerve lesions

25

(Asselman et al, 1975; Hennerici et al, 1977; Wilson, 1978). Although it is unusual to find reduced amplitude responses at normal latency after optic neuritis, such responses have nevertheless been reported (Matthews et al, 1977; Zeese, 1977; Blumhardt, 1982). In this context it should be noted that many authors, in an effort to increase their 'hit-rates' in suspected cases of MS, have included interocular amplitude comparisons (Shahrokhi et al, 1978) or estimates of 'waveform distortion or widening' (Collins et al, 1977), criteria which further emphasise the non-specificity of the VEP abnormalities reported in MS. Similarly, the small amplitudes, waveform variation and lability of the short latency BAEP and subcortical SEP's, preclude any clear pathological specificity of abnormalities of these responses, although attempts have been made to characterise typical features of the SEP in certain conditions (Jones, 1982).

Delayed EP's in MS have often been equated with decreased conduction velocity through demyelinated segments and this hypothesis has been extended by some authors to account for the delays found in, for example, B12 deficiency or chiasmal compression, where secondary demyelination can be invoked as the mechanism of the delay. However, the occurrence of delayed VEP's in such disparate conditions as the spinocerebellar degenerations (Carroll et al, 1980), posterior fossa tumours (Asselman et al, 1975), glaucoma (Huber & Wagner, 1978) and benign intracranial hypertension (Hume & Cant, 1976), requires a more cautious interpretation of the mechanism of the 'delay'.

THE 'DELAYED' EVOKED RESPONSE — A POTENTIALLY MISLEADING CONCEPT

In most clinical studies normal and abnormal EP's have been distinguished by establishing 'normal limits' for various waves (components) defined by their peak latencies and polarities. Most studies of the VEP in demyelinating disease have relied exclusively on comparisons between the peak latencies of a 'dominant' (i.e. the largest) surface-positive wave in patients' recordings and the P100 components recorded in healthy control subjects. The narrow latency range of this wave provides a sound platform for distinguishing normal from abnormal responses.* This technique in experienced hands is well established as a sensitive indicator of abnormality in the visual pathways. However, the interpretation of the apparent latency differences remains problematic.

The concept of a 'delayed response' rests on the assumption that the peak of a 'dominant positive wave' in an abnormal response is exactly analogous to the peak of a healthy P100 component. In fact the terms 'P100' and 'major positivity' are used interchangeably by many authors. This working hypothesis is based on recordings in the recovery phase of optic neuritis, of what appears to be a surprisingly intact waveform with near-normal amplitudes but delayed 'major

---

* Nevertheless, accurate P100 component peak identification requires half-field stimulation in up to 6% of healthy subjects who have bifid or 'W-shaped' positivities (Blumhardt & Halliday, 1979; Blumhardt et al, 1982b).

positivity' (Halliday & McDonald, 1977). On this basis it seems reasonable to conclude that the major cause of the abnormality is slowing of the propagated signal through demyelinated axons, an extrapolation that is automatically made by many authors.

This convenient concept results in estimations of latency prolongation that are difficult to account for on the data available from experimental studies of slowed conduction in demyelinated axons. Mean delays of the pattern VEP of the order of 40 ms and maximum delays in excess of 100 ms have been reported (Halliday et al, 1973; Asselman et al, 1975). However, theoretical calculations suggest that a single 'average' plaque of 1 cm can account for a maximum delay of only 24 ms* (McDonald, 1977). Delays even of this order have not been observed across experimental focally demyelinated lesions and McDonald has concluded that the present evidence is inadequate to allow slowing of conduction as the major scource of delay of EP's in demyelinating disease. Other mechanisms that have been considered as possible contributing factors include selective conduction block of faster fibres, delays at retinal level, delays in generation of the cortical response due to temporal dispersion of the afferent volley, and continuous non-saltatory conduction in demyelinated segments. Evidence to support a role for these mechanisms in the delayed human VEP is lacking and they remain hypothetical. A simpler explanation is that the basic assumption behind the measurements is in error.

The delays recorded due to demyelinating lesions in other sensory pathways (for example, the subcortical SEP or BAEP responses), are usually only several ms or less and the maximum delays encountered are of the order of 10 ms. The longer 'delays' seen with the cortical components of the SEP are associated with considerable broadening and temporal dispersion of the waveform (Halliday & Wakefield, 1963) so that the true response delay is difficult to determine. Similar waveform alterations of the cortical VEP, whose relative preservation may be more apparent than real, may account wholly or in part, for the discrepancy between the psychophysical and experimental data on the one hand and the VEP delays on the other. If a variety of psychophysical and EP tests are applied to patients with unilateral optic neuritis using the unaffected eyes as control, anomalously long delays are found only with the pattern VEP (e.g. average values of 31 ms versus 16 ms for subjective methods; Cook & Arden, 1977). We must examine the evidence that the VEP is merely *delayed* intact by a demyelinating lesion.

Is the EP waveform normal in multiple sclerosis?
Despite a vast literature on the subject, published illustrations of abnormal VEP's in patients with MS are surprisingly few and far between. Nevertheless, it is clear from these examples that responses which appear 'delayed' do not necessarily have normal amplitude and waveform. In fact, the relationship between response amplitude and latency in demyelinating disease appears to be

---

* Assuming propagation of a signal with maximum internodal conduction time across at least 50 internodes, a condition which may well cause conduction to fail altogether (Rasminsky & Sears, 1972).

controversial. Halliday et al (1972) reported recovery of the VEP amplitude to 'near normal levels' after optic neuritis, apparently in parallel with the return of visual acuity. The effects of demyelination on amplitude and latency thus appeared to be dissociated. Others, however, have found no clear relationship between VEP amplitude, latency, or acuity in MS, reporting markedly reduced amplitudes in association with normal or even *subnormal* latencies and normal acuities (Matthews et al, 1977). Some authors have noted that the 'delayed' responses tend to be those with the less well-defined and more variable waveforms (Zeese, 1977). This may be attributable to the highly significant association between increased latency and reduced amplitude of VEP's in demyelinating disease reported by Asselman et al (1975). In serial recordings in patients with MS, there appears to be a significant decline in amplitude irrespective of changes in latency (Matthews & Small, 1979).

While many authors have concentrated solely on response latency it is clear that the VEP can be so grossly and persistently attenuated after optic neuritis that no components can be identified (Milner et al, 1974; Shahrokhi et al, 1978; Nilsson, 1978). 'Absent responses', generally in association with marked residual visual deficits, have been reported in up to 14% of eyes following a single symptomatic attack of optic neuritis (Shahrokhi et al, 1978). Similarly, grossly attenuated, 'disorganised', or 'absent', responses are found in a minority of patients with MS (Lowitzsch et al, 1976; Collins et al, 1978). Thus one might expect to record a whole spectrum of amplitude changes from severe to minimal, depending upon the severity of the residual damage to the optic nerve. Lesser degrees of attenuation are undoubtedly obscured by the high intersubject amplitude variance, but are demonstrable by interocular comparisons when the pathology is unilateral. Thus a persisting 10–30% amplitude reduction of the 'major postitive wave' has been reported after optic neuritis (Bornstein, 1975). The addition of these interocular amplitude comparisons has slightly increased the 'abnormality detection rate' in some studies (Shahrokhi et al, 1978).

The frequency of pathological alterations in waveform morphology has been obscured by the use of full-field stimulation and single channel VEP recording. Nevertheless, from the earliest reports some authors have mentioned alterations in the 'form' of the VEP in patients with demyelination (Lowitzsch et al, 1976). Examination of the illustrated VEP recordings in some papers reveals obvious waveform differences between the responses from the affected and asymptomatic eyes in the same patient (Asselman et al, 1975; Shahrokhi et al, 1978). A common feature of the VEP in demyelinating disease is broadening of the triphasic response, particularly in the region of the major positive peak (Fig. 3.1). Various authors have referred to this feature as an 'increased duration', 'slurring', 'waveform widening', or 'temporal dispersion' (Collins et al, 1978; Nilsson 1978; Shahrokhi et al, 1978). The frequently associated loss of definition of the positive peak has obvious consequences for latency estimations (see Fig. 3.2). Some authors have used measurements between the negative peaks that preceed and follow the 'major positive wave' to demonstrate abnormal 'waveform widening' in 35% of clinically definite or suspected MS patients (Collins et al, 1978). Another common waveform alteration is the 'splitting' or 'breaking up' of the dominant positive wave into two or more small peaks (Hennerici et al, 1977;

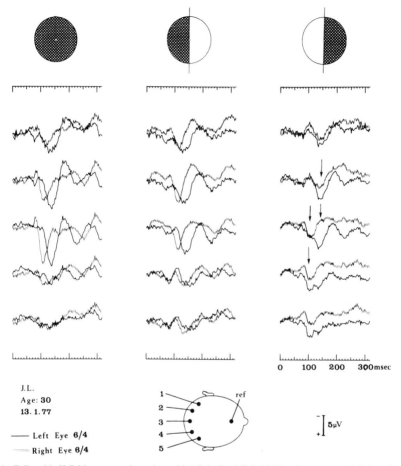

Fig. 3.1 Full and half-field responses in patient with 'clinically-definite' MS and asymptomatic left optic neuritis. LHF, left-half field, RHF, right-half field.

Abnormal midline full-field response from the affected left eye (heavy trace) appears characteristically well-preserved and delayed compared with the right eye response (light trace) which is within normal limits. Superimposition shows there are subtle waveform changes in left eye response. These include absent N75 wave (channel 3), prominent surface-negative peaks in lateral channels (i.e. at approx. 90 ms in channel 1 and 110 ms in channel 4), that are typical of 'scotomatous' waveforms, and an N145 wave that is delayed but *increased* in amplitude (left column).

Superimposed LHF responses (middle column) show N75 wave has identical *onset* latency (approx. 70 ms) in each eye, but peak is broad and dispersed in the abnormal response from the left eye (see channels 1 and 2). Onset of the first surface-negative wave in the left eye, LHF response in the mid-line is also 70 ms, but the peak latency at this electrode is about 105 ms. This is due to the abnormal projection of a slightly *enhanced* and delayed contralateral N105 wave into the mid-line. P100 wave from the left eye appears delayed in ipsilateral channels 1–3 but is dispersed and broadened, interacting near the mid-line with a prominent contralateral P135 wave. Peak delay of the mid-line positivity in the left eye response, which has both P100 and P135 contributions, is intermediate between the peak latencies of these 2 waves in the most lateral channels (c.f. the identical latencies of the LHF P100 waves in all 3 ipsilateral channels of the right eye response). Note descending 'leading' limb of the P100 is least delayed in channel 1 and increases in *gradient* and latency towards the mid-line due to interactions with the contralateral N105 and P135 waves.

RHF potentials from the left eye, including the P100 (first arrows), N105 and P135 (second arrows) not delayed, but the P135 wave enhanced relative to the potential from the right eye and projects into and across the mid-line. Its peak coincides with a second positive 'sub-component' in the abnormal, ipsilateral, 'W-shaped' positivity (right column).

Thus the full-field 'major positivity' in the mid-line response from the affected eye is composed mainly of a reduced but undelayed RHF P100 component and a *compound wave* from the LHF which has contributions from both P100 and P135 waves that are only slightly delayed. This major positivity also receives additional amplitude contribution from LHF contralateral N105 wave. By contrast the full-field 'major positivity' in the normal right eye response is composed entirely of ipsilateral P100 components.

29

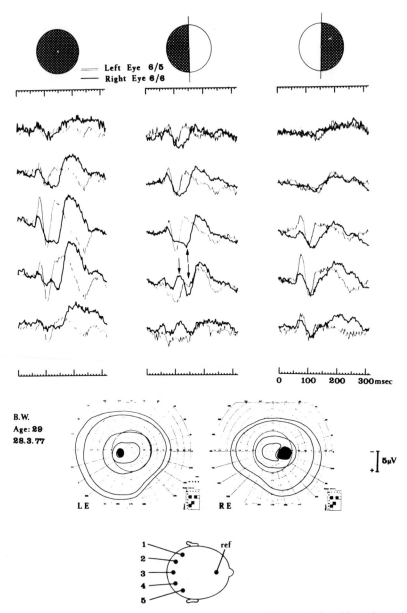

Fig. 3.2 Differential effects of demyelination on half-field components 20 months after right optic neuritis.

Full field response from affected eye (heavy trace) shows reduced amplitude N75 wave which has normal onset latency but *reduced* peak latency (approx. 10 ms earlier in the response from the affected eye). Major positive wave is broadened with a poorly defined peak. Lateral channels show 'scotomatous' 'W-shaped' waveforms (e.g. channel 4).

The left half-field N75 wave is similarly reduced in amplitude and latency in the response from the symptomatic eye. The descending 'leading' limb of the P100 is altered in slope but undelayed. Its reduced amplitude is more apparent near the midline where there is greater interaction with enhanced, undelayed contralateral PNP components (arrows). The abnormal mid-line projection of the P135 in the response from the right eye causes apparent widening of the ipsilateral positivity and a small, late positive peak (double arrow) which is also visible in the full field response. The responses from the right half-fields of the right eye also show 'scotomatous' features with a reduced amplitude, broadened and slightly *earlier* N75 wave and an insignificantly delayed P100 which shows some broadening and temporal dispersion when compared with the asymptomatic response from the left eye.

Full field response latency estimates taken either from the centre of the major positivity, or from the small late positive peak, will result in overestimation of the P100 delay due to the effects of the abnormal P135 distributions.

Bynke et al, 1977; Hoeppner & Lolas, 1978; Matthews & Small, 1979). This waveform has been shown to develop and persist without visual symptoms in serial recordings of patients with MS (Matthews & Small, 1979). As well as the appearance of 'new or displaced components' in the pathological response some authors have reported the loss of certain commonly-recorded waves (Lowitzsch et al, 1976; Duwaer & Spekreijse, 1978). Both the surface-negative wave (N78) which precedes the P100 in most healthy responses, as well as the 'trailing negative-going limb' of the P100, have been reported to be 'frequently missing' in MS responses (Shahrokhi et al, 1978). Only one study to date has made an attempt to classify the VEP waveforms in clinically definite or suspected MS (Hoeppner & Lolas, 1978). The waveform conventionally regarded as 'characteristic' of MS (i.e. a single well preserved and delayed positive wave), was found in only 38% of 104 patients. In 45% of patients the major positive deflection was bifid and in the remaining 17% there was a 'markedly distorted waveform in which there was no positive wave at the expected latency'. The example illustrated from this latter group showed a broad surface-negativity of the type usually associated with a central scotoma (Blumhardt et al, 1978).

These observations by many authors raise serious questions about the interpretation of latency estimations. It is clear that many patients with demyelinating disease have pathologically altered waveforms, with variable attenuation, temporal dispersion and both loss of some components and the appearance of other apparently 'new waves' in the response. Despite these observations few authors have mentioned any difficulties in estimating response latencies and yet most studies have produced very high 'abnormality detection rates', based predominantly, if not solely, on latency measurements of 'dominant positive waves'. In some published examples it can be seen that the choice of the 'major positivity' in a response waveform which shows a near-sinusodal series of positive and negative deflections, may be quite arbitrary (e.g. Bynke et al, 1977). Other authors have selected one or other peak in a bifid response on an entirely empirical basis, or even managed to estimate latencies in responses whose markedly distorted waveforms did not even contain an obvious positive wave (Hoeppner & Lolas, 1978).

While the technique of comparing the peak latencies of P100 waves in the responses of healthy subjects with the largest positive waves in the EP's of patients is a sensitive method for abnormality detection, data derived in this manner is virtually meaningless as a measure of the amount of conduction slowing in the visual pathways unless the P100 can be reliably identified in the abnormal responses.

The mechanisms of the waveform alteration in demyelinating disease
Most authors have regarded the 'clinically interpretable VEP' as a single positive wave (see review by Chiàppa & Ropper, 1982). However, the VEP to full-field stimulation is a compound response which, in most healthy subjects, contains a series of three major positive waves and three major negative waves from each hemisphere, each with distinctive mean latencies and scalp distributions (Blumhardt & Halliday, 1979). Both 'physiological scotomata' and pathological central field defects have variable and often profound differential effects on these multiple components (Blumhardt et al, 1977, 1978; Kriss et al, 1982; Blumhardt,

1982), yet no published study of the VEP in patients with MS has taken these facts into consideration.

Comparisons between the homonymous half-field responses from the affected and asymptomatic eyes after unilateral optic neuritis show that the effects of a single episode of demyelination are complex, due to the interaction between the variable density and extent of the pathological lesion and the premorbid half-field response waveform. The latter is determined by the marked variations in the cortical anatomy of each occipital lobe (Blumhardt, 1982). The commonly observed alterations include: amplitude changes which may be either reductions or increases of voltage depending on the particular component and the severity of the lesion; loss of wave peaks or replacement of single waves by multiple peaks; the appearance of new dominant waves not seen in the response from the asymptomatic eye; shifts in the distribution of potentials over the scalp; temporal dispersion, and component-dependent apparent latency changes, including reductions in peak latency, rather than a simple global response delay brought about by decreased conduction velocity.

Two to 71 months (mean 36·8 months) after a single episode of optic neuritis, all levels of disorganisation of the VEP may be found (Blumhardt, 1982). With moderate to severe residual optic nerve damage all components may appear equally attenuated. However, most responses contain some persisting evidence of the tendency for demyclination to cause disproportionate damage to macular (c.f. paramacular) fibres. Thus there is often some differential effect of the lesion on the ipsilateral and contralateral VEP (e.g. Figs. 3.1 and 3.3). The ipsilateral (negative-positive-negative or NPN) waves tend to be more attenuated and dispersed than the contralateral (positive-negative-positive or PNP) waves (Fig. 3.3), so that the latter tend to be more prominent than is the case in the average healthy response. Indeed the latter waves may only be seen in the responses from the eye with optic neuritis, as they tend to be 'masked' to a variable extent by the healthy ipsilateral components, which have relatively greater contributions from the macular regions of the visual field·(Blumhardt et al, 1978). Pseudo-delays may result when the relative sparing or even enhancement of the contralateral waves at the expense of the ipsilateral P100 causes the former to dominate in the algebraic summation that is the full-field response (Halliday, 1981; Blumhardt, 1982). Undelayed but prominent N105 and P135 waves may be responsible for the apparent preservation of near-normal amplitudes in some abnormal responses (Fig. 3.1) and may closely simulate the appearance of 'delayed' N75 and P100 waves.

Similar waveform changes occur in diseases other than MS. In a recent study of the VEP in 24 patients with toxic amblyopia, the group mean latency of the 'major full-field positive wave' was 130 ms (c.f. control mean of 104 ms; Kriss et al, 1982). Half-field recording showed that this wave was in fact made up of undelayed and unusually prominent P135 components arising from the relatively unaffected paramacular regions, while the P100 components were grossly attentuated or absent. Similar spurious delays may result from a variety of pathologies associated with central scotomata (Blumhardt, 1982). In optic neuritis these effects on the VEP waveform may be less obvious, due to the subtlety and complexity of component interactions. The so-called 'dominant positive wave' frequently turns out to be a compound wave made up of partially

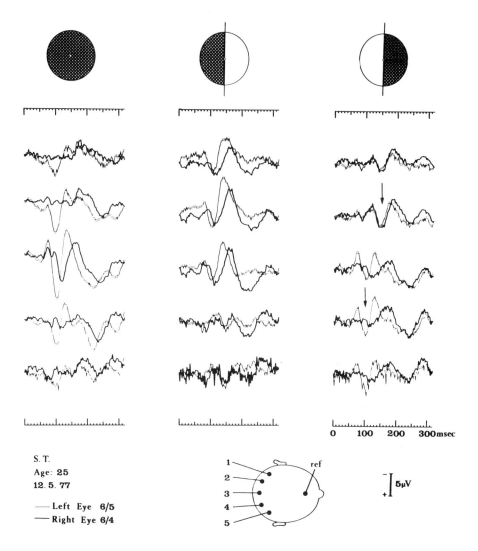

Fig. 3.3 Differential effects of demyelination on half-field components 71 months after right optic neuritis. The full field response waveform in the affected eye (heavy trace) is abnormal with reduced but undelayed N75 wave and a bifid major positivity in the midline. The grossly attenuated responses over the lateral scalp contain small but prominent negative waves at about 100 ms.

The left half-field responses from both eyes (middle column) are contaminated with muscle artefact but show contralateral PNP waves at normal latency. The ipsilateral P100 from the symptomatic right eye is reduced in amplitude and the descending, 'leading' limb and peak are delayed by approximately 12 ms.

Comparisons between the right half-field potentials (right column) show that the ipsilateral NPN complex from the eye previously affected by optic neuritis is grossly dispersed and attenuated with no clear component peaks. In contrast all the contralateral waves from the right eye are present and well defined including the P135 (arrow). The P75 wave appears to account for the first 'notch' in the full field positivity.

33

attenuated, dispersed and slightly delayed P100 waves, with varying contributions from abnormally distributed, prominent P135 components (Figs. 3.1, 3.2). This complex summation accounts for the 'broadening' and poor peak definition of the major positive deflection in many responses (Fig. 3.2), as well as the appearance of bifid positivities in others. The other contralateral waves may also project abnormally into or across the mid-line to contribute to distortions of the ipsilateral NPN waveform.

In patients with previous unilateral optic neuritis the frequent contribution of the contralateral P135 wave to the 'major positivity' of the full-field response (Figs. 3.1, 3.2) results in an approximately three-fold over-estimation of the actual P100 delays established by half-field recording (Blumhardt, 1982). In this study the mean interocular half-field P100 delays were of the order of only 6–7 ms. Furthermore, there is no universal response prolongation. The delays vary with each component. Not only do the ipsilateral P100 and N145 components show greater apparent delays (and more distortion and temporal dispersal) than the contralateral waves (Figs. 3.1, 3.3) but there may be a differential effect on peak latencies within the ipsilateral complex. For example, the latency shifts of the N75 wave are often negligible and the mean delays do not reach significance (Blumhardt, 1982). In some recordings from symptomatic eyes where this wave is attenuated, its peak latency appears to be reduced compared with the similar component from the asymptomatic eye (Fig. 3.2). The half-field P100 peak and trailing ascending limb which are frequently distorted by the mesially — projecting P135 wave, often appear more 'delayed' than the descending leading limb of the major positivity (Fig. 3.2).

These observations are more consistent with a persisting patchy conduction block with temporal dispersion preferentially affecting the activity arising from the macular regions of the visual field, than an overall decrease in response conduction velocity. Advocates of the latter hypothesis must explain how demyelination can result in apparent *increases* in conduction velocity. It has been reported that 'phase-shifts' of the 'steady-state' pattern reversal VEP in MS may result from the loss of certain pattern components or the appearance of new 'displaced' waves in the recorded activity (Duwaer & Spekreijse, 1978). Similarly, some if not most of the apparent delay of the transient pattern VEP in demyelinating disease may be due to alterations in relative component amplitudes and distributions. The observation of similar EP waveform alterations in a variety of pathologies further emphasises the non-specificity of the abnormal pattern VEP. While component latencies are more reliably estimated by multichannel recordings of half-field responses (Blumhardt & Halliday, 1979; Blumhardt et al, 1982b), it must be pointed out that this technique does not significantly increase the sensitivity of EP's for the detection of subclinical demyelinating lesions.

PREDICTIVE POWER OF EP'S VERSUS THE 'GOLD STANDARD'

Since no single test is specific for MS the diagnosis must be based on clinical grounds. In the early stages when the history is too short to be typical, or evidence is limited to a single lesion, the 'gold standard' against which the potential of a diagnostic test can be judged, is long-term follow-up. Follow-up needs to be prolonged as the mean relapse rate in early cases of MS is about 0·5 per annum. Although 10 years have elapsed since the introduction of the pattern VEP into routine clinical use, follow-up studies of patients with suspected MS are remarkably few and, as yet, too incomplete to assess fully the prognostic significance of 'clinically silent' EP abnormalities, or indeed of a normal EP.

One attempt has been made to follow up suspected cases of MS in whom BAEP's had been recorded 'blind' (Robinson & Rudge, 1980), but the numbers were very small and follow-up was incomplete. There was a high prevalence of false positives and·the subsequent development of MS in the few patients that were followed occurred, whether or not BAEP's were abnormal. Similarly, after a brief follow-up of patients who had presented with acute, isolated unilateral optic neuritis, one case with an abnormal SEP and two patients with normal SEP's developed MS (Matthews, 1978). The author concluded that the use of the SEP in this situation was unlikely to have any predictive value. In another study the VEP and SEP results were analysed with CSF IgG levels in patients with possible or probable MS who were then followed up for 2–4 years (Bottcher & Trojaborg, 1982). A combination of IgG levels and 'clinically silent' abnormalities of EP's appeared to justify the 're-classification' of cases to levels of greater diagnostic certainty. Thus 13 of 16 patients (81%) with abnormalities on both variables had progressed clinically whereas no changes occurred in 5 patients in whom one or other variable was normal. Deterioration appeared to correlate with 'moderate to large' increases in the IgG levels, but alterations in EP latency during the follow-up period did not parallel the course of the disease. However, the numbers in this study were small and no information was included on the fate of patients with normal EP's and IgG's.*

The clearest indication of the value of subclinical EP abnormalities is contained in two recent multi-modality studies, although the follow-up was a maximum of 38 months in one (Matthews et al, 1982) and from 2–52 months in the other (Deltenre et al, 1982; Table 3.4).

From the point of view of positive prediction, abnormal EP's in these selected patients impart a high risk of MS. Thus 67% of the Oxford patients and 68% of the Belgian patients, whose EP's suggested the presence of 'clinically silent' lesions, subsequently developed clinical evidence of MS during follow-up. This left 29% and 23%, respectively, of cases in each study who despite *abnormal* EP's had *not* developed clinically definite MS at the last clinical assessment.

The evaluation of the EP's as a diagnostic test must also take into account the proportion of 'false negatives' encountered. Thus 25% and 10%, respectively, of cases whose EP's failed to reveal 'clinically silent' lesions subsequently developed MS during follow-up. As the majority of cases in both studies who remained undiagnosed at follow-up had normal EP's (Table 3.4), the proportion of patients with definite MS which was successfully predicted by the tests in the early

---

* In this report and in the larger series from Belgium (Deltenre et al, 1982) the researchers unfortunately used a classification scheme which accepts the diagnostic test (EP's) under evaluation as evidence of MS (see McDonald & Halliday, 1977, section 5, p 8).

Table 3.4 Multi-modality follow-up studies in patients suspected to have MS.

Reference	Diagnostic classification	EP's	'Clinically silent' EP abnormality	Follow-up diagnosis	
Matthews et al (1982)	'Modified McAlpine' (1972) Probable Possible Acute not diagnosed	VEP, SEP, BAEP	Present 21/78 (27%)	Clinically definite MS Other disease Undiagnosed	14 1 6
			Absent 57/78 (73%)	Clinically definite MS Other disease Undiagnosed	14 6 37 (6)[a]
Deltenre et al (1982)	McDonald & Halliday (1972) Early probable or latent Progressive probable Progressive possible Suspected	VEP, SEP, BAEP and blink reflex	Present 53/133 (40%)	Clinically definite MS Other disease Undiagnosed	36 5 12
			Absent 80/133 (60%)	Clinically definite MS Other disease Undiagnosed	8 22 50

a Total includes 6 cases reclassified as McAlpine 'probable' or 'possible'.

stages must inevitably fall as the follow-up period lengthens and more cases reveal themselves. The group of patients with undiagnosed disease and normal EP's in the Oxford study already contains 6 patients re-classified into higher categories of diagnostic certainty (Table 3.5).

These results suggest that EP's are unable to predict the outcome in more than 50% of patients who develop unequivocal MS within about 3 years of presentation. In the early stages of the disease when 'hit-rates' are low the predictive value of the tests is even less reliable. Although the number of cases in the Oxford study with short histories (less than 3 months) is small, slightly more patients in this group with normal EP's (25%) went on either to clinically definite MS, or a higher level of diagnostic certainty, than did those with abnormal EP's (20%) (Table 3.5). It is clear that the absence of EP abnormalities is of no negative predictive value, as normal EP's can be found at all levels of diagnostic certainty.

The positive predictive power of 'clinically silent' EP abnormalities is encouraging but these results are achieved at the expense of a small number of 'false positives' (9% in the Belgian study to date). The proportion of these 'false positive' results differed in the two studies. One would expect the proportion of 'false positive' tests to decrease with the comprehensiveness of the work up to exclude other diseases before the patients were recorded and entered in the study. The number of 'other conditions' detected during the follow-up period in the Belgian series is more than double that of the Oxford study and the nature of the pathology in the few disclosed cases suggests that a policy of rigorous exclusion was not applied. The 'false positives' included abnormal VEP and/or SEP in one case each of B12 deficiency and Friedreich's ataxia, abnormal BAEP and SEP in

Table 3.5 Predictive value of 'clinically silent' EP abnormalities according to diagnostic certainty. (From Matthews et al, 1982.) *Key*: NYD, not yet diagnosed; AN, acute, not diagnosed. Cases of less than 3/12 duration at EP recording.

Classification	Probable MS ($n = 15$)		Possible MS ($n = 38$)		AN ($n = 25$)	
Subclinical EP abnormality	Present 6 (40%)	Absent 9 (60%)	Present 10 (26%)	Absent 28 (74%)	Present 5 (20%)	Absent 20 (80%)
Follow-up diagnosis (≤ 38 months)						
Clinically definite multiple sclerosis	5	6	8	5	1	3
Other disease	—	—	—	4	1	2
NYD	1	3[a]	2	19(2)[b]	3	15(4)[c]

a Including 2 cases lost to follow-up.
b Number of cases reclassified on clinical grounds as probable MS in parentheses.
c Number of cases reclassified on clinical grounds as possible or probable MS in parentheses.

frontal hygroma and abnormal BAEP in two patients with cervical spondylotic myelopathy. As abnormal EP's are common in other conditions and not specific for a particular pathology, there is little point in using EP's for the detection of possible subclinical demyelination until other likely diseases have been excluded. Despite this few authors have adequately described their entry criteria except in terms of the McAlpine et al (1972) or similar classification. The McAlpine progressive probable and progressive possible MS categories require the exclusion of other causes, yet few reports confirm that myelography was performed in all cases (see below).

It should also be borne in mind that some EP abnormalities recorded in patients who nevertheless progressed to clinically definite MS may also be falsely positive due to, for example, incidental ocular disease, poor quality recordings or too narrowly-defined normal parameters. It seems unlikely that 'slight delays' of the order of 1–2 ms over a 2·5 s.d. limit will prove to have the same predictive value as markedly abnormal responses, but follow-up studies have yet to correlate data of this type.

Other differences between these two follow-up studies may be due to a combination of technical factors, definitions of normality, and the selection of patients. Thus the difference in the overall 'hit-rates' (27% versus 40%) and the proportion of patients with definite MS at follow-up who had abnormal EP's (50% versus 82%), may have arisen from a larger percentage of acute cases in the Oxford study, or relatively more severe or long duration cases in the Belgian series. The latter investigators do not state whether abnormal EP's were considered diagnostic because there were no overt signs of cord or brain stem disease, or merely because there was no sensory loss. As an abnormal SEP was defined as an 'unsuspected lesion' in a case of Friedreich's ataxia, it appears that the latter criterion was applied. This policy would clearly inflate the proportion of 'clinically silent' EP's in this study. Other workers have more realistically proposed that abnormal SEP's in patients with signs of cord disease should be regarded as merely confirmatory and not indicative of a separate subclinical lesion (Purves et al, 1981; Matthews et al, 1982).

The ultimate criterion for a diagnostic test is whether the patient benefits from it. It has been suggested that the early detection of patients with MS by EP methods may have important therapeutic implications, but this remains a hypothetical consideration as no treatment capable of preventing progression exists at present. If an effective, and safe drug was available would we withhold it from the majority of patients whose EP results were normal despite symptoms or signs highly suggestive of early demyelination and in whom appropriate investigations had ruled out other possibilities? On the other hand, if the treatment was toxic or unpleasant but capable of arresting progression, the positive predictive ability of abnormal EP's in suspected MS may then be a useful method of selecting at least some patients for treatment,* but again, only if other diseases had been excluded by prior tests thus avoiding the risk of treating 'false positives'.

A further potential 'benefit' of abnormal VEP's for the patient who has disease clinically limited to the spinal cord, is the possible avoidance of myelography (Halliday et al, 1977; Mastaglia et al, 1980). This practice has become commonplace although no prospective study has been reported. The potential saving in X-rays is unlikely to be dramatic as subclinical VEP abnormalities are much less frequent when demyelination presents in this way, particularly in early cases where the 'hit-rate' is 10% or less (Blumhardt et al, 1982a). In one retrospective survey of 129 patients with suspected MS, the 22 patients who had had negative myelograms performed, included only 15 who had either a VEP or an electro-oculographic abnormality which the authors considered could have prevented the X-ray (Mastaglia et al, 1980). No data were presented on the patients with abnormal myelograms. In this clinical situation the false positive VEP's reported with Arnold-Chiari malformation have lead some authors to propose CT scanning to exclude hydrocephalus (which may cause a delayed response) and myelography despite the abnormal VER, if 'typical' oligoclonal bands are not present in the CSF (Halliday & McDonald, 1977)..Although this complicated strategy may correctly avoid myelography in most cases, delays in the diagnosis of treatable lesions could result when, for example, false positives occur in association with cord compression from a thoracic disc (Blumhardt et al, 1982a), or cervical spondylosis (Deltenre et al, 1982; Blumhardt et al, 1982a), or in the other conditions discussed above. Without prospective studies the fate of patients who did not get myelograms on the basis of abnormal VEP's cannot be determined. Moreover, once a diagnosis of MS has been made on the basis of an abnormal EP it may actually discourage further investigations despite clinical deterioration.

---

* Whether early subclinical EP abnormalities combined with raised CSF IgG levels indicate a 'malignant' form of MS (e.g. Bottcher & Trojaborg, 1982), remains to be established.

Finally, what is the point of doing these tests at all in short duration disease if the 'hit-rate' is poor despite characteristic symptoms and findings, if years may elapse before further episodes of demyelination may occur, if no treatment is available, if the abnormalities found are non-specific and the occurrence of false positives requires the exclusion of all other likely possibilities? Despite these severe limitations in the use of these tests for early diagnosis, there is no denying that EP's have a useful *confirmatory* role in many patients. Depending on the sensitivity of the technique they can provide an objective method of establishing an organic basis for complaints in the face of equivocal signs or symptoms. However, in atypical cases when abnormal EP's provide unsuspected clues, it is clearly even more important to rigorously exclude other conditions.

CONCLUSIONS

It has been said that a delayed VEP has the status of a positive Babinski reflex. This is a fine analogy if extended to encompass the often vicarious behaviour of the hallux valgus. The plantar response like the EP is not pathology-specific and may be positive, negative, absent, or impossible to interpret in the presence of unequivocal pathology, or spuriously positive when no organic lesion exists! The elicitation and interpretation of EP's and plantar responses depends on the skill of the person carrying out the test. The abnormal EP, like the Babinski reflex, is a valuable clinical sign, provided its limitations are recognised.

REFERENCES

Aminoff M J, Ochs A L 1981 Pattern-onset visual evoked potentials in suspected multiple sclerosis. Journal of Neurology, Neurosurgery and Psychiatry 44: 608–614
Asselman P, Chadwick D W, Marsden C D 1975 Visual evoked responses in the diagnosis and management of patients suspected of multiple sclerosis. Brain 98: 261–282
Bauer H J 1974 Communication to: Judgment of the validity of a clinical MS-diagnosis. In: The International Symposium on Multiple Sclerosis, Goteborg 1972. Acta Neurologica Scandinavica 50: suppl. 58
Blumhardt L D 1982 Topography of normal and abnormal pattern evoked potentials in man. M.D. Thesis, University of Otago, University Microfilms International, Ann Arbor
Blumhardt L D, Barrett G, Halliday A M 1982a The pattern evoked potential in the clinical assessment of undiagnosed spinal cord disease. In: Courjon J, Mauguière F, Revol M (eds) Advances in neurology, Vol 32, Clinical applications of evoked potentials in neurology. Raven Press, New York, p 463–471
Blumhardt L D, Barrett G, Halliday A M, Kriss A 1977 The contralateral negativity of the half field response and its association with central scotomata. Electroencephalography and Clinical Neurophysiology 43: 286
Blumhardt L D, Barrett G, Halliday A M, Kriss A 1978 The effect of experimental 'scotomata' on the ipsilateral and contralateral responses to pattern-reversal in one half-field. Electroencephalography and Clinical Neurophysiology 45: 376–392
Blumhardt L D, Barrett G, Kriss A, Halliday A M 1982b The pattern-evoked potential in lesions of the posterior visual pathways. Annals of the New York Academy of Sciences 388: 369–387
Blumhardt L D, Halliday A M 1979 Hemisphere contributions to the composition of the pattern-evoked potential wave-form. Experimental Brain Research 36: 53–69
Bodis-Wollner I, Yahr M D 1978 Measurement of visual evoked potentials in Parkinson's disease. Brain 101: 661–671
Bornstein Y 1975 The pattern evoked response (VER) in optic neuritis. Archives of Opthalmology 197: 101–106
Bøttcher J, Trojaborg W 1982 Follow up of patients with suspected multiple sclerosis: a clinical and electrophysiological study. Journal of Neurology, Neurosurgery and Psychiatry 45: 809–814

Brooks E B, Chiappa K H 1982 A comparison of clinical neuro-ophthalmological findings and pattern shift visual evoked potentials in multiple sclerosis. In: Courjon J, Mauguière F, Revol M (eds) Advances in neurology, Vol. 32: Clinical applications of evoked potentials in neurology. Raven Press, New York, p 453–458

Bynke H, Olsson J E, Rosén I 1977 Diagnostic value of visual evoked response, clinical eye examination and CSF analysis in chronic myelopathy. Acta Neurologica Scandinavica 56: 55–69

Cant B R, Hume A L, Shaw N A 1978 Effects of luminance on the pattern visual evoked potential in multiple sclerosis. Electroencephalography and Clinical Neurophysiology 45: 496–504

Cappin J M, Nissim S 1975 Pattern visual evoked responses in the detection of field defects in glaucoma. Archives of Ophthalmology 93: 9–18

Carroll W M, Kriss A, Baraitser M, Barrett G, Halliday A M 1980 The incidence and nature of visual pathway involvement in Friedreich's ataxia: a clinical and visual evoked potential study of 22 patients. Brain 103: 413–434

Carroll W M, Kriss A, Halliday A M 1982 Improvements in the accuracy of pattern visual evoked potentials in the diagnosis of visual pathway disease. Neuro-opthalmology 2: 237–253

Carroll W M, Mastaglia F L 1979 Leber's optic neuropathy: a clinical and visual evoked potential study of affected and asymptomatic members of a six generation family. Brain 102: 559–580

Chiappa K H, Ropper A H 1982 Evoked potentials in clinical medicine. New England Journal of Medicine 306: 1140–1150

Cohen S N et al 1982 Improved diagnostic yield in evaluation of multiple sclerosis using critical frequency of photic driving with pattern reversal evoked potentials. In: Courjon J, Mauguière F, Revol M (eds) Advances in neurology, vol 32, Clinical applications of evoked potentials in neurology. Raven Press, New York, p 459–462

Collins D W K, Black J L, Mastaglia F L 1978 Pattern reversal visual evoked potential: method of analysis and results in multiple sclerosis. Journal of Neurological Sciences 36: 83–95

Cook J H, Arden G B 1977 Unilateral retrobulbar neuritis: a comparison of evoked potentials and psychophysical measurements. In: Desmedt J E (ed) Visual evoked potentials in man: new developments. Clarendon Press, p 450–457

Deltenre P, van Nechel C, Vercrusse A, Strul S, Capon A, Ketelaer P 1982 Results of a prospective study on the value of combined visual, somatosensory, brainstem auditory evoked potentials and blink reflex measurements for disclosing subclinical lesions in suspected multiple sclerosis. In: Courjon J, Mauguière F, Revol M (eds) Advances in neurology, vol 32, Clinical applications of evoked potentials in neurology. Raven Press, New York, p 463–471

Dorfmann L J, Nikoskelainen E, Rosenthal A R, Sogg R L 1977 Visual evoked potentials in Leber's hereditary optic neuropathy. Annals of Neurology 1: 565–568

Duwaer A L, Spekreijse H 1978 Latency of luminance and contrast evoked potentials in multiple sclerosis patients. Electroencephalography and Clinical Neurophysiology 45: 244–258

Eggermont J J, Don M, Brackman D E 1980 Electroencephalography and auditory brain stem electric responses in patients with pontine angle lesions. Annals of Otology, Rhinology and Laryngology 89: (Suppl. 75) 1–19

Fine E J, Hallet M 1980 Neurophysiological study of subacute combined degeneration. Journal of Neurological Sciences 45: 331–336

Ganes T 1980 Somatosensory conduction times and peripheral, cervical and cortical evoked potentials in patients with cervical spondylosis. Journal of Neurology, Neurosurgery and Psychiatry 43: 683–689

Halliday A M 1981 Visual evoked potentials in demyelinating disease. In: Waxman S G, Ritchie J M (eds) Demyelinating disease: basic and clinical electrophysiology. Raven Press, New York, p 201–215

Halliday A M, McDonald W I 1977 Pathophysiology of demyelinating disease. British Medical Bulletin 33: 21–27

Halliday A M, McDonald W I, Mushin J 1972 Delayed visual evoked response in optic neuritis. Lancet 1: 982–985

Halliday A M, McDonald W I, Mushin J 1973 Visual evoked response in diagnosis of multiple sclerosis. British Medical Journal 4: 661–664

Halliday A M, McDonald W I, Mushin J 1977 Visual evoked potentials in patients with demyelinating disease. In: Desmedt J E (ed) Visual evoked potentials in man: new developments. Clarendon Press, Oxford, p 438–449

Halliday A M, Wakefield G S 1963 Cerebral evoked potentials in patients with dissociated sensory loss. Journal of Neurology, Neurosurgery and Psychiatry 26: 211–219

Hennerici M, Wenzel D, Freund H J, 1977 The comparison of small size rectangle and checkerboard stimulation for the evaluation of delayed visual evoked responses in patients suspected of multiple sclerosis. Brain 100: 119-136

Hoeppner T, Lolas F 1978 Visual evoked responses and visual symptoms in multiple sclerosis. Journal of Neurology, Neurosurgery and Psychiatry 41: 493-498

Huber C, Wagner T 1978 Electrophysiological evidence for glaucomatous lesions in the optic nerve. Ophthalmological Research 10: 22-29

Hume A L, Cant B R 1976 Pattern visual evoked potentials in the diagnosis of multiple sclerosis and other disorders. Proceedings of the Australian Association of Neurology 13: 7-13

Hutchinson W M 1976 Acute optic neuritis and the prognosis for multiple sclerosis. Journal of Neurology, Neurosurgery and Psychiatry 39: 283-289

Ikeda H, Tremain K E, Sanders M D 1978 Neurophysiological investigation in optic nerve disease: combined assessment of the visual evoked response and electroretinogram. British Journal of Ophthalmology 62: 227-239

Jones S J 1982 Clinical applications of short latency somatosensory evoked potentials. Annals of the New York Academy of Sciences 388: 369-387

Jones S J, Baraitser M, Halliday A M 1980 Peripheral and central somatosensory nerve conduction defects in Friedreich's ataxia. Journal of Neurology, Neurosurgery and Psychiatry 43: 495-503

Khoshbin S, Hallett M 1981 Multimodality evoked potentials and blink reflex in multiple sclerosis. Neurology 31: 138-144

Kjaer M 1980 The value of brainstem auditory, visual and somatosensory evoked potentials and blink reflexes in the diagnosis of multiple sclerosis. Acta Neurologica Scandinavica 62: 220-236

Kriss A, Carroll W, Blumhardt L D, Halliday A M 1982 Pattern and flash evoked potential changes in toxic (nutritional) optic neuropathy. In: Courjon J, Mauguière F, Revol M (eds) Advances in neurology, vol 32, Clinical applications of evoked potentials in neurology. Raven Press, New York, p 11-19

Krumholz A, Weiss H D, Goldstein P J, Harris K C 1981 Evoked responses in vitamin B_{12} deficiency. Annals of Neurology 9: 407-409

Lancet 1982 Editorial i: 1445-1446

Lowitzsch K, Kuhnt U, Sakmann Ch, Maurer K, Hopf H C, Schott D, Thäter K 1976 Visual evoked responses and blink reflexes in assessment of multiple sclerosis diagnosis. Journal of Neurology 213: 17-32

McAlpine D, Lumsden C E, Acheson E D 1972 Multiple sclerosis: a re-appraisal. Churchill Livingstone, Edinburgh

McDonald W I 1977 Pathophysiology of conduction in central nerve fibres. In: Desmedt J E (ed) Visual evoked potentials in man: new developments. Clarendon Press, Oxford p 427-437

McDonald W I, Halliday A M 1977 Diagnosis and classification of multiple sclerosis. British Medical Bulletin 33: 4-8

Marshall J 1955 Spastic paraplegia of middle age: a clinicopathological study. Lancet i: 643-646

Mastaglia F L, Black J L, Cala L A, Collins D W K 1977 Evoked potentials, saccadic velocities and computerised tomography in diagnosis of multiple sclerosis. British Medical Journal 1: 1315-1317

Mastaglia F L, Black J L, Cala L A, Collins D W K 1980 Electrophysiology and avoidance of invasive neuroradiology in multiple sclerosis. Lancet i: 144

Mastaglia F L, Black J L, Collins D W K 1976 Visual and spinal evoked potentials in diagnosis of multiple sclerosis. British Medical Journal 2: 732-733

Matthews W B 1978 Somatosensory evoked potentials in retrobulbar neuritis. Lancet i: 443

Matthews W B, Small D G 1979 Serial recordings of visual and somatosensory evoked potentials in multiple sclerosis. Journal of Neurological Sciences 40: 11-21

Matthews W B, Small D G, Small M, Pountney E 1977 The pattern reversal evoked visual potential in the diagnosis of multiple sclerosis. Journal of Neurology, Neurosurgery and Psychiatry 40: 1009-1014

Matthews W B, Wattam-Bell J R B, Pountney E 1982 Evoked potentials in the diagnosis of multiple sclerosis: a follow up study. Journal of Neurology, Neurosurgery and Psychiatry 45: 303-307

Mauguière F, Brudon F, Challet E, Maraval G, Courjon J 1982 Delayed visual evoked potentials in multiple sclerosis: interpretation of VEP latencies for follow up studies. In: Courjon J, Mauguière F, Revol M (eds) Advances in neurology, vol 32, Clinical applications of evoked potentials in neurology. Raven Press, New York, p 443-452

Meador C K 1965 The art and science of non-disease. New England Journal of Medicine 272: 92-95

Milner B A, Regan D, Heron J R 1974 Differential diagnosis of multiple sclerosis by visual evoked potential recording. Brain 97: 755–772

Nilsson B Y 1978 Visual evoked responses in multiple sclerosis: comparison of two methods for pattern reversal. Journal of Neurology, Neurosurgery and Psychiatry 41: 499–504

Oepen G, Brauner C, Doerr M, Thoden U 1982 Visual evoked potentials by central foveal and checkerboard reversal stimulation in multiple sclerosis. In: Courjon J, Mauguière F, Revol M (eds) Advances in neurology, vol 32, Clinical applications of evoked potentials in neurology. Raven Press, New York, p 427–431

Pedersen L, Trojaborg W 1981 Visual, auditory and somatosensory pathway involvement in hereditary cerebellar ataxia, Friedreich's ataxia and familial spastic paraplegia. Electroencephalography and Clinical Neurophysiology 52: 283–297

Purves S J, Low M D, Galloway J, Reeves B 1981 Comparison of visual, brainstem, auditory and somatosensory evoked potentials in multiple sclerosis. Canadian Journal of Neurological Science 8: 15–19

Rasminsky M, Sears T A 1972 Internodal conduction in undissected demyelinated nerve fibres. Journal of Physiology (London) 227: 323–350

Robinson K, Rudge P 1980 The use of the auditory evoked potential in the diagnosis of multiple sclerosis. Journal of Neurological Science 45: 235–244

Rosen I, Bynke H, Sandberg M 1980 Pattern reversal VEP after unilateral optic neuritis. In: Barber C (ed) Evoked potentials. M.T.P. Press, Lancaster, p 567–574

Selters W A, Brackman D E 1977 Acoustic tumour detection with brainstem electric response and audiometry. Archives of Otolaryngology 103: 181–187

Shahrokhi F, Chiappa K H, Young R R 1978 Pattern shift visual evoked responses: two hundred patients with optic neuritis and/or multiple sclerosis. Archives of Neurology 35: 65–71

Small D G, Matthews W B, Small M 1978 The cervical somatosensory evoked potential (SEP) in the diagnosis of multiple sclerosis. Journal of Neurological Sciences 35: 211–224

Stevens R A, Newman N M 1981 Abnormal visual evoked potentials from eyes with optic nerve head drusen. American Journal of Ophthalmology 92: 857–862

Streletz L J, Chambers R A, Sung H B, Israel H L 1981 Visual evoked potentials in sarcoidosis. Neurology 31: 1545–1551

Tackman W, Radu E W 1980 Pattern shift visual evoked potentials in Charcot-Marie-Tooth disease, HMSN Type 1. Journal of Neurology 224: 71–74

Trojaborg W, Petersen E 1979 Visual and somatosensory evoked cortical potentials in multiple sclerosis. Journal of Neurology, Neurosurgery and Psychiatry 42: 323–330

Troncoso J, Mancall E L, Schatz N J 1979 Visual evoked responses in pernicious anaemia. Archives of Neurology 36: 168–169

Walsh J C, Garrick R, Cameron J, McLeod J G 1982 Evoked potential changes in clinically definite multiple sclerosis: a two-year follow up study. Journal of Neurology, Neurosurgery and Psychiatry 45: 494–500

Wanger P, Nilsson B Y 1978 Visual evoked responses to pattern reversal stimulation in patients with amblyopia and/or defective binocular functions. Acta Ophthalmologica 56: 617–627

Wenzel W, Camacho L, Claus D, Aschoff J 1982 Visually evoked potentials in Friedreich's ataxia. In: Courjon J, Mauguière F, Revol M (eds) Advances in neurology. Vol 321, Clinical applications of evoked potentials in neurology. Raven Press, New York, p 131–140

Wilson W B 1978 Visual evoked response differentiation of ischaemic optic neuritis from the optic neuritis of multiple sclerosis. American Journal of Ophthalmology 86: 530–535

Zeese J A 1977 Pattern visual evoked responses in multiple sclerosis. Archives of Neurology 34: 314–316

4. Do anticoagulants prevent embolism from the heart to the brain?

David de Bono

'Oh, Let us never, never doubt,
The things that we are sure about.'

H. Belloc

This chapter examines the pathogenesis of embolism from the heart to the brain and, briefly, the mode of action of anticoagulants. It will try to define the present indications for the use of anticoagulants in the prophylaxis of cerebral embolism, the extent to which these are based on objective clinical trials, and the fields in which there is a particular need for fresh information.

THE PATHOLOGY OF EMBOLISM FROM THE HEART TO THE BRAIN

Embolic stroke accounted for 5–8% of the fatal cases of stroke in the United States National Survey of Stroke (Walker, Robins & Weinfeld, 1981). The authors concluded that this was probably an underestimate, since the prevalence of embolic stroke was higher in centres which performed a greater number of necropsies. The incidence of embolic stroke peaked at an earlier age than that of thrombotic cerebral infarction; in other words embolism was relatively more common in younger patients. Emboli from heart to brain do not necessarily consist of thrombus, but may include calcific and tumour emboli or portions of endocarditic vegetations (see de Bono, 1982 for further review).

Intracardiac thrombus forms under a variety of conditions, and its appearance, components and consistency will reflect this (Fig. 4.1). There is evidence from animal models that platelet anti-aggragant drugs may be more effective than coumarins in preventing the formation of platelet thrombi under rapid flow conditions in damaged arteries, whereas coumarin derivatives may be more effective in preventing fibrin-rich 'red thrombi' forming under conditions of sluggish flow. Extension of these observations to the human heart is speculative. It is not unusual at necropsy to see different varieties of thrombus in the same heart.

Clinically it is almost impossible to be sure that a given embolic event was due

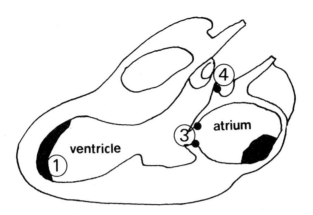

Fig. 4.1 Sketch of left-sided cardiac chambers (corresponding to echocardiographic 'long axis view') to show sites of thrombus formation. 'Red' thrombus, rich in fibrin with many red cells and leucocytes, tends to form at sites of left ventricular aneurysms (1) and in the left atrium (2). Platelet thrombi, usually small and friable, may form on damaged cusps of the mitral valve (3) or aortic valve (4). Both types of thrombus may form in patients with artificial heart valves.

to a particular type of thrombus or to other material, except in the case of retinal embolism where the embolus may be seen opthalmoscopically. Two dimensional echocardiography has now made it possible to visualise different sorts of intracardiac thrombus during life (Mikell et al, 1979: Schweizer et al, 1981), but at present this technique has not been put to large scale epidemiological use, and its sensitivity is not absolute.

There have been numerous reports on the occurrence of thromoembolic complications in patients with chronic rheumatic heart disease, particularly mitral valve disease. For example, Fleming & Bailey (1971) found 32% of patients with mitral stenosis and atrial fibrillation who were not on anticoagulants had had presumed emboli, as had 8% of patients with mitral stenosis and sinus rhythm, and 22% of patients with mitral incompetence and atrial fibrillation. Unfortunately, it is not possible with an 'open' population of patients to determine a true incidence rate: on one hand patients may die from a stroke without the presence of valvular heart disease being appreciated, on the other thromboembolism may cause the presentation of patients whose heart disease is otherwise asymptomatic. Myocardial infarction, which may lead to cerebral embolism as a result of the detachment of mural thrombus, has also been extensively studied. Mural thrombus is common, affecting up to 50% of patients (Hilden et al, 1971), but symptomatic cerebral embolism is relatively rare, accounting for only 0.5% of mortality in the first year after infarction (Ebert et al, 1969).

Prosthetic heart valve replacement, particularly in the mitral position, carries a high risk of thrombotic and embolic complications in patients who are not anticoagulated. This seems to be partly related to thrombosis on the surface of mechanical prostheses, and partly to left atrial stasis. 'Tissue' valves, usually mounted, preserved pig aortic valves, were expected to be relatively free of embolic risk in non-anticoagulated subjects, but this hope has not been fully realised. Lakier et al (1980) reported a 9.5% incidence of thromboembolic events in patients with porcine xenograft valves followed up for 60–89 months, and others have similar experiences. Many of the patients with thromboembolic complications also had atrial fibrillation, which may have contributed.

Atrial fibrillation in the absence of valve abnormalities is itself associated with an increased risk of cerebral ischaemic events. Kannel et al (1982) were able to show a five-fold excess of strokes in a cohort of patients with atrial fibrillation followed up in the Framingham study, but nearly half the patients also had evidence of hypertension or ischaemic heart disease. Thromboembolism is almost certainly the cause of stroke in patients who develop it immediately after cardioversion from atrial fibrillation to sinus rhythm (Turner & Towers, 1965), but Lavy et al (1980) have shown that many patients with atrial fibrillation have reduced cerebral regional blood flow compared with age-matched controls, and the possibility that some strokes in patients with atrial fibrillation are thrombotic rather than embolic cannot be ignored.

Over the past few years considerable interest has been shown in the possible association between stroke and mitral leaflet prolapse (Barnett et al, 1980). Cerebral ischaemic events affect only a tiny minority of the large number of people with this condition, and the potential mechanisms are probably as diverse as its clinical spectrum. Some at least of the ischaemic events may be related to an associated platelet abnormality rather than to the mitral lesion itself. Platelet abnormalities leading to a 'hypercoagulable state' have also been suggested as a complement or alternative to the traditional view that left atrial stasis is the principal reason for intracardiac thrombosis in patients with mitral valve lesions (Steele et al, 1974).

THE MECHANISM AND CONTROL OF ANTICOAGULATION

For practical purposes, anticoagulants can be divided into warfarin and its congeners (coumarin-type anticoagulants), platelet anti-aggregants, and heparin.

Warfarin

Warfarin antagonises vitamin K and impairs the formation of active varieties of plasma clotting factors, principally factors V, VII and X. Total inhibition would cause fatal bleeding, and it is important to control the dose of anticoagulant so as to reduce but not abolish blood clotting ability. This first became practicable when Quick invented the prothrombin time test, in which citrated plasma was activated with a rabbit brain thromboplastin and the time taken for it to clot after recalcification was measured (Quick, 1961). The result was expressed as a 'prothrombin time' in seconds, and in Quick's hands was very reproducible. Unfortunately other workers 'improved' the test by introducing their own thromboplastins made from different tissues and species. These gave different 'prothrombin times', and results began to be expressed either as a ratio compared to normal plasma (prothrombin time ratio or PTR) or by reference to a standard curve (result usually expressed as a percentage). A great deal of clinical work was done in attempting to define 'optimal ranges' for anticoagulation in terms of prothrombin time, PTR, or percentage prothrombin activity. Since each study usually involved a single centre and its own thromboplastin, results were internally consistent, but problems tended to arise when optimal ranges were transferred from centre to centre. Only gradually was it appreciated that different thromboplastin preparations made a striking difference to the sensitivity of the test: thus a patient with a PTR of 2.0 might be underanticoagulated at one centre, while in a hospital using a less sensitive thromboplastin a PTR of 2.0 might be associated with dangerous haemorrhage. It is only in the last decade that the need for national and international standardisation of thromboplastins has been widely recognised and appropriate action taken (Loeliger, 1979; Poller, 1982).

Failure to appreciate the problems of anticoagulant control has had far-reaching consequences: in the majority of clinical trials involving anticoagulants before about 1975 we know very little about the level or quality of anti-coagulation achieved. Even now, it is depressingly common to encounter studies which are critically dependent on the level of anticoagulation reached but which neglect to specify the standardisation of the thromboplastin used or the proportion of patients who actually maintain the desired levels of anticoagulation. The problems of interpretation which ensue have been elegantly discussed by Mitchell (1981).

At present, most British laboratories aim at prothrombin time ratios of between 2.0 and 4.0 standardised against a national reference thromboplastin (BCR) which in turn is closely comparable with the WHO international reference thromboplastin (Poller, 1971; Ingram & Hills, 1976; Duxbury, 1982). This is a slightly more conservative level of anticoagulation than that attempted in some continental and American centres, but most British units are not yet convinced that the case has been made for different levels of anticoagulation in patients with different problems.

Platelet anti-aggregants

Platelet anti-aggregant drugs, or 'anti-platelet drugs', have recently attracted attention for three reasons: increased awareness of the role of the platelets in arterial thrombosis, better understanding of the pharmacology of platelet aggregation, and a wish, possibly unrealistic, to confer the benefits of anticoagulation without the hazards.

Platelets exposed to thrombogenic stimuli release, among other things, thromboxane A_2 — an arachidonic acid derivative which is a powerful aggregant stimulus to other platelets. Pharmacological antagonists to thromboxane A_2 have been developed, but clinical experience with them is as yet minimal. However, a number of commonly used anti-inflammatory agents such as aspirin will prevent thromboxane A_2 production by inhibiting the enzyme cyclo-oxygenase, which converts arachidonic acid to one of the thromboxane precursors. Unfortunately, cyclo-oxygenase is also part of a synthetic pathway in endothelial cells leading to the production of the potent platelet anti-aggregant prostacyclin (PG I_2). Indiscriminate cyclo-oxygenase inhibition will therefore suppress both pro-aggregatory thromboxane A_2 and anti-aggregatory prostacyclin. Certain stratagems have been used to avoid this impasse. One may use a very weak cyclo-oxygenase inhibitor such as sulphinpyrazone, which blocks platelet but not endothelial cyclo-oxygenase. Alternatively, both the dose and the interval between doses of the more potent inhibitors might be manipulated to block the platelet enzyme but leave functional the more resilient endothclial system. In theory the latter approach is attractive, but a major snag is the lack of agreement on what constitutes an appropriate dose. Extrapolation of animal data to man suggested that a daily dose of 600–1000 mg might be appropriate. Such doses are known to prolong the bleeding time, but incidentally they also affect the vitamin K dependent plasma coagulation factors. Saltzmann (1982) has summarised a number of trials (not all relevant to cardiac thromboembolism) using this sort of dose, and points out that though a modest effect is sometimes apparent, it seems, rather oddly, to be confined to males. The validity and implications of this observation are still open to question. More recent studies have indicated that the human endothelial cyclo-oxygenase system is much more sensitive than animal experiments would have predicted, and that aspirin doses of 600–1000 mg per day probably block both thromboxane and prostacyclin production. Dosage schedules which in theory should inhibit thromboxane but preserve prostacyclin production range from 3.5 mg per kg every third day (Masotti et al, 1979) to 40 mg on alternate days (Hanley et al, 1982). Sadly, these observations were made too late for incorporation into the first generation of clinical trials of antiplatelet agents.

There is no 'simple' test which can measure the efficacy with which platelet aggregation is being inhibited in vivo. This is a major snag both to studies with aspirin and sulphinpyrazone and in the use of a different antiplatelet drug, dipyridamole (Persantin) which is reputed to work by increasing the platelet concentration of cyclic AMP. Probably the best way of showing that platelet anti-aggregants actually do something to platelets is by demonstrating their ability to restore to normal a shortened platelet survival time, but this is a cumbersome technique ill-suited to long-term control of therapy.

Heparin
Heparin is a powerful inhibitor of the plasma coagulation system. Its effects on platelet behaviour are complex but in vivo it probably has some platelet-inhibiting effect. The need for parenteral administration limits its usefulness, although the long-term use of intermittent subcutaneous heparin is being explored.

CLINICAL TRIALS OF ANTICOAGULANTS

Rheumatic heart disease
An ideal trial would compare prospectively two randomised groups of patients, well matched for age, sex and diagnosis. One group would be given anticoagulants, and the level of anticoagulation well controlled. The groups would be assessed without prior knowledge of therapy at predetermined intervals using 'hard' endpoints such as death or objective evidence of cerebral infarction. There have been a number of trials of anticoagulants in chronic rheumatic heart disease, but all of them fall short of this ideal in several respects. The trend in favour of anticoagulation is such however that it would now probably be regarded as unethical to conduct a 'good' trial in high risk patients.

One of the most influential studies was that of Owren (1963). In a group of 17 patients with recurrent thromboembolic episodes, there were 35 major embolic events before starting anticoagulation, but only 4 in 94 patient-treatment-years after anticoagulation. In a second study 15 patients were treated after a first embolic episode and between them had only one further embolus in 90 patient treatment years, while in a non-randomised control group of 17 untreated patients there were 22 episodes over 81 patient-treatment-years. Anticoagulation in these patients was controlled using the 'P&P' method aiming at a level of 15% (range 10–20%). These levels are roughly comparable with the present day recommendation for a corrected PTR between 2.0 and 4.0 (Owren, personal communication). The widespread prophylactic use of anticoagulation in patients with rheumatic heart disease, and particularly mitral stenosis, was further fostered by the retrospective survey of Fleming & Bailey (1971), which showed a much lower incidence of thromboembolism in patients receiving anticoagulation, although the difficulties of precise comparison in this type of study are immense. The problem was examined from a different angle by Michaels (1970) who studied the incidence of thromboembolism in patients with rheumatic heart disease once anticoagulants were withdrawn. This had the advantage of being a 'closed' study, and he concluded that anticoagulants did indeed reduce an embolic risk, the size of which was related to the nature of the underlying disease rather than to the timing of anticoagulant withdrawal. Despite their demerits, the vast majority of 'trials' published over the past two decades suggest that warfarin-type anticoagulants are effective in preventing, or at least inhibiting, cerebral embolism in patients with rheumatic mitral valve disease. One of the few dissenting voices has been a small but recent study by Steele & Rainwater (1980) in which sulphinpyrazone, but not warfarin, appeared to prevent transient ischaemic attacks in a group of patients with mitral valve disease. However, the numbers were small, details of warfarin therapy scanty, and the study had not been primarily designed to assess the efficacy of warfarin.

Satisfactory studies of platelet anti-aggregant drugs used on their own in rheumatic heart disease are presently lacking, perhaps because of the ethical problem of witholding 'established' therapy with anticoagulant drugs in high risk patients.

Myocardial infarction
There have been trials of both coumarin anticoagulants and antiplatelet agents in patients who have had acute myocardial infarction; the object has usually been the prevention of further infarction, but a certain amount of evidence has emerged about effects on TIA or stroke. The American Veterans Administration study (1965) disclosed 12 episodes of 'cerebrovascular accident' in 359 patients on placebo and 8 episodes in 355 treated patients. The level of anticoagulation actually achieved in this study was very modest, and this also applies to the British MRC anticoagulation trial (1969). In addition to these were the experiences of the Dutch 60-plus reinfarction study group (1982). They took a group of patients already established on anticoagulants after myocardial infarction, and randomised them to stopping or continuation of therapy. 'Adequate' levels of anticoagulation were reached. Of 878 patients in each group,

'intracranial events' occurred in 12 on anticoagulants and 20 on placebo. Eight of the 12 events in the anticoagulated group were due to haemorrhage, as was 1 of the 20 in the placebo group. This is one of the few true controlled studies to show that anticoagulation can reduce the risk of cerebral infarction, albeit at the cost of an increased risk of haemorrhage. It can be argued, however, that continuing or stopping an anticoagulant may not be equivalent to starting anticoagulant therapy from scratch.

Artificial heart valves

Patients receiving the earliest artificial mitral valves (Starr & Edwards, 1961) were anticoagulated because previous experience with dogs had suggested there was a thrombosis risk. Starr and colleagues later started a double-blind trial of anticoagulation, but curiously abandoned it in favour of routine anticoagulation because the incidence of embolic events was so small that they anticipated a long delay before a definitive result. This was not a universal experience: Moggio et al (1978) compared results within a single institution where the surgeons had different ideas on postoperative anticoagulation and found a four-fold increase in embolic events in patients not anticoagulated compared to those receiving warfarin. With aortic Starr-Edwards prostheses, anticoagulation also reduced thromboembolic complications, albeit in a consecutive rather than a randomised trial (Bonchek & Starr, 1975). Sullivan, Harken & Gorlin (1971) suggested that adding the anti-platelet agent dipyridamole to warfarin would further reduce the embolic risk after valve replacement, but results with dipyridamole alone or dipyridamole plus aspirin were disappointing. Butt et al (1981) found a 20% incidence of thromboembolic complications (8.7 per 100 patient-years) in patients with aortic Starr-Edwards prostheses receiving aspirin and dipyridamole. When they were changed to warfarin there were only 2 embolic episodes in 2132 patient-months of treatment (1.1 per 100 patient-years). Results with other mechanical prostheses have in general been similar to those with the Starr-Edwards valve.

Tissue valves were introduced in the hope that they would be non-thrombogenic, and certainly the embolic risk in patients with tissue valves in the aortic position is very small. Tissue valves in the mitral position in patients with atrial fibrillation are associated with an increased risk of embolism, but whether this is greater than the risks of anticoagulation may depend critically on the standards of anticoagulant control available and the degree of cooperation of the patient (Hill et al, 1982).

HAZARDS OF ANTICOAGULANT THERAPY

There are few other clinical situations where the potential benefits have to be weighed so carefully against the risks. There are two components to the latter: a 'predictable' component relating to the level of anticoagulation aimed at, and an 'unpredictable' component resulting, for example, from the inadvertent prescribing of drugs which upset anticoagulant control. It would be best to call the former a theoretically predictable risk, as quantitative data comparing the risks of different levels of anticoagulation are scanty. A 'therapeutic range' is inevitably a compromise and Duxbury (1982) has pointed out how uncertain anticoagulant control can be unless rigorous quality control is enforced. Forfar (1979) surveyed the complications of anticoagulant therapy over 7 years in a clinic dealing mainly with 'cardiac' patients. The anticoagulation level aimed at was slightly conservative by present standards. There were 2 deaths and 51 serious complications in 501 patients followed for 1199 treatment years. Risk was greatest in patients whose anticoagulant control had been difficult to establish from the start, and there was some increased risk between the 4th and 7th years of treatment, possibly because of complacency. In this study the PTR was beyond the therapeutic range in 23 of 24 patients with life-threatening haemorrhage, but within it in 26 of 27 patients with 'minor' complications.

Of the platelet anti-aggregants, dipyridamole probably carries the smallest risk of precipitating haemorrhage either alone or in combination with warfarin. Aspirin therapy is associated with a significant risk of gastrointestinal haemorrhage, although the risks of very low dose therapy (e.g. 40 mg every third day) have not yet been evaluated. Aspirin potentiates warfarin, and although combined therapy gives efficient anticoagulation there is a considerable risk of haemorrhage. Sulphinpyrazone alone is well tolerated, although it may cause abdominal symptoms and there is a small risk of blood dyscrasias. Sulphinpyrazone potentiates warfarin by a differential effect on the metabolism of its R and L enantiomers (O'Reilly, 1981) and the combination is perhaps best avoided.

CURRENT POLICY

Practical decisions about anticoagulant therapy have to be made, at present, on the basis of incomplete data, intelligent guesswork, and clinical 'feel'. My current policy is outlined below:

Rheumatic heart disease
Patients with mitral stenosis, of whatever severity, together with atrial fibrillation should be anticoagulated with warfarin unless there are compelling reasons to the contrary. Anticoagulation should be *considered* in all patients with mitral stenosis in sinus rhythm, and in all patients with mitral regurgitation in atrial fibrillation, i.e. the potential benefit of anticoagulation should be weighed against its potential risk in the individual patient. The ease of anticoagulant control, and patient compliance, are often unpredictable, so there may be a case for a trial of anticoagulants in individual patients.

The timing of the introduction of anticoagulation in patients who have valvular disease and experience a presumed cerebral embolus has been controversial. On one hand, emboli are frequently multiple (Szekely, 1964), on the other, there is a fear that anticoagulation may precipitate secondary haemorrhage into an infarcted area (Lieberman et al, 1978). Part of the problem is the difficulty of distinguishing between cerebral infarction and intracranial haemorrhage. Ideally, all patients with presumed cerebral embolism should have an urgent computerised tomographic scan before starting anticoagulation, even if this involves their transfer to a specialist centre. If no haemorrhage is demonstrated, anticoagulation can be started using heparin followed by warfarin. Heparin should be given by continuous slow intravenous infusion using a motorised syringe or equivalent, and the dose should be carefully controlled by estimation of the plasma thrombin time.

Replacement heart valves
All patients with mechanical prostheses, e.g. Starr-Edwards or Bjork-Shiley valves, should be anticoagulated. It has been claimed that these patients should be anticoagulated at a higher PTR level than rheumatic heart disease patients, but I remain to be convinced that the benefits would outweigh the risks, and the logistic problems would be considerable. In our experience major embolic episodes are very rare if PTR is scrupulously maintained in the range 2.0–4.0 (standardised against BCR), but some patients do have minor embolic episodes and for these we would add dipyridamole 100 mg thrice daily. Patients with 'tissue' valves in the aortic position, or with mitral tissue valves and sinus rhythm, probably do not need anticoagulants, but all patients with mitral valve replacement who are in atrial fibrillation should be considered for anticoagulation.

Ischaemic heart disease
The risk of stroke after acute myocardial infarction is not large enough in itself to warrant routine anticoagulation. The ability to detect left ventricular thrombus echocardiographically may enable a group of patients at particular risk to be identified. Patients with left ventricular aneurysms or dilated cardiomyopathies should be considered for anticoagulation.

Mitral prolapse
Mitral prolapse is so common that universal prophylaxis for the small risk of embolism would be counter-productive. My present policy is to treat patients with mitral prolapse who have had recurrent TIA with platelet anti-aggregants.

Atrial fibrillation
Although I accept that 'lone' atrial fibrillation is associated with an increased embolic risk, I am not aware that the benefits of prophylactic anticoagulation have been shown to outweigh the risks. There would seem to be scope here for a controlled trial. I would anticoagulate a patient with atrial fibrillation who had had a cerebral embolus, and I would recommend anticoagulation before elective cardioversion.

Endocarditis
The possibility of infective endocarditis needs to be remembered in patients presenting with a heart lesion and presumed cerebral embolism (Pruitt et al, 1978). Blood cultures remain the mainstay of diagnosis, but echocardiography can help. Anticoagulant treatment in active endocarditis carries an increased risk of cerebral haemorrhage from 'mycotic' aneurysms: however, once adequate antibiotic therapy has been instituted it is probably safe to continue

anticoagulants if there is a major risk of thromboembolism, e.g. in patients with prosthetic valves.

FUTURE PLANS

The present consensus on the use of anticoagulants in mitral valve disease, or in patients with replacement heart valves, will not be abandoned lightly, in spite of the inadequacy of some of the evidence on which it is based. There is no convincing evidence yet that platelet anti-aggregants are effective in preventing embolism under these circumstances, and a comparative trial of anticoagulants against antiplatelet agents in high risk patients would probably not be acceptable at present. There are, however, sufficient patients with high risk lesions and contraindications to anticoagulation for a trial of antiplatelet agents in this subgroup to be feasible. Of the lower-risk lesions, where there is continuing uncertainty about optimal management, chronic atrial fibrillation would be the most suitable for a prospective controlled trial of either anticoagulants or platelet anti-aggregants. There is still scope for improvements in anticoagulant control and the concept of different therapeutic ranges for different conditions requires further investigation. New anticoagulants, and in particular antiplatelet drugs are about to be introduced, including stable prostacyclin analogues and thromboxane inhibitors. They will need proper evaluation and this would be greatly helped by a reliable measure of platelet function. It would be a pity if the hard-won lessons of the warfarin saga went unheeded.

REFERENCES

Barnett H J M, Baughner D R, Taylor D W, Cooper P E, Kostuk W J & Nichol P M 1980 Further evidence relating mitral valve prolapse to cerebral ischaemic events. New England Journal of Medicine 302: 139–144
Bonchek L I, Starr A 1975 Ball valve prostheses-current appraisal of late results. American Journal of Cardiology 35: 843–853
Brott W H, Zajtchuk R, Bowen T E, Davia J, Green D C 1981 Dipyridamole — aspirin as thromboembolic prophylaxis in patients with aortic valve prostheses. Journal of Thoracic and Cardiovascular Surgery 81: 632–635
de Bono D P 1983 Cardiac causes of stroke. In: Russell R W R (ed) Vascular disease of the central nervous system, 2nd edn. Churchill Livingstone, Edinburgh
Duxbury B McD 1982 Therapeutic control of anticoagulant treatment. British Medical Journal 284: 702–704
Ebert R V, Borden C W, Hipp H R, Holzman D, Lyon A F, Schnaper H 1969 Long term anticoagulant therapy after myocardial infarction. Journal of the American Medical Association 207: 2263–2267
Fleming H A, Bailey S M 1971 Mitral valve disease, systemic embolism and anticoagulants. Postgraduate Medical Journal 47: 599–604
Forfar J C 1979 A 7 year analysis of haemorrhage in patients on long term anticoagulant treatment. British Heart Journal 42: 128–132
Hanley S P, Bevan J, Cockbill S R, Heptinstall S 1981 Differential inhibition by low dose aspirin of human venous prostacyclin synthesis and platelet thromboxane synthesis. Lancet i: 969–971
Hilden T, Raaschou F, Iversen K, Schwartz M 1971 Anticoagulants in acute myocardial infarction. Lancet ii: 327–331
Hill J D et al 1982 Risk benefit analysis of warfarin therapy in Hancock mitral valve replacement. Journal of Thoracic and Cardiovascular Surgery 83: 718–723
Ingram G I C, Hills M 1976 Reference method for the one-stage prothrombin time test on human blood. International committee for standardization in haematology. Thrombosis and Haemostasis 36: 237–238

Kannel W B, Abbott R D, Savage D I, McNamara P M 1982 Epidemiological features of chronic atrial fibrillation: the Framingham study. New England Journal of Medicine 306: 1018–1021

Lakier J B, Khaja F, Magilligan D J, Goldstein S 1980 Porcine xenograft valves — long term (60–89) month) follow-up. Circulation 62: 313–318

Lavy S, Storm S, Melamed M D, Cooper G, Keren A K, Levy P 1980 Effect of chronic atrial fibrillation on regional cerebral blood flow. Stroke 11: 35–38

Lieberman A et al 1978 Intracranial haemorrhage and infarction in anticoagulated patients with prosthetic heart valves. Stroke 9: 18–24

Loeliger E A 1979 The optimal therapeutic range in oral anticoagulation. Thrombosis and Haemostasis 42: 1141–1152

Masotti G, Galanti G, Poggesi L, Abbate R, Neri-Serneri G S 1979 Differential inhibition of prostacyclin production and platelet aggregation by aspirin. Lancet ii: 1213–1215

Michaels L 1970 Recurrence of thromboembolic disease after discontinuing anticoagulant therapy. British Heart Journal 32: 335–342

Mikell F L, Asinger R W, Rourke T, Hodges M, Sharma B, Francis G S 1979 Two dimensional echocardiographic demonstration of left atrial thrombus in patients with prosthetic mitral valves. Circulation 60: 1183f1187

Mitchell J R A 1981 Anticoagulants in coronary heart disease — retrospect and prospect. Lancet i: 257–262

Moggio R A, Hammond G I, Stansel H C, Glen W W L 1978 Incidence of emboli with cloth covered Starr-Edwards valve without anticoagulation and with varying forms of anticoagulation. Journal of Thoracic and Cardiovascular Surgery 75: 296–299

O'Reilly R A 1982 Stereo-selective interaction of sulfinpyrazone with racemic warfarin and its separated enantiomorphs in man. Circulation 65: 202–207

Owren P A 1963 The results of anticoagulant therapy in Norway. Archives of Internal Medicine 111: 240–247

Poller L 1971 The British national thromboplastin. British Journal of Haemoatology 20: 359–362

Poller L 1982 Oral anticoagulants reassessed. British Medical Journal 284: 1425–1426

Pruitt A, Rubin R, Korchmer A, Duncan G W 1978 Neurological complications of bacterial endocarditis. Medicine (Baltimore) 57: 329–343

Quick A (1961) Clinical interpretation of the one-stage prothrombin time. Circulation 24: 1422–1428

Report of the working party on anticoagulant therapy in coronary thrombosis to the Medical Research Council 1969 Assessment of short-term anticoagulant therapy after cardiac infarction. British Medical Journal i: 335–342

Saltzman E 1982 Aspirin to prevent arterial thrombosis. New England Journal of Medicine 307: 113–115

Schweizer P, Bardos P, Erbel R, Meyer J, Merx W, Messmer B J, Effert S 1981 Detection of left atrial thrombi by echocardiography. British Heart Journal 45: 148–156

Sixty-Plus Reinfaction Study Research Group 1982 Risks of long term oral anticoagulant therapy in elderly patients after acute myocardial infarction. Lancet i: 64–67

Starr A, Edwards D E 1961 Mitral replacement : Clinical experience with a ball valve prosthesis. Annals of Surgery 154: 726–740

Steele P P, Weily H S, Davies H, Genton E 1974 Platelet survival in patients with rheumatic heart disease. New England Journal of Medicine 290: 537–540

Steele P P, Rainwater J 1980 Favorable effect of sulfinpyrazone on thromboembolism in patients with rheumatic heart disease. Circulation 62: 462–468

Sullivan J M, Harken D E, Gorlin R 1971 Pharmacologic control of thromboembolic complications of cardiac valve replacement. New England Journal of Medicine 284: 1391–1394

Szekely P 1964 Systemic embolism and anticoagulant prophylaxis in rheumatic heart disease. British Medical Journal i: 1209–1212

Turner J R B, Towers J R H 1965 Complications of cardioversion. Lancet ii: 612–614

Veterans Administration Co-operative Study 1965 Long term anticoagulant therapy after acute myocardial infarction. Journal of the American Medical Association 193: 929–933

Walker A E Robins R, Weinfeld F D 1981 The national.survey of stroke: Ch 3 Clinical findings. Stroke 12: suppl I, 12–44

Walsh P N, Kansu T A, Corbett J J, Savino P J, Goldbergh W P, Schatz W J 1981 Platelets, thromboembolism and mitral valve prolapse. Circulation 63: 552–559

5. Should spontaneous cerebral haematomas be evacuated and if so when?

John Marshall

The incidence of cerebral haemorrhage has been falling during the last half century for reasons which remain obscure. Because cerebral haemorrhage is strongly associated with hypertension it might be thought that the introduction of effective therapy was responsible. This cannot be the entire explanation because the decline had begun long before. Yates (1964), in a careful examination of the pattern of death certification during the period 1932 to 1960, showed that whereas in the 1930s cerebral hacmorrhage was three times as common as infarction, by the 1960s cerebral infarction was more common.

Death certification is of course subject to error particularly in distinguishing between different pathological causes of a stroke. Dalsgaard-Nielsen (1956) followed 1000 cases of stroke to autopsy and found that the hospital clinical diagnosis was confirmed in only 65% of cases of cerebral haemorrhage and 58% of cerebral infarctions. Yates (1964) was fully aware of this difficulty which he met by examining the necropsy records of three large hospitals where he found the same reversal of the ratio of cerebral haemorrhages to cerebral infarcts.

A reversal of the ratio between cerebral haemorrhage and cerebral infarction does not mean there must have been a decline in the number of haemorrhages. The same effect could have resulted from a rise in infarctions. Close examination of the data showed that though infarcts had increased there had also been a decline in the number of cerebral haemorrhages.

The decline in the number of deaths from cerebral haemorrhage has not, however, entirely eliminated an important medical and social problem. Inspection of epidemiological data shows that the incidence rises with age beginning as early as the fourth decade. Bread-winners may therefore be eliminated by the condition. Nor is mortality the only consideration. The effects of a stroke caused by cerebral haemorrhage may be devastating leading to a life-long handicap involving motor power, speech and other functions. It is therefore entirely appropriate to pose the question which forms the title of this chapter.

PATHOLOGY

Cerebral haemorrhage can occur from a variety of causes. Whilst berry aneurysms commonly rupture into the subarachnoid space, they may, particularly if there have been previous minor bleeds so that the fundus of the aneurysm has become attached to the brain, rupture into the parenchyma giving an intracerebral haematoma. Head injury is another example of a condition which may be associated with intracerebral haematoma. In both these situations the management of the primary condition — the berry aneurysm or the traumatised brain — dominates the situation. For this reason cerebral haemorrhage from these causes will not be considered further here.

What is meant by 'spontaneous' in this context? In fact the haemorrhage is not truly spontaneous but occurs because arteries are diseased. The commonest form of the disease is that produced by hypertension. This causes fibrinoid necrosis of the walls of small arteries and arterioles and the formation of miliary aneurysms of the Charcot-Bouchard type. The work of Ross Russell (1963) and Cole & Yates (1967a, b) has clearly demonstrated the association between miliary aneurysms on the one hand and hypertension and advancing years on the other, and the predilection for the aneurysms to form on the small, deep penetrating arteries. Rupture of one or more of this type of aneurysm is believed to be the cause of 'spontaneous' intracerebral haemorrhage.

Because of the 'spontaneous' occurrence of the haemorrhage there has been little opportunity to study events at the precise moment of rupture. Circumstantial evidence such as the association with coitus and other events which are known to give rise to abrupt rise in blood pressure suggest this is at least one precipitating factor.

Cryptic arteriovenous malformations
Not all people who develop a 'spontaneous' cerebral haemorrhage are hypertensive hence there must be another cause. Dorothy Russell (1954) in a classic paper gave a detailed account of what she called cryptic arteriovenous hamartomas which had been first described by Margolis, Odom et al (1951). These are often destroyed by the haematoma when they rupture, but in some instances it is possible to identify the remnants of a hamartoma and so establish the cause of the haemorrhage. It is probable that 'spontaneous' cerebral haemorrhage in non-hypertensive people springs from a cryptic hamartoma. The lesions are however so small that their existence does not materially influence the management of the haematoma in the way the presence of a large arteriovenous malformation would. The maximum size has never been strictly defined. Dorothy Russell (1954) accepted lesions up to 2 or 3 cm as coming into this category. They can sometimes be seen on angiography as shadows a few millimetres in size.

EXPERIMENTAL PATHOLOGY

In deciding about the value of a treatment it is important not only to consider pragmatically controlled or uncontrolled clinical experience but also to take into account the underlying pathology. A treatment is most likely to succeed if it is on a rational basis.

Experimental haematomas in the dog produced by injecting 2 ml of autologous blood into the brain show at about 3 hours, the haematoma surrounded by a thin layer of brain described as in status spongiosus (Suzuki & Ebina, 1980). Over the succeeding 24 hours the picture evolves so that the haematoma becomes surrounded by a layer of necrotic tissue, outside of which is a layer of perivascular bleeding which is in turn enclosed by the layer of status spongiosus. The point to note is that though the production of the haematoma was instantaneous, the changes in the surrounding brain evolved over a period extending up to 48 hours. This provides an argument for intervention, if it is to be undertaken at all, to be early before the changes have had time to develop. There is, of course, the possibility that though the histologically observable changes take time to evolve they are irreversibly initiated at the onset. This possibility would have to be tested by comparing the results following early removal with those following later evacuation of experimental haematomas.

Suzuki & Ebina (1980) also studied the effect of injecting 2 ml of oil-wax into the brain. Changes comparable with those following injection of autologous blood were found but they were much less severe and there was the noteworthy difference that the surrounding perivascular bleeding was much less marked. This suggests that the effect of the haematoma is not solely attributable to the fact that it occupies space; reaction to the presence of blood seems also to be important and constitutes another argument for removal independent of whether the haematoma is producing a mass effect.

One other feature which it is important to note is that oedema was not a prominent feature either in the blood or the oil-wax experiments. There was some oedema but it was not a major feature of the lesions.

The conclusion from this experimental work is that one is endeavouring to treat a lesion which not only occupies space but produces a reaction in the brain to the constituents of the lesion, the reaction not being associated with massive oedema.

NATURAL HISTORY

Before deciding about treatment it is important to know what happens to haematomas which are left in patients who survive. CT scanning has made it possible to answer this question in a more precise way than was previously possible. Clearly haematomas are absorbed but leave a detectable abnormality on the scan. About the second or third day the haematoma is surrounded by a zone of reduced density which, in view of experimental pathological observations, is probably the area of necrosis or status spongiosus rather than being oedema. Haematomas of less than 2 cm diameter have usually been reabsorbed in about 5 weeks whereas larger haematomas may take 8 or 9 weeks (Grumme, et al1980). When the haematoma has been of sufficient size to produce a mid-line shift this does not return to normal before 3 weeks at the earliest and usually requires about 5 weeks. There is therefore a considerable period of time during which changes are occurring which might be expedited by removal of the haematoma.

Natural history studies also throw light on the features of a haematoma which influence mortality. Size is of course of prime importance. Location is of equal importance and has a determining influence on mortality. Haemorrhage into the frontal, temporal or occipital pole — usually described as lobar haemorrhage —

carries a mortality of up to 20 %, whereas with haemorrhage into the basal ganglia mortality may reach 90 % (Regli & Jeanmonod, 1980). Displacement of mid-line structures is also a bad sign largely because it usually involves distortion of the brain stem with all its consequences.

Rupture into the ventricle might be thought to be helpful by effecting a form of internal decompression. In fact it proves not to be the case, intraventricular rupture being associated with higher mortality. Whether this is an effect of blood in the ventricles per se or whether it reflects the fact that bigger and deeper haematomas — both features carrying a worse prognosis — are more likely to rupture into the ventricles is hard to say.

MANAGEMENT

A landmark in the scientific evaluation of surgical treatment of spontaneous cerebral haematomas was the paper of McKissock et al (1961) which reported a controlled trial of surgical versus conservative treatment in 180 cases. The diagnosis was based on a combination of clinical history and examination, examination of the cerebrospinal fluid and angiography. Haemorrhages in the posterior fossa were excluded. The patients were randomised between conservative treatment and surgery. In the surgically treated group the haematoma was evacuated by craniotomy. In the conservative group there was vigorous attention to the airway etc. but no specific drug regime.

In the event the surgically treated cases did not fare better than those managed conservatively; in some sub-groups, such as hypertensive women without displacement of mid-line structures on the angiogram, they did worse. The authors expressed the intention of continuing to study the subject by selecting sub-groups in whom surgery appeared to have more to offer. Some 20 years later a monograph on *Spontaneous Intracerebral Haematomas* (Pia et al, 1980), which reported a number of operative series, showed what little progress has been made in deciding the issue.

What has emerged is a better definition of the clinically detectable factors which influence the outcome. First among these is the level of consciousness of the patient. In one series (Kanaya et al, 1980) mortality after surgery in patients who were alert or merely confused was 2% whereas in patients in deep coma was 87%. This has been the general experience; patients in coma fare badly with or without surgery. In determining who, if anyone, should have their cerebral haematoma evacuated, the level of consciousness should be the first criterion to be taken into account. Patients who are alert, confused, drowsy or in stupor should be considered; patients in coma should be left alone. (Patients in coma from a cerebellar haemorrhage will be considered later.)

The factor of next importance is the site of the lesion. Lobar haematomas are a good risk; capsular and, even more so, basal ganglia haematomas are a bad risk. Size also comes into the equation. Small haematomas, which before CT scanning might well not have been recognised as such, do well both in terms of mortality and residual disability. This being so there seems little argument in favour of adding even the minimal damage to the brain involved in surgical evacuation of the clot.

Drawing these main points together it would seem that patients who are not in coma who have a lobar haematoma of more than 3–4 cm are ideal subjects. The difficulty then arises in deciding whether what is obviously a better risk group do any better with surgery than they would with only conservative measures.

Conservative treatment

This clearly raises the question, 'Of what should conservative treatment consist?' There can be no doubt that general measures properly applied make a significant difference to the outcome. First and foremost is the securing and maintenance of an adequate airway to maintain oxygenation and to reduce the risks of pulmonary complications. Similarly, maintaining an appropriate water and electrolyte balance is essential. Here the margin is a narrow one. Space occupying lesions in the head are traditionally managed by a degree of dehydration. There is no surer way of hastening the demise of elderly people (who are often the victims of cerebral haemorrhage) than to allow them to become dehydrated. The aim therefore should be to keep patients in normal balance leaning towards the dehydration end rather than the overhydration end of the normal range. These measures together with physiotherapy would be applied equally to surgically and medically managed cases.

The role of hypotensive drugs

Since cerebral haemorrhage is closely associated with hypertension it may be expected that many patients will have a raised blood pressure. There are two problems involved in reducing the blood pressure. Firstly the patient may not be truly hypertensive; the elevated blood pressure may be a response to raised intracranial pressure — the so-called Cushing effect. It is a necessary factor in the maintenance of normal cerebral blood flow in the face of raised intracranial pressure. Lowering the blood pressure in these circumstances lowers perfusion and so may further harm the damaged brain.

Even if the patient is truly hypertensive, autoregulation is invariably damaged temporarily by a stroke, so again lowering blood pressure lowers blood flow. In these circumstances, unless the patient has evidence of malignant hypertension, it is better to wait until the patient is on the way to recovery before embarking on blood pressure reduction.

SURGICAL EVACUATION OR NOT?

The alternative to surgical evacuation is so-called conservative management which, as outlined in the preceding section, comprises measures which would be applied equally to surgically treated cases. There is no specifically medical therapy as such. The essential difference between the two approaches is therefore the removal of the clot. The clinical studies to date do not permit a definitive answer to be given to the question as to the value of this procedure. Apart from the study by McKissock et al (1961) there has been no prospective randomised controlled trial of surgery versus no surgery, the patients being treated identically in all other respects. Kanaya et al (1980) have summarised the results of surgery in three large series from Japan, Mitsuno (1971), Kanaya & Handa (1974) and

Kanaya et al (1978), but comparison was made with separate series of cases treated in neurological departments. Surgical mortality was slightly less in patients who were alert or only somnolent, but the difference was not statistically significant. Mortality was significantly less in patients in stupor or semi-coma who were treated surgically. Patients in coma did badly in either group.

On the basis of this evidence it could be argued that in alert or somnolent patients surgery is unnecessary because they do well medically. Patients in coma do badly whatever is done. It is patients in stupor or semi-coma in whom surgery appears to have something to offer. It could of course be argued that patients in coma have nothing to lose by surgery as the mortality with conservative measures alone is extremely high, nearing 100% in some series. Surgery might offer some chance however slender. This line of argument is fallacious because it is wrong to tie up surgical skills and facilities on procedures which offer little hope and, more important, any survivors are left severely handicapped.

If those who are stuporose are to be operated the question arises when? Guidetti & Gagliardi (1980) found that 7 of 22 patients operated on within 3 days died whereas only 9 of 85 patients operated later succumbed. This type of evidence is however difficult to interpret as waiting eliminates some bad risk patients and so favours the results of late surgery. The evidence from experimental pathology would certainly favour early intervention.

In summary, patients who are stuporose would seem to be the prime target for early surgery. The question of patients who are alert and have lobar haematomas is debatable. They do well when managed conservatively but whether their long-term disability would be less if the clot were removed is not known. Patients in coma are best left alone.

CEREBELLAR HAEMATOMAS

Haematomas in the cerebellum must be considered separately from those above the tentorium. They are not uncommon, constituting between 5 and 10% of all intracranial haematomas. The added factor of brain stem compression makes for a high mortality in this group. McKissock et al (1960) reported 34 consecutive cases, 14 of whom were treated surgically, 9 surviving. Sano & Yoshida (1980) reported 39 cases, 18 of whom were operated, with a 39% mortality. This occurred in patients who were stuporose or comatose prior to surgery. Arseni & Gontea (1980) reported 25 cases operated with only 1 death, but 12 of the cases were chronic haematomas. Klinger & Kunze (1980) found 109 cases in the literature, most of whom were treated surgically with a mortality of 30%

Though the operative mortality in patients who are comatose or stuporose is high it is still worth while undertaking surgery because the outlook is otherwise hopeless.

This may seem to be in complete opposition to the philosophy outlined for cerebral haematomas. The situation is however different for coma in cerebellar haematomas is frequently due to brain stem compression, relief of which is followed by dramatic improvement. Moreover disability in survivors is in no way comparable to that following a cerebral haemorrhage; the ability to compensate for damage to one cerebellar hemisphere is considerable.

Patients who are drowsy and deteriorating should have their clot removed. For patients who are alert and stable a policy of close observation has been suggested (Klinger & Kunze, 1980). However these patients can deteriorate quite quickly hence it may be better to operate early unless the haematoma can be seen on CT scan to be very small. The encouraging feature about surgical removal of cerebellar haematomas is that survivors are usually left with little or no deficit.

THE WAY AHEAD

None of the policies outlined in this chapter are beyond dispute. The way ahead lies with prospective randomised controlled trials of specific sub-groups. A large scale trial, including all types of cerebral haemorrhage, would increase our present uncertainties. A sub-group worth studying is lobar haemorrhage in alert patients, the question to be answered being, does surgery reduce the degree of long term disability? Another group is the stuporose patient with lobar or capsular haemorrhage, the question there being does surgery reduce mortality as has been suggested by uncontrolled trials? Study of other groups should wait on some advance which gives hope that a trial would be worth while.

REFERENCES

Arseni C, Gontea A 1980 In: Pia HW, Langmaid C, Zierski J (eds) Spontaneous intracerebral haematomas. Springer-Verlag, Berlin, p 287
Cole F M, Yates P O 1967a The occurrence and significance of intracerebral micro-aneurysms. Journal of Pathology and Bacteriology 93: 393–411
Cole F M, Yates P O 1967b Intracerebral aneurysms and small cerebrovascular lesions. Brain 90: 759–768
Dalsgaard-Neilsen T 1956 Some clinical experience in the treatment of cerebral epoplexy (1000 cases). Acta Psychiatrica Scandinavica Suppl 108: 101–19
Grumme T, Kretzschmar K, Lanksch W 1980 In: Pia H W, Langmaid C, Zierski J (eds) Spontaneous intracerebral haematomas. Spinger-Verlag, Berlin, p 216
Guidetti B, Gagliardi F 1980 In: Pia H W, Langmaid C, Zierski J (eds) Spontaneous intracerebral haematomas. Springer-Verlag Berlin p 247
Kanaya H, Handa K 1974 The surgical treatment of hypertensive intracerebral hemorrhage on the cooperative study in Japan. Thirty ninth Annual Meeting of the Japan Neurosurgical Society
Kanaya H et al 1978 A neurological grading for patients with hypertensive intracerebral hemorrhage and a classification for hematoma location on computed tomography. In: Proceedings of the 7th Conference of Surgical Treatment of Stroke, p 265–70
Kanaya H et al 1980 In: Pia HW, Langmaid C, Zierski J. (eds) Spontaneous intracerebral haematomas. Springer-Verlag, Berlin, Heidelberg, New York, p 268
Klinger M, Kunze S 1980 In: Pia HW, Langmaid C, Zierski J. (eds) Spontaneous intracerebral haematomas. Springer-Verlag, Berlin p 358
McKissock W, Richardson A, Walsh L 1960 Spontaneous cerebellar haemorrhage. A study of 34 consecutive cases treated surgically. Brain 83: 1–9
McKissock W, Richardson A, Taylor JC 1961 Primary intracerebral haemorrhage. A controlled trial of surgical and conservative treatment in 180 unselected cases. Lancet 2: 221–226
Margolis G, Odom GL, Woodhall B, Bloor BM 1951 The role of small angiomatous malformations in the production of intracerebral hematomas. Journal of Neurosurgery 8: 564–575
Mitsuno T 1971 Surgical management of apoplexy. The 18th General Assembly of the Japanese Medical Congress, Tokyo
Pia H W, Langmaid C, Zierski J (eds) 1980 Spontaneous cerebral haematomas. Springer-Verlag, Berlin
Regli F, Jeanmonod D 1980 In: Spontaneous intracerebral haematomas. Springer-Verlag, Berlin, p 233

Ross Russell R W 1963 Observations on intracerebral aneurysms. Brain 86: 425–442

Russell D S 1954 The pathology of spontaneous intracranial haemorrhage. Proceedings of the Royal Society of Medicine 47: 689–704

Sano K, Yoshida S 1980 In: Spontaneous intracerebral haematomas. Springer-Verlag, Berlin, p 348

Suzuki J, Ebina T 1980 In: Spontaneous intracerebral haematomas. Springer-Verlag, Berlin, p 121

Yates P O 1964 A change in the pattern of cerebrovascular disease. Lancet 1: 65–69

6. Is shrinking the brain a good thing after cerebral infarction?

M. J. G. Harrison

Swelling of the brain occurs after cerebral infarction. Approximately 30% of the early mortality after ischaemic stroke is due to the effect of this swelling causing raised intracranial pressure and herniation of the temporal lobe or brain stem. Most early deaths from coning after cerebral infarction occur after an interval of 2–10 days (Fig. 6.1) and are due to oedematous swelling associated with a necrotic

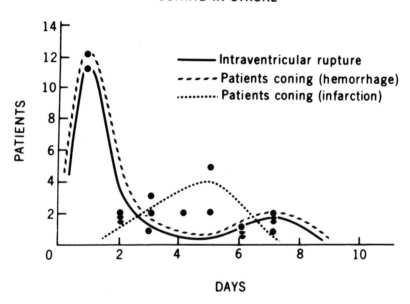

CONING IN STROKE

— Intraventricular rupture
- - - - Patients coning (hemorrhage)
·········· Patients coning (infarction)

Fig. 6.1 Time of deaths from coning after stroke from White et al (1979) with permission of the authors and the editor of Stroke.

infarct (White et al, 1979; Fig. 6.2) Deterioration of stroke patients, which is seen in as many as 1 in 3 is also due to swelling in some 25% of instances (Hachinski et al, 1981).

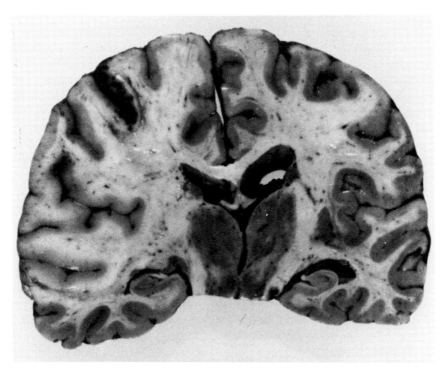

Fig. 6.2 Swelling of infarcted hemisphere with shift of mid-line structures.

PATHOPHYSIOLOGY

Swelling of ischaemic and infarcted brain occurs by a number of mechanisms. Congestion of the brain (increased cerebral blood volume) may occasionally contribute, for example when blood flow is restored by dissolution of an embolus and blood re-enters a vascular bed which, due to a period of ischaemia, has lost vasoreactivity and is vasodilated by ischaemic metabolites. Venous infarcts may also be congested. More important, however, is the development of oedema (an increase in the water content of the tissue).

Klatzo (1972) has suggested that oedema is basically of two types. Cytotoxic oedema consists of an increase in cell water (cellular hydrops) due to impaired osmoregulation across cell membranes, usually a sign therefore of metabolic cell damage. Grey and white matter are both affected. This type of oedema is seen for example with trimethyltin or hexachlorophene toxicity. Morphologically cytotoxic oedema is manifest in swelling of mitochondria and of astrocytic processes. The passage of water across the cell membrane may be simply due to osmotic forces, or through 'pores'. There is however evidence that the permeability to water is under neurogenic control and it is, therefore, possible that selective changes in water movement may be created by a neural lesion (Raichle et al, 1976).

Vasogenic oedema is defined as an increase in extracellular water due to a breakdown of the blood brain barrier with egress of plasma constituents. Vasogenic oedema is produced experimentally by cold injury and occurs around cerebral tumours. The leaked plasma fluid spreads preferentially through the cerebral white matter to a distance that is determined by the hydrostatic pressure. Tissue swelling due to vasogenic oedema can be accompanied by a reciprocal decrease in regional cerebral blood flow (c.b.f.) (Reulen & Tsuyumu, 1981), probably due to passive compression of the microcirculation (Little, 1976). Expansion of the extracellular space by the ingress of fluid will also increase intervascular distances and might affect energy supply to the tissues. Cerebral blood flow may be reduced in areas in which the water content is not markedly elevated (e.g. quite distant from the site of maximal vasogenic oedema due to experimental cold injury) and these changes may be caused by the elevated tissue pressure secondary to the volumetric increase due to the oedematous area. The extent of oedema will tend to be limited by increasing tissue pressure but its resolution will be delayed in areas with an intact blood brain barrier by the presence of extracellular proteins with osmotic effects on the transcapillary movement of water. There is some evidence that the proteins in spreading vasogenic oedema may have local deleterious effects (Tanaka et al, 1981). Thus direct local infusions of serum cause greater reduction in c.b.f. than do equal volumes of dialysed serum. The resolution of this type of oedema depends at least in part on the intracytoplasmic uptake of extravascated proteins by astrocytes.

Oedema fluid is also thought to gain access to c.s.f. spaces through the ependyma. The spread of vasogenic oedema through the hemisphere may thus be checked when it reaches the ventricular system. This may explain the common clinical observation of limitation of the peritumourous oedema to the frontal or occipital area. Spread through the whole hemisphere is unusual (Fig. 6.3).

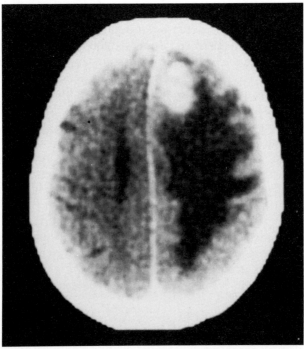

Fig.6.3 CT scan showing right hemisphere oedema affecting white matter due to a frontal tumour.

In experimental models of cerebral ischaemia both types of oedema are seen. With models of total global ischaemia no net increase in water content occurs during arrest of the circulation (no inflow) but water moves from extracellular to intracellular compartments. When the circulation is restored a net increase in water content occurs the severity of which is predetermined by the severity of the preceeding ischaemic insult. Osmotic forces may well be involved in this early phase of cytotoxic post-ischaemic oedema (Hossman, 1976). The degree of water retention in the ischaemic tissue is proportional to the rise in tissue lactate but the rise in tissue osmolarity is not simply due to lactate ions. At this stage there may be an increase in pinocytosis but the blood brain barrier is intact. After restoration of the circulation the ionic and osmotic gradients slowly return to normal with resolution of the 'cytotoxic' oedema. This stage of ischaemic oedema preceeds evidence of necrosis in the tissue. Necrosis when it occurs will be expected to be accompanied by release of more osmotically active substances.

In focal ischaemia (e.g. middle cerebral artery (MCA) occlusion) the situation is a little different. Cerebral blood flow does not fall to zero so there is a supply of water, and the net water content of the tissue may rise, particularly in the grey matter, as soon as 5 minutes after the onset of ischaemia. The rise in tissue osmolarity is however less severe. Oedema develops at flow levels at which energy metabolism is only partially suppressed. It has been suggested that some activities (e.g. ion homeostasis) may be affected not only by energy failure but by accumulation of inhibiting compounds such as glutamate, or by shut down of cortical activity. In the first few hours after the onset of MCA occlusion the oedema is of this cytotoxic type with no change in the blood brain barrier. (Hossman & Scheier, 1980).

The barrier 'opens' to different materials at different times after the onset of ischaemia (Fujimoto et al, 1976; Klatso et al, 1981). Thus at 1 hour some serum protein can be detected extracellularly by the peroxidase method whereas albumin-bound Evans Blue is not seen outside blood vessels until several hours later. The barrier damage first appears at the periphery of the ischaemic area. Extravasated proteins appear in grey matter initially and spread through the extracellular space. Severe breakdown of the blood brain barrier occurs 6–18 hours after carotid occlusion in the gerbil or MCA occlusion in the cat (Fig. 6.4). It is associated with an increase in oedema which spreads through the white matter. Although the breakdown of the blood brain barrier may only be transient, fluid continues to accumulate due to the trapped extracellular plasma derived macromolecules. The protein is eventually cleared by proteolytic digestion in necrotic tissue, and by uptake by glia. It is this second phase of vasogenic oedema that leads to the peak of swelling after 2–3 days. Water content falls at the end of the first week. The cytotoxic and vasogenic phases of ischaemic oedema overlap. Thus Scuccimarra et al (1980), using a method of measuring cortical impedance, showed a rise after carotid clamping in dogs which reached a peak at 2 hours associated with cell swelling. Thereafter impedance fell as the extracellular space filled with extravascated protein-rich fluid. With models in which cerebral ischaemia is produced by multiple emboli, the blood brain barrier breakdown occurs at once and vasogenic oedema predominates with widened extracellular spaces in areas where there is no cellular swelling.

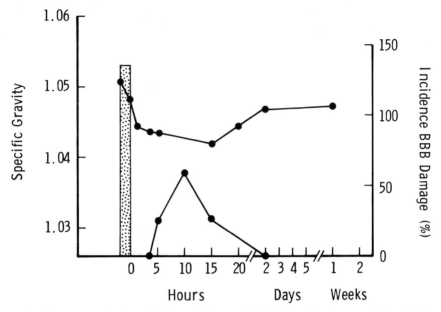

Fig. 6.4 Time course of oedema (falling specific gravity) and increasing damage of blood brain barrier after experimental infarction redrawn from Fujimoto et al (1976).

There is evidence that there is a gradual decrease in c.b.f. in the presence of ischaemic oedema. For example Hossman & Scheier (1980) showed that when MCA occlusion caused a fall of c.b.f. to the critical levels at which oedema developed flow fell further, but in animals in which the initial fall did not trigger oedema formation flow tended to recover (Fig. 6.5). There is little direct evidence that the presence of oedema per se causes an increase in the area of infarction, however. Nonetheless, volumetric increase may cause tentorial herniation.

Kogure et al (1981) has recently demonstrated the crucial role of the hydrostatic pressure on the severity of ischaemic oedema. An elevated perfusion pressure increased early cytotoxic oedema especially when collateral flow was good into the ischaemic area (as with cerebral ischaemia due to vessel occlusion by an embolus). Hypertension also increased macromolecular extravasation through the blood brain barrier.

This experimental evidence suggests that cerebral ischaemia initially causes cytotoxic oedema related to metabolic changes, and later quantitatively more important vasogenic oedema occurs. The presence of oedema may affect the local microcirculation and is certainly of pathological relevance when its volumetric effect causes tentorial herniation. The severity of the oedema is dependent on the severity of the initial ischaemic insult, but is aggravated by an elevated hydrostatic pressure. The retention of water in ischaemic tissue probably depends on the rate of clearing of osmotically active materials, initially lactate and other catabolites, and of extravasated macromolecules (proteins).

Hossman et al (1980) used the model of MCA occlusion in the cat to assess possible therapies. Grey matter water content rose after 2 hours from 80.1 ± 0.2 to 83.2 ± 0.8 ml/100 g net weight at which time blood flow in the MCA territory

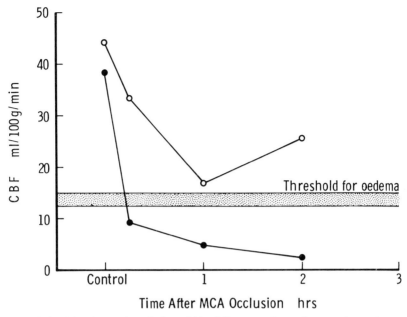

Fig. 6.5 Relationship of secondary decline of blood flow to oedema after experimental infarction. Redrawn from Hossman & Scheier (1980).

was down to about 15% of the control level. 1.5 g/kg of 20% mannitol, given at 15 minutes after MCA occlusion, elevated the blood osmolarity and was the only regime that limited oedema (water content only reached 81.3 ± 0.6 ml/100 g). Hypothermia, barbiturates and haemodilution proved ineffective. Corticosteroids were assessed in the same model by Lee et al (1974). They proved ineffective in limiting the size of the infarction or in improving the neurological deficit (Table 6.1). This proved to be due to the fact that dexamethasone only affected the leak of an albumin bound marker and the associated water content in necrotic infarcted areas, while failing to affect ischaemic non-necrotic areas.

The relevance of these animal models to human cerebral infarction must be considered before translating the foregoing conclusions and using them as the

Table 6.1 Effect of dexamethasone on MCA occlusion in cats. (From Lee et al, 1974.)

Group	Neurological deficit at 2 weeks (graded 0–4)	Size of infarct marked by 2 observers
No dexamethasone (*n* = 5)	1.6	8.0
Dexamethasone before and after occlusion (*n* = 5)	1.8	7.8
Dexamethasone after occlusion (*n* = 5)	1.6	8.2

rationale for therapy. The animals used have much smaller cranial cavities and c.s.f. space volumes. They are more vulnerable to the effects of elevated tissue pressure therefore. Also the infarcts produced experimentally are commonly huge when considered as a percentage of the hemisphere affected.

In man there is little information about the oedema occurring immediately after the onset of ischaemia (before necrosis has occurred). That oedema does develop in the first hours after carotid or middle cerebral occlusion is however clear from the swelling of an affected cerebral hemisphere as seen on a CT scan taken within a few hours of the onset of hemiplegia. Swelling, seen in up to 70% of cases, is most marked on scans taken 2–4 days later however and may be expected to have resolved by 25 days. The time course suggests that this later oedema is vasogenic in nature, and there is some evidence of a disturbed blood brain barrier in such patients. Thus, though isotope scans are only markedly positive at the end of the first week, Harrison & Ell (1981) obtained evidence that some movement of Technetium could be detected after 24 hours: the more striking isotope scan pictures obtained later may relate to reactive vascular changes, and not just blood brain barrier effects. Though some of the oedema around an infarct is thought to be vasogenic therefore, there are differences from that associated with cerebral tumours, which may be important when discussing therapy. Thus, as readily seen on CT scans, the swelling of ischaemic brain affects grey and white matter with a homogenous appearance (Fig. 6.6), whilst peritumourous oedema is confined to the white matter which it follows giving rise to the familiar digital pattern (Fig. 6.3). Also it should be recalled that some of

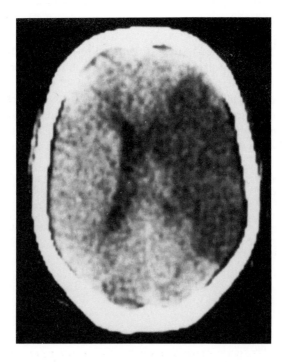

Fig. 6.6 CT scan showing right hemisphere oedema related to infarction.

the ischaemic tissue swelling will be due to cytotoxic oedema, and some to congestion.

THERAPY

If swelling of cerebral infarcts accounts for some 30% of their mortality and oedema has adverse effects on the microcirculation in ischaemic areas, there would seem to be a clear rationale for the use of anti-oedema therapies in stroke victims. The clearcut success of corticosteroids in patients with cerebral tumours led to the conclusion that vasogenic oedema could be reduced or resolved by their use. Reulen et al (1972) showed that the water content of perifocal oedematous areas associated with tumours was lower in the patients who were given dexamethasone prior to operation (Table 6.2). The effect was greatest in the

Table 6.2 Perifocal oedema surrounding brain tumours. (From Reulen et al, 1972.)

| | No. | Water content (g/100 g fresh weight tissue) | |
		Cortex	White matter
Untreated	18	81.0 ± 0.7	79.0 ± 1.3
Dexamethasone	16	80.3 ± 0.9	75.7 ± 1.2[a]

a $P < 0.05$

white matter. Pappius (1972), however, advanced some evidence that suggested that the dramatic clinical benefit in patients with pure vasogenic oedema might not be due to the reduction in water content. Thus in an animal model (cold injury in the cat) dexamethasone produced a modest reduction in hemisphere water content, but a dramatic improvement in the e.e.g. By contrast the diuretic frusemide had a greater dehydrating effect on the brain but no beneficial effect on the e.e.g. (Table 6.3).

Table 6.3 Cold injury (cat) 48 hours. (From Pappius, 1972.)

	Difference in hemisphere weight (g)	Ratio low/high frequency in e.e.g. (normal — 0.8)
Untreated	0.72 ± 0.29	5.0
Dexamethasone	0.56 ± 0.21	2.1
Fruosemide 3 mg/kg/day	0.48 ± 0.14	7.5

In stroke victims corticosteroids have been disappointing (Table 6.4). Dyken & White (1956) treated 17 patients with cortisone while 19 acted as controls.

Table 6.4 Steroids in acute stroke.

Reference	Number in trial	Treated group Mortality %	Control group Mortality %
Dyken & White (1956)	36	76	53
Bauer & Tellez (1973)	54	18	35
Norris (1976)	53	27	18
Mulley, Wilcox & Mitchell (1978)	118	41	47

Treatments were simply alternated on admission. Treatment began within 24 hours and involved a decreasing 21 day schedule commencing with 300 mg of cortisone a day, but it made no difference to mortality. Patten et al (1972) randomised 31 patients and gave dexamethasone or placebo within 24 hours. A small difference suggested a benefical effect of treatment but haemorrhage and infarction, carotid and basilar territories were not equally represented in the two small groups invalidating the comparison. Bauer & Tellez (1973) carried out a double-blind study of dexamethasone (120 mg in 10 days) in 54 patients admitted within 48 hours of their stroke who were nearly all affected by clouding of consciousness. At 14 days both morbidity and mortality were lower in the treated group. In a double-blind study of similar size Norris (1976) assessed the use of steroids in 53 patients treated within 24 hours. Five of 27 died on placebo, 7 of 26 on dexamethasone, within 29 days. Larger trials by Candelise et al (1975) and Santanbrogio et al (1978) used only historical controls. The best trial to date was carried out in Nottingham and reported by Mulley, Wilcox & Mitchell (1978). One hundred and eighteen patients received dexamethasone (192 mg over 15 days) or placebo. Patients were randomised within 72 hours of the onset of their stroke (mean 5.5 hours). The mortality (41% treated 47% placebo) showed no evidence of a therapeutic effect, nor did assessments of function in hospital or at follow-up, 1 year later. They concluded, as one must from these studies, that there is no clear indication to treat all stroke victims with steroids. Hachinski (personal communication) is currently carrying out a trial of high dose dexamethasone. It is of course true that none of the published studies had CT scan control and there has yet to be a trial in which dexamethasone has been assessed in patients whose CT scan shows swelling related to cerebral infarction.

The alternative approach, which has theoretical justification because of the cytotoxic element in ischaemic oedema, is to use hyperosmolar materials. Mannitol, and glycerol have been assessed. Unfortunately mannitol, which dehydrates the normal contralateral hemisphere and lowers intracranial pressure in tumour cases, has only been tested in stroke victims in inadequate trials. These were the same two non-blind, non-randomised surveys using historical controls and already mentioned in their use of steroids (Candelise et al, 1975; Santanbrogio et al, 1978).

In the case of glycerol there have been three placebo controlled studies (Table 6.5). Mathew et al (1972) randomised 54 patients with assumed cerebral infarcts and 8 with cerebral haemorrhage to intravenous glycerol (50 g/day) for 4–6 days, or to placebo. Trial end points, including a clinical score, were assessed at 14 days. Patients were entered within 4 days of ictus so some were at the stage of maximal oedema before treatment began. The clinical scoring suggested that more patients improved and less stayed unchanged or deteriorated over 2 weeks.

Table 6.5 Use of glycerol in acute stroke.

| Authors | Number | Treated group | | Control group | |
		Mortality %	Clinically improved %	Mortality %	Clinically improved %
Mathew et al (1972)	54	7	76	8	56
Larsson et al (1976)	27	33	25	33	27
Fritz & Werner (1975)	106	28	a	41	a

a See text

Larsson et al (1976) repeated this study with the same protocol but included patients within 6 hours, theoretically improving the chances of seeing a beneficial effect of a regime aimed at limiting oedema formation. No difference in mortality or in the rate of improvement in clinical status up to 10 days was seen. Sadly, haemorrhage cases were included and accounted for most deaths, and the study was very small ($n = 27$). Fritz & Werner (1975) reported a larger study. Fifty patients received a glycerol infusion (50 g a day for 6 days) and 56 served as controls. Patients were included if they were admitted within 24 hours of the onset of their stroke. The authors chose to allocate to treatment or control status on the basis of the day of birth (even dates treated, uneven dates controls). The 6 day clinical rating suggested that mild and severe cases had not benefited from glycerol. The moderately affected group showed a tendency to stabilise if treated.

Gilsanz et al (1975) tried to compare dexamethasone and glycerol. Unfortunately the 30 patients treated for 6 days with glycerol were compared only with 31 'similar' patients on dexamethasone. The clinical rating used demonstrated a greater proportion of glycerol treated patients improving and a smaller number dying but the lack of randomisation makes the study unconvincing, and the patients were not well matched for severity prior to treatment.

CONCLUSIONS

One must sadly conclude that the case for osmotherapy is at best unproven either because it really is ineffective or because the trials were too small and too poorly designed to demonstrate modest clinical usefulness. Measurements of cerebral blood flow and c.s.f. pressure in patients within 36 hours of stroke show that glycerol treatment can reduce pressure and raise c.b.f. (Battistini et al, 1976) so this appraoch warrants further clinical study. There are theoretical reasons for studying the use of isovolaemic infusions of hyperosmolar albumin. This would have the advantage of having the required osmotic effect without the difficulties of glycerol (which can disturb diabetic control). It would also reduce whole blood viscosity by haemodilution, and thereby increase cerebral blood flow.

There is a further problem in this field. Thus, it may be that those patients whose deterioration is due to massive oedema are the only ones who would benefit from its prevention, but that they are the very individuals who have extensive necrotic infarcts. 'Successful' treatment may move them from the fatal outcome category into the group with devastating residual disability.

REFERENCES

Battistini N, Fieschi C, Nardini M, Ciacci C 1976 Effects of glycerol treatment on CSF pressure and rCBF in patients with cerebral infarction. In: Pappius H M, Feindel W (eds) Dynamics of brain edema. Springer Verlag, Berlin, p 326–329

Bauer R, Tellez H 1973 Dexamethasone as treatment in cerebrovascular disease 2. A controlled study in acute cerebral infarction. Stroke 4: 547–555

Candelise L, Colombo A, Spinnler H 1975 Therapy against brain swelling in stroke patients. A retrospective Study on 227 patients. Stroke 5: 353–356

Dyken M, White P T 1956 Evaluation of cortisone in the treatment of cerebral infarction. Journal of the American Medical Association 162: 1531–1534

Fritz G, Werner I 1975 The effect of glycerol infusion in acute cerebral infarction. Acta Medica Scandinavica 198: 287–289

Fujimoto T, Walker J T, Spatz M, Klatzo I 1976 Pathophysiological aspects of ischemic edema. In: Pappius H M, Feindel W (eds) Dynamics of brain edema. Springer Verlag, Berlin, p 171–180

Gilsanz V, Rabollar J L, Buencuerpo J, Chantres M T 1972 Controlled trial of glycerol versus dexamethasone in the treatment of cerebral oedema in acute cerebral infarction. Lancet i: 1049–1051

Hachinski V C, Norris J W 1981 The deteriorating stroke. In: Meyer J S, Lechner H, Ott E O, Aranibar A (eds) Cerebral vascular disease 3. 10th Saltzburg Conference. Excerpta Medica, p 315–318

Harrison M J G, Ell P J 1981 Ischaemic edema. Stroke 12: 888

Hoppe W E, Waltz A G, Jordan M M, Jacobson R L 1974 Effects of dexamethasone on distributions of water and pertechnetate in brains of cats after middle cerebral artery occlusion. Stroke 5: 617–622

Hossman K A 1976 Development and resolution of ischemic brain swelling. In: Pappius H M, Feindel W (eds) Dynamics of cerebral edema. Springer Verlag, Berlin, p 21–227

Hossman K A, Scheier F J 1980 Experimental brain infarcts in cats. 1, Pathological observations. Stroke 11: 583–592

Hossman K A, Matsuoka Y, Bloink M, Fitzgerald G, Hossman V 1980 Treatment of experimental infarction of the cat brain. Proceedings of the International Symposium on Experimental and Clinical Methodologies for Study of Acute and Chronic Cerebrovascular Disease, Pergamon Press, p 375–381

Klatzo L 1972 Neuropathological aspects of brain edema. Journal of Neuropathology and Experimental Neurology 26: 1–14

Klatzo L, Chui E, Fujiwara K 1981 Aspects of the blood brain barrier. In: de Vlieger M, de Lange S A, Bebs J W F (eds) Brain edema. Wiley Medical, p 11–18

Kogure K, Busto R, Scheinberg P 1981 The role of hydrostatic pressure in ischemic brain edema. Annals of Neurology 9: 273–282

Larsson O, Marinovich N, Barber K 1976 Double blind trial of glycerol therapy in early stroke. Lancet 1: 832–834

Lee M C, Mastri A G, Waltz A G, Loewenson R B 1974 Ineffectiveness of dexamethasone for treatment of experimental cerebral infarction. Stroke 5: 216–218

Little J R 1976 Microvascular alterations and edema in focal cerebral ischaemia. In: Pappius H M, Feindel W (eds) Dynamics of brain edema. Springer Verlag, Berlin, p 236–243

Mathew N T, Meyer J S, Rivera V M, Charney J Z, Hartmann A 1972 Double blind evaluation of glycerol therapy in acute cerebral infarction. Lancet ii: 1327–1329

Mulley G, Wilcox R G, Mitchell J R A 1978 Dexamethasone in acute stroke. British Medical Journal 2: 994–996

Norris J W 1976 Steroid therapy in acute cerebral infarction. Archives of Neurology 33: 69–71

Pappius H M 1972 Effects of steroids on cold injury edema. In: Reulen H J, Schurmann K (eds) Steroids and brain edema. Springer Verlag, Berlin, p 57–63

Patten B M, Mendell J, Brunn B, Curtin W, Carter S 1972 Double blind study of the effects of dexamethasone on acute stroke. Neurology 22: 377–383

Raichle M E, Eichling J O, Grubb R L Hartman B K 1976 Central noradrenergic regulation of brain microcirculation. In: Pappius H M, Feindel E (eds) Dynamics of brain edema. Springer Verlag, Berlin, p 11–17

Reulen H J, Tsuyumu M 1981 Pathophysiology of formation and natural resolution of vasogenic brain edema. In: de Vlieger M, de Lange S A, Bebs J W F (eds) Brain edema. Wiley Medical, 31–48

Reulen H J, Hadjudimos A, Schurmann K 1972 The effect of dexamethasone on water and electrolyte content and on rCBF in perifocal brain edema in man. In: Reulen H J, Schurmann K (eds) Steroids and brain edema. Springer Verlag, Berlin, p 239–252

Santanbrogio S, Martinotti R, Sardella J, Porro F, Randazzo A 1978 Is there a real treatment for stroke: clinical and statistical comparison of different treatments in 300 patients. Stroke 9: 130–132

Scuccimarra A, Pensabene V, Pandolfo N, de Blasi F 1980 Study of various types of experimental brain edema using the electrical impedence technique and the electron microscope. Advances in Neurosurgery 9: 332–336

Tanaka K, Marmarou A, Shulman K 1981 Regional cerebral blood flow changes associated with direct infusion edema. Journal of Cerebral Blood Flow Metabolism 1: Suppl 1 S156–157

White O B, Norris J W, Hachinski V C, Lewis A 1979 Death in early stroke. Causes and mechanisms. Stroke 10: 743

7. Are antifibrinolytic agents useful after subarachnoid haemorrhage?

Stephen J. Haines

It has been estimated that of all patients suffering subarachnoid haemorrhage from a ruptured intracranial aneurysm, approximately one-third are dead or disabled as a result of the initial haemorrhage, and of the two-thirds remaining, 45% will die or be disabled, some from medical and surgical complications but most from recurrent haemorrhage and vasospasm (Kassel & Drake, 1982). The ultimate objective of the surgical treatment of aneurysmal subarachnoid haemorrhage is to prevent rebleeding. Initial experience with direct surgical treatment shortly after the initial haemorrhage was quite discouraging and was responsible for the standard recommendation to delay surgery for 2 to 3 weeks. However, the Cooperative Study of Aneurysmal Subarachnoid Haemorrhage figures indicate that approximately 25% of patients will suffer a second haemorrhage during those 2 weeks (Locksley, 1966). Attention naturally turned to a search for ways to reduce that risk. It was suggested that therapy to delay the natural process of clot lysis might prevent or delay the second haemorrhage. Therefore, drugs that inhibit the normally active fibrinolytic system were administered to patients with subarachnoid haemorrhage.

CLINICAL EVALUATION OF ANTIFIBRINOLYTIC THERAPY

Three review articles have examined the papers reporting clinical use of antifibrinolytic agents after subarachnoid haemorrhage (Ramierez-Lassepas, 1981; Vermeulen & Muizelaar, 1980; Warlow 1981). For detailed discussion of the papers, the reader is referred to these reviews. The following tables and discussion are intended to highlight this information.

Suggestive data

The earliest suggestive clinical data came in the late 1960s from Gibbs & O'Gorman (1967), Mullan & Dawley (1968), and Norlen & Thulin (1969). Gibbs & O'Gorman (1967) did not find any overall benefit but concluded that there was a suggestion that if the whole blood clot lysis time could be raised to the level of 40 hours, the risk of recurrent haemorrhage might be reduced. Mullan & Dawley (1968) found only 2 recurrent haemorrhages in 13 patients. Both groups felt that this was a much lower rate of rebleeding than they would have expected from previous experience.

Supportive data

This information stimulated others to try such therapy. Two drugs were in common use, epsilon amino caproic acid and tranexamic acid. The uncontrolled trials are listed in Table 7.1. As might be expected, the authors overwhelmingly concluded that antifibrinolytic therapy was a valuable addition to the treatment of subarachnoid haemorrhage. The reports of these uncontrolled series leave much to be desired. Many are in the form of letters. In most reports it is impossible to determine the criteria used for diagnosis of subarachnoid haemorrhage, either initial or recurrent. There was variation in the drug dose, duration of therapy, laboratory control of drug administration, and other features of the treatment protocols.

Controlled data

Non-random controls. These favorable reports stimulated attempts at controlled evaluation of antifibrinolytic therapy. A number of authors, beginning with Gibbs & O'Gorman (1967), selected their control groups with patients who, for various reasons, did not receive antifibrinolytic therapy. These reports are listed in Table 7.2. In none of these reports was the control group selected by a random allocation scheme; some were consecutive series of patients, in some the use of drug was at the surgeon's preference, in others a day of the week allocation scheme was used. The report of Profeta et al (1975) contains so little information that it is not evaluable. Of the remaining studies, three concluded that antifibrinolytic therapy was beneficial while the other four concluded that it was not. In two of the studies concluding that the therapy was not beneficial, the recurrent haemorrhage rate in the drug treated group was approximately 50% of that in the control group, although the differences were not statistically significant (Gelmers, 1980; Ameen & Illingworth, 1981). This will be discussed later. The treatment and control groups in the study of Shucart et al (1980) differed so greatly in clinical grade that the results are uninterpretable. These studies do not clarify the role of antifibrinolytic therapy because the results are contradictory and the variation in method of selecting controls, drug doses, treatment regimens and diagnostic criteria make the results difficult to compare and interpret.

Randomised controls. One would hope that randomised clinical trials of antifibrinolytic therapy would provide more useful information. Eight have been carried out and are listed in Table 7.3. In contrast to the uncontrolled and non-randomly controlled studies, most of these studies have been done in European centres using tranexamic acid. Although the authors are evenly split in their conclusion regarding the effectiveness of antifibrinolytic therapy, Chandra's results, showing four times as many recurrent haemorrhages in the untreated group, did not attain statistical significance. In addition, each of these studies has significant design flaws. Only three studies used a placebo and blinding procedure. Two showed no beneficial effect and the third was Chandra's (1978) study suggesting, but not statistically proving, benefit. Although the diagnosis of

Table 7.1 Uncontrolled series.

Reference	Treatment effective[a]	Dose g/day	Objective diagnosis[b]	Objective endpoint[b]	Number of pts	No. (%) rebleeding	Deaths, (%) analyzed?
			Epsilon amino caproic acid				
Mullan & Dawley (1968)	Yes	24	?	?	35	2 (6)	Yes
Norlen & Thulin (1969)	Yes	16–20	?	?	3	0 (0)	?
Nibbelink et al (1975)	Yes	24–36	Yes	Yes	471	60 (13)	55 (12)
Post et al (1977)	Yes	36	Yes	?	100	10 (10)	15 (15)
Corkill (1974a)	Yes	24	?	?	60	2 (3)	2 (3)
Corkill (1974b)	Yes	24	?	?	20	0 (0)	2 (10)
Uttley & Richardson (1974)	Yes	24	?	?	45	8 (18)	7 (16)
Mullan (1975)	Yes	24	?	?	117	8 (7)	31 (26)
Shaw & Miller (1974)	No	36	?	?	9	5 (55)	3 (33)
			Tranexamic acid				
Norlen & Thulin (1969)	Yes	30–40 mg/kg/day	?	?	11	0 (0)	?
Tovi (1973)	Yes	4–6	Yes	?	34	6 (18)	7 (21)
Schisano (1975)	Yes	1–1.5	?	?	42	2 (5)	No
Uttley & Richardson (1974)	Yes	12	?	?	182	22 (12)	14 (8)

a In opinion of author of study
b LP or CT scan

Table 7.2 Non-random controlled studies.

Reference	Treatment effective[a]	Dose g/day	Blinding	Objective diagnosis[b]	Objective endpoint[b]	Patients drug/control	No. (%) rebleed drug/control	No. (%) dead drug/control
				Epsilon amino caproic acid				
Sengupta et al (1976)	Yes	24	No	Yes	No	66/76	0 (0)/17 (22)	?
Chowdhary et al (1979)	Yes	36	No	Yes	No	83/82	3 (4)/22 (27)	?
Shucart et al (1980)	No	36	No	Yes	Yes	45/55	12 (27)/5 (9)	?
Profeta et al (1975)	No	10–15	?	?	?	135/166	?	?
Ameen & Illingworth (1981)	No	24	No	Yes	Yes	100/100	8 (8)/15 (15)	13 (13)/11 (11)
Gibbs & O'Gorman (1967)	No	36	No	Yes	No	32/24	9 (28)/7 (29)	13 (41)/10 (42)
				Tranexamic acid				
Gibbs & Corkill (1971)	Yes	3	No	Yes	?	25/22	1 (4)/4 (18)	2 (8)/9 (40)
Gelmers (1980)	No	4	No	Yes	No	31/26	5 (16)/9 (35)	4 (13)/4 (15)

a In opinion of author of study
b LP or CT scan

Table 7.3 Randomized studies.

References	Treatment effective[a]	Dose g/day	Blinding	Objective diagnosis[b]	Objective endpoint[b]	Patients drug/control	No. (%) rebleed patients drug/control	No. (%) dead drug/control
					Epsilon amino caproic acid			
Nibbelink et al (1975)	Yes	24–36	No	Yes	Yes	85/69	5 (6)/15 (22)	5 (6)/20 (29)
Girvin (1973)	No	24	No	Yes	?	39/27	14 (36)/4 (15)	7 (18)/4 (15)
					Tranexamic acid			
Fodstad et al (1978)	Yes	4–6	No	Yes	Yes	23/23	1 (4)/9 (39)	5 (22)/5 (22)
Chandra (1978)	Yes	6	Yes	Yes	?	20/19	1 (5)/4 (21)	1 (5)/5 (26)
Maurice-Williams (1978)	Yes	6	No	Yes	No	25/25	6 (24)/14 (56)	3 (12)/11 (44)
Fodstad et al (1981)	No	4–6	No	Yes	Yes	30/29	6 (20)/7 (24)	10 (33)/7 (24)
van Rossum et al (1977)	No	4	Yes	Yes	?	26/25	5 (19)/4 (16)	15 (58)/11 (44)
Kaste & Ramsey (1979)	No	6	Yes	Yes	No	32/32	7 (22)/6 (19)	4 (13)/4 (13)

a In opinion of author or study
b LP or CT scan

the initial subarachnoid haemorrhage was confirmed objectively in all studies, in half of them there was no objective evidence of recurrent haemorrhage. Nibbelink's (1975) study compared antifibrinolytic therapy to hypotensive therapy and there was no true placebo group. Antifibrinolytic therapy alone was superior either to hypotension alone or to hypotension plus antifibrinolytic therapy. Whether the results would have been superior to those in patients treated with neither hypotension not antifibrinolytic agents is not known. Girvin's (1973) study is not reported in sufficient detail to assess its design adequately. He recently updated his report to 164 patients and states that no beneficial effect has been seen (Girvin, 1982).

The two studies by Fodstad et al (1978, 1981) seem to be contradictory. In the second study, although the number of patients rebleeding in the treated and control groups is nearly identical, because of multiple recurrent haemorrhages there were nearly twice as many recurrent haemorrhages in the untreated group as the treated group. Fodstad concluded that tranexamic acid should continue to be administered following initial subarachnoid haemorrhage until surgical treatment was carried out, but should be discontinued after recurrent haemorrhage and in patients with symptoms of delayed cerebral ischaemia. He raised the possibility that increased delayed cerebral ischaemia in the treated group might counterbalance the supposed benefit of reducing the rebleeding risk. Fodstad's studies used no blinding procedure.

Chandra's (1978) study has been mentioned already. Although double-blind and randomised, the criteria for diagnosis of recurrent haemorrhage were not clear and the sample was so small that statistical significance was not reached. Maurice-William's (1978) study used no blinding procedures and confirmation of recurrent haemorrhage was inadequate. The study of van Rossum et al (1977) and that of Kaste & Ramsey (1979) did not document objective criteria for the diagnosis of recurrent haemorrhage.

All studies were handicapped by the lack of a rapid and clinically useful method of assaying either blood or c.s.f. antifibrinolytic levels.

The randomised studies do not seem to establish or refute the value of antifibrinolytic therapy after subarachnoid haemorrhage. This has led the authors of the previously mentioned reviews to conclude that the value of antifibrinolytic therapy is not established, and there has been a swing away from its routine use in many centres. In addition to the previously mentioned problems, reviewers cite the variation in time between haemorrhage and onset of therapy, variation in duration of therapy, variation in clinical grades between treatment and control groups lack of 'blinding', and failure to analyse total mortality and morbidity rather than recurrent haemorrhage, as reasons for the inadequacy of the published studies.

Statistical power analysis
There is one more piece of information which may help to make some sense of the conflicting results reported in the literature. All of the published studies are rather small, the largest being the consecutive series of Ameen & Illingworth (1981) with 100 patients in each of the control and treatment groups. The largest placebo controlled study has only 64 patients evenly divided between drug and placebo. While the question of statistical significance of the results has been

addressed by these authors, it is also fair to ask what chance these small studies had to demonstrate an important clinical effect if it really exists. To begin to answer this question, the statistical power of each controlled study has been estimated according to the methods of Lachin (1981). The estimate is expressed as the probability of finding in the drug treated group a 50% reduction from the rebleeding rate reported in the control group. This probability is known as the statistical power of the study. A 50% reduction was chosen because it is a substantial and clinically important effect and is approximately the effect that most of the successful studies have reported. Using a smaller reduction, such as 25%, would result in a lower statistical power estimate for each study.

The estimate of statistical power is shown in Tables 7.4 and 7.5. An interesting fact emerges. Among the randomised studies, all of the studies concluding that there is no benefit to antifibrinolytic therapy have a statistical power of 0.33 or less. This means that if antifibrinolytic therapy actually reduces rebleeding by 50%, these studies have no better than a 1 in 3 chance of finding that difference. All studies with a power of greater than 0.4 (or 2 chances in 5) of finding such a difference did, in fact, find a significant reduction in rebleeding in patients treated with antifibrinolytics. Chandra's (1978) study appears to be an exception in proclaiming benefit with a lower power, but the proclaimed benefit cannot be statistically supported.

Table 7.4 Statistical power. Non-random studies.

Reference	Treatment effective[a]	Patients drug/control	Rebleed drug/control	Estimated power
Gibbs & Corkill (1971)	Yes[c]	25/22	1/4	0.22
Shucart et al (1980)	No	45/55	12/5	0.22
Gibbs & O'Gorman (1967)	No	32/24	9/7	0.35
Gelmers (1980)	No[b]	31/26	5/9	0.43
Ameen & Illingworth (1981)	No[b]	100/100	8/15	0.56
Sengupta et al (1976)	Yes	66/76	0/17	0.56
Chowdhary et al (1979)	Yes	83/82	3/22	0.67

a In opinion of author of original study
b The rebleeding rate in the treated groups is about half that in the untreated group
c Not significant, Fisher's exact test, P = 0.12

Table 7.5 Statistical power. Randomised studies.

Reference	Treatment effective[a]	Patients drug/control	Rebleed drug/control	Estimated power
van Rossum et al (1977)	No	26/25	5/4	0.22
Chandra (1978)	Yes[b]	20/19	1/4	0.25
Girvin (1973)	No	39/27	14/4	0.26
Kaste & Ramsey (1979)	No	32/32	7/6	0.30
Fodstad et al (1981)	No	30/29	6/7	0.33
Fodstad et al (1978)	Yes	23/23	1/9	0.40
Nibbelink et al (1975)	Yes	85/69	5/15	0.58
Maurice-Williams (1978)	Yes	25/25	6/14	0.65

a In opinion of author of original study
b Not statistically significant, Fisher's exact test, P = 0.13

Looking at the non-random controlled studies, the situation is very similar. Gibb's & Corkill's (1971) study, with a very low power, claims benefit but again the results are not statistically significant. The studies of Gelmers (1980) and Ameen & Illingworth (1981) claim no benefit. However, in both cases the incidence of rebleeding in the drug treated group was approximately one-half that in the control group. The results fail to reach statistical significance because of the small sample size. Each study has only approximately a 50–50 chance of detecting such a difference. The remaining two studies of equal or greater power did find a significant reduction in rebleeding in the treated group.

This information does help to clarify the results of controlled studies. In every randomised trial where there was at least a 50–50 chance of finding a clinically important effect of antifibrinolytic therapy on incidence of rebleeding, such an effect has been found. The negative studies may have failed because they were simply too small to detect an important therapeutic effect.

What conclusion can be drawn? I believe that the current data adequately support the hypothesis that antifibrinolytic therapy in the few weeks after subarachnoid haemorrhage reduces the incidence of rebleeding by approximately 50%

COMPLICATIONS OF ANTIFIBRINOLYTIC THERAPY

When antifibrinolytic agents first came into clinical use in neurosurgery, the major concern was that there would be thrombotic complications such as cerebral thrombosis or pulmonary embolism. While there are scattered reports of such events, their frequency has not been so high as to discourage use of these agents.

Of greater concern is the possibility that the neurological complications of subarachnoid haemorrhage may be worsened by antifibrinolytic therapy. There are theoretical reasons why this might be so. To the extent that hydrocephalus is related to the presence of blood in the subarachnoid space occluding cerebrospinal fluid pathways, the prolongation of clot lysis will lengthen the period of risk for the development of hydrocephalus. Using the same reasoning, the component of vasospasm that is related directly to the presence of blood in the cerebrospinal fluid around blood vessels will be prolonged by antifibrinolytic agents. In addition, plasmin which is the catalyst for the hydrolysis of fibrin also catalyses reactions leading to the formation of kinins (McNicol & Douglas, 1976). Kinins are known to be vasodilatory and to be activated after subarachnoid haemorrhage. Antifibrinolytic agents, by blocking the formation of plasmin, may reduce the concentration of kinins in the cerebrospinal fluid after subarachnoid haemorrhage. This might remove a vasodilatory effect that counteracts vasospasm and in this way lead to an increased incidence of vasospasm.

Hydrocephalus

Ewald et al (1971) evaluated the administration of epsilon amino caproic acid (EACA) to dogs with blood in the subarachnoid space. No increased incidence of hydrocephalus or arachnoiditis was found. Park (1979) reviewed 94 patients with subarachnoid haemorrhage 46 of whom had received EACA. Selection was made in a retrospective, non-random fashion. He found that 31% of the patients receiving EACA as opposed to 10% of the controls developed symptomatic hydrocephalus. The retrospective nature of the study and the introduction of CT scanning late in the series when most of the patients were being treated with EACA make interpretation of these suggestive results difficult. Schisano (1978) found only 1 case of symptomatic hydrocephalus in 38 patients treated with tranexamic acid. The incidence of hydrocephalus requiring shunting in the patients in the randomised clinical trials cited previously is shown in Table 7.6. The numbers are quite small but do not suggest an increased risk of hydrocephalus requiring shunting in treated patients.

Cerebral ischaemia

Kagstrom & Palma (1972) first raised the question of the effect of antifibrinolytic therapy on cerebral ischaemia when they found an increased incidence of ischaemic complications in their treated patients. Schisano (1978) found angiographically detectable vasospasm in 52% of his 58 patients , but clinically detectable cerebral ischaemia in only 17%.

The reporting of clinically important cerebral ischaemic complications in the randomised trials of antifibrinolytic therapy is quite variable. Some authors report only deaths due to cerebral infarction while others report delayed cerebral ischaemic symptoms not attributable to cerebral haemorrhage. Criteria for making the diagnosis are variable and not well specified. Therefore, the incidence figures reported in the studies are not necessarily comparable. The best available information is shown in Table 7.6. There does seem to be a tendency for an

Table 7.6 Hydrocephalus and cerebral ischaemia in randomised trials of antifibrinolytic therapy.

Reference	No. (%) shunts drug/control	No. (%) symptomatic cerebral ischaemia drug/control
Girvin (1973)	?	3 (8)/1 (4)
Nibbelink (1975)	?	?
van Rossum et al (1977)	?	?
Chandra (1978)	?	?
Maurice-Williams (1978)	0 (0)/0 (0)	8 (32)/2 (8)
Fodstad et al (1978)	0 (0)/1 (4)	2 (8)/1 (4)
Kaste & Ramsey (1979)	0 (0)/1 (3)	0 (0)/1 (3)
Fodstad et al (1981)	2 (7)/0 (0)	7 (23)/3 (10)

increased incidence of cerebral ischaemia in the treated patients. Table 7.3 shows the gross mortality in the randomised trials and one sees that in only three trials does the mortality appear to be substantially lower in the treated than in the untreated group. In two trials the mortality is identical in the drug and placebo group and in these the drug treated groups have a slight and statistically insignificant excess mortality. On the basis of these results, many have concluded that antifibrinolytic therapy may increase cerebral ischaemic complications following subarachnoid haemorrhage and that this increase in morbidity and mortality may counteract any benefit conferred by a reduction in rebleeding.

However, a recent report from the cooperative aneurysm study (Adams et al, 1981) did not find increased mortality in patients treated with antifibrinolytic agents. The quality of the available data is such that this hypothesis cannot be considered to be well established.

CONCLUSIONS

Careful consideration of the available data, recognising all of the design and statistical flaws of the best published studies, leads to the conclusion that antifibrinolytic therapy after subarachnoid haemorrhage probably reduces the risk of recurrent haemorrhage by about 50% during the first few weeks of therapy. The same data do not clearly demonstrate a reduction in mortality and morbidity in those patients treated with antifibrinolytic agents. The data further suggest that a possible explanation for the lack of effect on total mortality and morbidity, in spite of a significant reduction in recurrent haemorrhage, is that ischaemic complications of subarachnoid harmorrhage may be increased in the antifibrinolytic treated patients. As these uncertainties cannot be resolved on the basis of currently available information, there is a clear need for further clinical trials of antifibrinolytic therapy. Such trials must recognise and correct the serious design flaws present in all of the previously published studies. Careful attention must be given to objective diagnosis of initial and recurrent haemorrhages, to precise and consistent clinical grading of patients, precise clinical definitions of cerebral ischaemic complications must be used, angiographic confirmation of delayed vasospasm should be obtained, and attention must be paid to multiple endpoints including recurrent haemorrhage, cerebral ischaemic complications and total management mortality and morbidity. Such a study must be large enough so that there is a reasonably high probability of detecting important differences in the endpoints. This implies a multicentre study. Indeed, assuming 33% mortality in the control group, to have an 80% chance of detecting a 25% difference in mortality between treated and control patients, nearly 1000 patients would have to be entered into the study. Further trials not meeting these criteria will only add to the confusion.

The clinician is left in a rather uncomfortable position by these data. On the one hand, there is a fairly strong suggestion that antifibrinolytic therapy will decrease his patients' risk of recurrent haemorrhage with its high attendent morbidity and mortality. On the other hand, by using these agents he may have no impact on the patient's ultimate chance of a satisfactory outcome. My current practice is to use antifibrinolytic agents in patients with subarachnoid haemorrhage due to a ruptured intracranial aneurysm. Therapy is continued until the time of definitive surgery. Antifibrinolytic agents are discontinued in patients who develop signs of cerebral ischaemia accompanied by angiographically demonstrated cerebral vasospasm. One might reasonably consider withholding antifibrinolytic therapy from patients judged to be at high risk of vasospasm on the basis of their initial CT scan.

It is important to separate the value of antifibrinolytic agents in preventing recurrent haemorrhage from their value in the total management of subarachnoid haemorrhage. Future advances in the treatment or prevention of vasospasm may allow us to confidently take advantage of the decreased incidence of rebleeding without the risk of increased cerebral ischaemia.

REFERENCES

Adams H P, Nibbelink D W, Torner J C, Sahs A L 1981 Antifibrinolytic therapy in patients with aneurysmal subarachnoid hemorrhage. A report of the cooperative aneurysm study. Archives of Neurology 38: 25–29

Ameen A A, Illingworth R 1981 Antifibrinolytic treatment in the preoperative management of subarachnoid hemorrhage caused by ruptured intracranial aneurysm. Journal of Neurology, Neurosurgery and Psychiatry 44: 220–226

Chandra B 1978 Treatment of subarachnoid hemorrhage from ruptured intracranial aneurysm with tranexamic acid: a double-blind clinical trial. Annals of Neurology 3: 502–504

Chowdhary U M, Carey P C, Hussein M M 1979 Prevention of early recurrence of spontaneous subarachnoid hemorrhage by E-amino-caproic acid. Lancet 1: 741–743

Corkill G 1974a Epsilon-aminocaproic acid and subarachnoid hemorrhage. Lancet 2: 1319 (letter)

Corkill G 1974b Earlier operation and antifibrinolytic therapy in the management of aneurysmal subarachnoid hemorrhage. Review of recent experience in Tasmania. The Medical Journal of Australia 1: 468–470

Ewald T, Mahaley S, Goodrich J, Wilkinson R, Silver D 1971 Experimental epsilon-aminocaproic acid (EACA) administration in the presence of subarachnoid blood. Journal of Neurosurgery 35: 657–663

Fodstad H, Liliequist B, Schannong M, Thulin C A 1978 Tranexamic acid in the preoperative management of ruptured intracranial aneurysms. Surgical Neurology 10: 9–15

Fodstad H, Forssell A, Liliequist B, Schannong M 1981 Antifibrinolysis with tranexamic acid in aneurysmal subarachnoid hemorrhage: a consecutive controlled clinical trial. Neurosurgery 8: 158–165

Gelmers J H 1980 Prevention of recurrence of spontaneous subarachnoid hemorrhage by tranexamic acid. Acta Neurochirurgica 52: 45–50

Gibbs J R, Corkill A G L 1971 Use of an antifibrinolytic agent (tranexamic acid) in the management of ruptured intracranial aneurysms. Postgraduate Medical Journal 47: 199–200

Gibbs J R, O'Gorman P 1967 Fibrinolysis in subarachnoid hemorrhage. Postgraduate Medical Journal 43: 779–784

Girvin J P 1973 The use of antifibrinolytic agents in the preoperative treatment of ruptured intracranial aneurysms. Transactions of the American Neurological Association 98: 150–152

Girvin J P 1982 The use of antifibrinolysis in the treatment of ruptured intracranial aneurysms. Presented at the American Association of Neurological Surgeons meeting, Honolulu, Hawaii April, 1982

Kagstrom E, Palma L 1972 Influence of antifibrinolytic treatment on the morbidity in patients with subarachnoid hemorrhage. Acta Neurologica Scandinavica 48: 257–258 (abstract)

Kassell N F, Drake C G 1982 Timing of aneurysm surgery. Neurosurgery 10: 514–519

Kaste M, Ramsay M 1979 Tranexamic acid in subarachnoid hemorrage. A double-blind study. Stroke 10: 519–522

Lachin J M 1981 Introduction to sample size determination and power analysis for clinical trials. Controlled Clinical Trials 2: 93–113

Locksley J B 1966 Report of the cooperative study of intracranial aneurysms and subarachnoid hemorrhage. Section V, part II. Natural history of subarachnoid hemorrhage, intracranial aneurysms and arteriovenous malformations. Based on 6368 cases in the cooperative study. Journal of Neurosurgery 25: 321–368

Maurice-Williams R S 1978 Prolonged antifibrinolysis: an effective non-surgical treatment for ruptured intracranial aneurysms? British Medical Journal 1: 945–947

McNicol G P, Douglas A S 1976 The fibrinolytic enzyme system. In: Biggs R (ed) Human blood coagulation, haemostasis and thrombosis. Blackwell Scientific, Oxford, ch 14, p 339–435

Mullan S 1975 Conservative management of the recently ruptured aneurysm. Surgical Neurology 3: 27–32

Mullan S, Dawley J 1968 Antifibrinolytic therapy for intracranial aneurysms. Journal of Neurosurgery 28: 21–23

Nibbelink D W 1975 Cooperative aneurysm study: antihypertensive and antifibrinolytic therapy following subarachnoid hemorrhage from ruptured intracranial aneurysm. In: Whisnat J P, Sandok B A (eds) Ninth conference. Cerebral vascular disease. Grune and Stratton, New York, p 155–173

Nibbelink D W, Turner J C, Henderson W G 1975 Intracranial aneurysms and subarachnoid hemorrhage. A cooperative study. Antifibrinolytic therapy in recent onset subarachnoid hemorrhage. Stroke 6: 622–629

Norlen G, Thulin C A 1969 The use of antifibrinolytic substances in ruptured intracranial aneurysms. Neurochiurgica 12: 100–102

Park B E 1979 Spontaneous subarachnoid hemorrhage complicated by communicating hydrocephalus: epsilon amino caproic acid as a possible predisposing factor. Surgical Neurology 11: 73–80

Post K D, Flamm E S, Goodgold A, Ransohoff J 1977 Ruptured intracranial aneurysms. Case morbidity and mortality. Journal of Neurosurgery 46: 290–295

Profeta G, Castellano F, Guarnieri L, Cigliano A, Ambrosio A 1975 Antifibrinolytic therapy in the treatment of subarachnoid hemorrhage caused by arterial aneurysms. Journal of Neurosurgical Sciences 19: 77–78

Ramierez-Lassepas M 1981 Antifibrinolytic therapy in subarachnoid hemorrhage caused by ruptured intracranial aneurysm. Neurology 31: 316–322

Schisano G 1975 Antifibrinolytics in the treatment of subarachnoid hemorrhage due to ruptured aneurysms. Journal of Neurosurgical Sciences 19: 79–80

Schisano G 1978 The use of antifibrinolytic drugs in aneurysmal subarachnoid hemorrhage. Surgical Neurology 10: 217–222

Sengupta R P, So S C, Villarejo-Ortega F J 1976 Use of epsilon aminocaproic acid (EACA) in the preoperative management of ruptured intracranial aneurysms. Journal of Neurosurgery 44: 479–484

Shaw M D M, Miller J D 1974 E-aminocaproic acid and subarachnoid hemorrhage. Lancet 2: 847–848 (letter)

Shucart W A, Hussain S K, Cooper P R 1980 Epsilon-aminocaproic acid and recurrent subarachnoid hemorrhage. A clinical trial. Journal of Neurosurgery 53: 28–31

Tovi D 1973 The use of antifibrinolytic drugs to prevent early recurrent aneurysmal subarachnoid hemorrhage. Acta Neurologica Scandinavica 49: 163–175

Uttley D, Richardson A E 1974 E-aminocaproic acid and subarachnoid hemorrage. Lancet 2: 1080–1081 (letter)

van Rossum J, Wintzen A R, Endtz L J, Schoen J H R, de Jonge H 1977 Effect of tranexamic acid on rebleeding after subarachnoid hemorrhage: a double-blind controlled clinical trial. Annals of Neurology 2: 242–245

Vermeulen M, Muizelarr J P 1980 Do antifibrinolytic agents prevent rebleeding after rupture of a cerebral aneurysm? A review. Clinical Neurology and Neurosurgery 82: 25–30

Warlow C P 1981 Cerebrovascular disease. Clinics in Haematology 10: 645–647

8. When should ruptured berry aneurysms be operated upon?

Michael Briggs

INTRODUCTION

Thirty years ago the title of this chapter might well have been 'do we operate on berry aneurysms' rather than when do we operate on aneurysms. The neurosurgeons who attempted to answer the first question recognised that the answer to it lay in a broad understanding of the natural history of aneurysmal subarachnoid haemorrhage, with which the results of attempts at surgical treatment could be compared. The present question arose from the mass of information collected and partly analysed in an effort to discover the cause of surgical mortality and morbidity in patients with berry aneurysms.

Two major factors influence the outcome of patients following aneurysmal subarachnoid haemorrhage: the natural history of the disease, in particular the risk of recurrent haemorrhage, and the occurrence of cerebral hypoxia and infarction possibly resulting from arterial vasospasm.

The natural history of aneurysmal subarachnoid haemorrhage
Many of the earlier statistics relating to the outcome of patients treated conservatively following subarachnoid haemorrhage came from neurosurgical studies which attempted to assess the possible advantage of surgical management (Logue, 1956; McKissock et al, 1960 & 1965; Sahs et al, 1969). Logue described 36 patients with aneurysms of the anterior cerebral or anterior communicating arteries treated by the conservative methods in vogue at that time, the follow-up period ranging between 17 months and 9 years. Twenty (55%) suffered recurrent haemorrhage, which was fatal in 14 (70%), the mortality from recurrent haemorrhage being 41% in the survivors from the first bleed. Seven of these recurrences occurred during the first week after the initial bleed, 4 others during the second week.

The observations of McKissock et al (1958) that 'at the present time there is no evidence indicating the natural death rate in a large series of unselected cases of ruptured intracranial aneurysms and so there can be no proof of the value of surgical treatment in this condition', stimulated a series of trials from the Atkinson Morley's Hospital (McKissock et al, 1960, 1965) which greatly influenced medical opinion on the subject at that time. In their study of haemorrhage from ruptured posterior communicating artery aneurysms, 83% of patients in poor clinical condition at the time of admission and treated conservatively died, while 36% of those in good condition died. These patients were compared with those treated surgically (mainly common carotid ligation) in whom the mortality rate was 100% for those in poor condition but only 8% for those in good condition. In this publication the deleterious effect on prognosis of poor clinical state, age over 50, and pre-existing arterial hypertension, were recognised.

Further insight into the fate of such patients was obtained from studies in Scandanavia. Tappura (1962) analysed 120 patients treated conservatively following ruptured intracranial aneurysms, contact with the survivors being maintained for $1\frac{1}{2}$–25 years. He found a recurrence rate of 55% in the survivors from the initial haemorrhage, 76% of those suffering a recurrent haemorrhage dying, giving a mortality rate of 41% of those surviving the first bleed. Importantly he observed that the second haemorrhage occurred within 8 weeks of the initial haemorrhage in 62%, but even those surviving the first 8 weeks had a 28% chance of dying from recurrent haemorrhage. This risk of death or deterioration in the early stages following subarachnoid haemorrhage is found time and again in the literature (Pakarinen, 1967; Brosman & Norlén, 1963). Those patients who died before getting to hospital were necessarily excluded from many series but Brosman & Norlén (1963) found that 16.5% (of 145 patients) did just this, and a further 27.3% died from the initial haemorrhage in hospital — death occurring within 24 hours in more than 50% and very rarely after 2 weeks. Pakarinen (1967) found a death rate from the first haemorrhage due to ruptured aneurysms of 43.0% occurring rapidly within 24 hours in 31.7%. Recurrent haemorrhage occurred in 51.7% of the survivors, within 8 weeks in 40.1%. McKissock's (1965) non-surgical group of patients with anterior communicating artery aneurysms provide further information about the natural history of conservatively treated aneurysmal subarachnoid haemorrhage; 64 out of 153 suffered recurrent haemorrhage, more than 50% of those occurring within 2 weeks of the presenting haemorrhage. In the report of the Co-operative Study (Sahs et al, 1969) a mortality rate of 38% within 14 days of haemorrhage and 68% at the end of 1 year is quoted in non-surgically treated patients. In their up-dated publication Sahs et al (1981) stated that in a mean follow-up period of 6.5 years the mortality rate of their 'bed rest group' was 55.1, 34.2% of those dying from a proven re-bleed.

It can be seen from this brief outline of studies, which are probably as near to the natural history of aneurysmal subarachnoid haemorrhage as one can get, that there is a high initial mortality which is probably in most cases outside the influence of medical or surgical treatment. There is, however, a high risk of further damage from recurrent haemorrhage which is at its greatest in the few weeks immediately following the first haemorrhage, but which persists at a lesser degree for years. The prevention of this recurrent haemorrhage is the aim of treatment provided this can be achieved with an acceptable mortality and morbidity when compared with the natural history. The main problem is not 'the surgical management of the patients referred a few weeks after bleeding; it was as Richardson and Hyland reminded us in 1951 "the prevention of recurrent bleeding during the first 3 weeks after initial haemorrhage" (Gillingham, 1979). A second quotation, this time from McKissock et al (1965) leads into the main surgical problem: of all causes of death, infarction, often related to angiographic evidence of vasospasm has been the greatest problem and has so far resisted any therapeutic measure'.

Arterial vasospasm

While the natural history of aneurysmal subarachnoid haemorrhage outlined above is generally accepted, the position regarding the significance of vasospasm is less certain. Angiographic evidence of narrowing of the intracranial vessels following subarachnoid haemorrhage is extensive (duBoulay, 1963; Allcock & Drake, 1965; Adams et al, 1978) but agreement on its importance in relation to clinical state is not universal. Allcock & Drake (1965) studied a series of 175 patients with ruptured aneurysms who were treated surgically, 83 of whom had adequate pre and postoperative angiograms. They found that although the presence of preoperative vasospasm had no convincing correlation with the clinical grading of patients, its presence postoperatively was associated with a poor outcome. They noted that the average interval between haemorrhage and surgery in a group with postoperative vasospasm was 5.1 days compared with 10.7 days for those patients who did not develop this complication, suggesting to them that earlier operation had played some part in the genesis of vasospasm.

The time of onset of vasospasm is obviously important and evidence relating to this comes from various sources. Wilkins et al (1968) found preoperative vasospasm in 36.7% of 120 patients with aneurysmal subarachnoid haemorrhage. Of 19 patients who had carotid angiograms within 24 hours of the haemorrhage none showed any evidence of vasospasm, whereas 9 patients with normal angiograms on day 1 had developed vasospasm by day 8. In the light of these findings they suggested that surgery should be delayed when preoperative vasospasm was present. Weir et al (1978) reported that no vasospasm was found in 160 patients having angiograms on day 1 following haemorrhage and reported a greatest incidence at 10 days after the initial bleed. They described a correlation between vasospasm and death; the more vasospasm, the greater risk there was of death. Support for this delayed development of vasospasm can be found in the Co-operative Study (Sahs et al, 1979) where it is reported that localised and diffuse vasospasm occurred most frequently between the sixth and fourteenth day following the last haemorrhage. Sano & Saito (1979) agreed with the relationship described between vasospasm and morbidity, 'vasospasm exerts a crucial influence on the mortality and morbidity of patients with intracranial aneurysms, whether preoperative or postoperative'. They found that between days 7 and 14 following subarachnoid haemorrhage it was the most important cause of impaired consciousness in 80.6% of their patients and that severe generalised vasospasm always caused depression in the conscious level. In their study it was never seen before day four. Adams et al (1978) studying purely postoperative vasospasm also found that when present to a significant degree it was always associated with clinical deterioration.

So much for the agreement. The main voice against the significance of vasospasm comes from Millikin (1975), who in an extensive review of the

88

literature complained that there was no evidence that vasospasm was harmful and was not even always present when it was thought to be. In support of these views he presented data from his own series of 198 patients of whom 41% had evidence of vasospasm. 52.2% of those without vasospasm had neurological signs whereas they were present in only 45.7% of those with vasospasm. More deaths occurred in patients without vasospasm than with, whether treated surgically or conservatively. He formed the opinion that 'known cerebral vasospasm had no effect on the mortality of subarachnoid haemorrhage due to ruptured aneurysm'. Maurice-Williams (1982), however, took a diametrically opposite view being of the opinion that many patients whose preoperative deterioration was previously ascribed to small recurrent haemorrhage were in fact suffering from the effect of vasospasm, and suggested that the risks of vasospasm were higher and the risks of re-bleeding lower than previously thought.

It has been demonstrated earlier that one of the main factors influencing the outcome of patients following subarachnoid haemorrhage is cerebral hypoxia and infarction, which may occur either as a result of the initial haemorrhage or perhaps the later development of vasospasm. The presence or absence of this complication may be recognised clinically and from the earliest analytical studies neurosurgeons have realised the significance of the clinical condition of the patient in determining prognosis following surgery. McKissock et al (1960) reported 100% surgical mortality for those patients in their category A (poor condition). Since then various grading systems have been suggested in an attempt to standardise classification (Botterell et al, 1956; Nishioka, 1966; Hunt & Hess, 1968) all of which have five point scales on which grade I patients are in the best clinical condition. All these sources reported an increasing operative mortality with a worsening clinical grade.

It is now possible to recognise the main problems involved in treating patients following aneurysmal subarachnoid haemorrhage:

1. It is a disease which carries a high initial mortality. The maximum risk of recurrence is during the first 2 weeks after presentation.

2. The main cause of death and disability other than recurrent haemorrhage is cerebral infarction probably related to arterial vasospasm which can be worsened by surgery and has a peak incidence 4–14 days after haemorrhage, and for which there is as yet no effective remedy, i.e. the two main causes of mortality and morbidity both have a peak incidence during the first 2 weeks after the initial bleed: one can be prevented and the other made worse by surgery.

3. The clinical grade of the patient at the time of surgery is the single most important factor in determining surgical outcome.

What is the solution?

Timing of surgery

There is no doubt that delaying surgery on ruptured intracranial aneurysms until the patient is in clinical grade I–II and 3 weeks have elapsed from the day of haemorrhage, results in very low surgical mortality rates. Almost 30 years ago Norlén & Olivercrona (1954) quoted a mortality rate of less than 4% in patients treated surgically between 3 and 4 weeks after the haemorrhage, but did not consider the management mortality, i.e. surgical mortality plus those patients who died awaiting surgery. Kaftan & Hamby (1969) suggested monitoring the intracranial pressure and delaying surgery until it was normal in an attempt to reduce surgical mortality and rationalise the timing of surgery. Adams et al (1972) in a review of 100 patients with aneurysmal subarachnoid haemorrhage reported an overall management mortality of 19% compared with 37% in the conservative group of McKissock et al (1960). When the figures were broken down the mortality of those patients operated upon in the first week was 22% and only 5% in the second and 1% after 3 weeks. Mullan et al (1978) delayed surgery for at least 10 days (until the patient was alert) and reported no surgical mortality. Despite intensive medical management while awaiting surgery, including hypotension and antifibrinolytics, 15 of his patients died in this period.

These samples from the literature indicate clearly that surgical treatment of ruptured intracranial aneurysms is effective and safe when performed on patients in good clinical condition after the risk of vasospasm and infarction has passed. This, however, does not take into account those patients who deteriorated and die before surgery is undertaken. Adams et al (1981) studied 249 patients admitted following subarachnoid haemorrhage within 3 days of haemorrhage in whom surgery was delayed by 2 weeks. Compared to a management mortality of 36.2% the operative mortality was 14%. They ended their paper by remarking 'one promising approach under investigation is early intracranial operation, but its superiority over delayed intracranial operation must still be proven'.

Hunt & Hess (1968) were among the earlier protagonists of early surgery but even then not for everyone. They noted a mortality rate following surgery of 14% for grades I and II patients combined, but that for grade I patients was 1.4% and grade II patients 22%, and suggested some delay for grade II patients. Early surgery was not recommended for grade III patients. Drake (1968) in his printed comments on this paper quoted his own figures at that time of 35% mortality when surgery was in the first week and 17% in the second, and remarked 'it is probably true that if we could learn how to keep patients safe from re-bleeding for a week or longer in obtunded patients with cerebral symptoms, the problems of surgery of ruptured intracranial aneurysms would be solved'. While awaiting this solution some neurosurgeons have attempted earlier, or even per-acute surgery, that is within 48 hours following haemorrhage (Hori & Suzuki, 1979; Suzuki, 1979; Hugenholtz & Elgie, 1982).

Hori & Suzuki (1979) described a large series of 346 patients with anterior communicating artery aneurysms. Their overall mortality was 5.5% and 82% of those operated upon after 3 weeks had good or excellent results, a figure mirrored by those patients operated upon within the first 48 hours. By far the worst figures relate to those patients undergoing surgery 3–7 days after the last haemorrhage. Despite their enthusiasm for per-acute surgery, study of their tables reveals that only 20 of 338 patients underwent surgery within 48 hours, including 3 out of 186 grade I patients, in 141 of whom surgery was delayed for longer than 22 days. Similarly Suzuki (1979), an often quoted champion of per-acute surgery, in an impressive personal series on 1000 patients with aneurysms with an overall mortality of 6.1% delayed surgery by more than 8 days in 837. Even between 1971 and 1975 when a policy for early surgery was adopted, 138 patients underwent operation between 8 and 14 days and 370 after 15 days delay. In those patients undergoing early surgery the mortality rate was 17% in the 0–48 hour group and 20% for the 3–7 day group. Elsewhere Suzuki (1979) analysed 635 cases, of whom 122 were operated upon within 48 hours with a mortality rate of 15.6%, compared to 3.7% of 136 undergoing surgery between days 8 and 14, and 2.7% if the delay was more than 2 weeks. He recommended that the conscious level of the patient should be normal or improving before surgery was undertaken.

It can be interpreted from these figures that even in centres where per-acute surgery is recommended circumstances are such that often surgery is not performed until after a delay of 1 week or more. The attraction of per-acute surgery is obvious — aneurysms can be made safe before a period of high re-bleeding risk and potential treatment of vasospasm, such as induced hypertension (Koswik & Hunt, 1976) can be undertaken safely. However, if this policy were adopted the timing would be crucial and the leeway minimal. All series quoted earlier recognised that surgery between days 3 to 7 carries a higher risk than either per-acute or delayed operation. It can be deduced from the large numbers of patients undergoing delayed operation, even in centres promoting per-acute surgery, that there are problems in carrying out such a policy in practice. In many neurosurgical units in Great Britain, where resources such as bed numbers and emergency facilities may be limited, these problems may well outweigh any possible advantage. Good surgical management of patients following subarachnoid haemorrhage demands the cooperation and coordination of a highly skilled team of neuroradiologist, anaesthetist, surgeon, radiographer and theatre staff. Most members of this team are already heavily involved in providing an emergency service to patients with head injuries and other neurosurgical emergencies, and others may be required to provide emergency service to other hospital departments. In many hospitals the resources are already stretched almost to breaking point. If per-acute surgery to aneurysm patients was unarguably shown to be a significantly superior method of management then pressure would need to be applied to obtain adequate facilities for its general adoption. The situation, however, is not so clear cut and consideration must be given to local facilities and existing commitments when deciding the optimum treatment of such patients. Whereas it was noted earlier that the advantages of per-acute surgery were obvious, there are also attractions to the surgeon of delayed surgery — time to plan investigation and treatment, good operating conditions and low surgical mortality among them. When one recommends this method of management, however, it must be recognised that one is not treating the disease of subarachnoid haemorrhage but a selection of surviving patients with that disorder.

Current practice
My own method of management of patients with aneurysmal subarachnoid haemorrhage is as follows:

1. I attempt early surgery where it is possible within the facilities available, both in my unit and in the referring hospitals, on patients in good clinical state (grade I and II), who are under 50 years of age, and have no history of arterial

hypertension. Even this is not entirely straightforward because observer variations in grading recently reported by Lindsay et al (1982) at times leads to inappropriate transfer.

2. Patients in grades I and II who cannot be transferred, investigated and operated upon within the first 48 hours following haemorrhage, and patients in grades I and II who are over 50 years of age and/or hypertensive, are assessed at the time of referal from the receiving hospital shortly after haemorrhage, and investigation and surgery where appropriate is planned for 7 to 10 days later.

3. Investigation and surgery on patients in grade III is delayed until they have either improved to a higher grade or they have a stable neurological deficit without impairment of conscious level.

REFERENCES

Adams C B T, Fearnside M R, O'Laoire S A 1978 An investigation with Serial angiography into the evolution of cerebral arterial spasm following aneurysm surgery. Journal of Neurosurgery 45: 805–815

Adams C B T, Loach A B, O'Laoire S A 1972 Intracranial aneurysms: Analysis of results of microsurgery. British Medical Journal 2: 607–609

Adams H P Jnr, Kassell N F, Turner J C, Nibbelink D W, Sahs A L 1981 Early management of aneurysmal subarachnoid haemorrhage. A report of the Co-operative Aneurysm Study. Journal of Neurosurgery 54: 141–145

Allcock J M, Drake C G 1965 Ruptured intracranial aneurysms: the role of arterial spasm. Journal of Neurosurgery 22: 21–29

Botterell E H, Lougheed E M, Scott J W, Vandewater S L 1956 Hypothermia and interuption of carotid, or carotid and vertebral circulation, in the management of intracranial aneurysms. Journal of Neurosurgery 13: 1–42

Brosman T, Norlén G 1963 Subarachnoidalblödaringar, Det Neurologiska sjukomsparoramat i Goteborg. Nord Med 69: 645–646

duBoulay G 1963 Distribution of spasm in the intracranial arteries after subarachnoid haemorrhage. Acta Radiologica 1: 257–266

Gillingham F J 1979 Cerebral aneurysms: Advances in diagnosis and therapy. Springer-Verlag, Berlin

Hori S, Suzuki J 1979 Early and late results of intracranial direct surgery of anterior communicating artery aneurysms. Journal of Neurosurgery 50: 433–440

Hugenholtz H, Elgie R G 1982 Considerations in early surgery on good risk patients with ruptured intracranial aneurysms. Journal of Neurosurgery 56: 180–185

Hunt W E, Hess R M 1968 Surgical risk as related to time of intervention and the repair of intracranial aneurysms. Journal of Neurosurgery 28: 14–20

Kaftan L A, Hamby W B 1969 Significance of CSF pressure in determining the time for repair of intracranial aneurysms. Journal of Neurosurgery 31: 217–219

Koswik E J, Hunt W E 1976 Post-operative hypertension in the management of patients with intracranial aneurysm. Journal of Neurosurgery 45: 148–154

Lindsay K W, Teasdale G, Knill-Jones R P, Murray L 1982 Observer variability in grading patients with subarachnoid haemorrhage. Journal of Neurosurgery 56: 628–633

Logue V 1956 Surgery in spontaneous subarachnoid haemorrhage: operative treatment of aneurysms on the anterior cerebral and anterior communicating artery. British Medical Journal 1: 473–479

McKissock W, Paine K, Walsh L 1958 Further observations on subarachnoid haemorrhage. Journal of Neurology, Neurosurgery and Psychiatry 21: 239–48

McKissock W, Richardson A, Walsh L 1960 'Posterior communicating' aneurysms: controlled trial of the conservative and surgical treatment of ruptured aneurysms on the internal carotid artery at or near the point of origin of the posterior communicating artery. Lancet 1: 1203–1206

McKissock W, Richardson A, Walsh L 1965 'Anterior communicating' aneurysms. Trial of conservative and surgical treatment. Lancet 1: 873–876

Maurice-Williams R S 1982 Ruptured intra-cranial aneurysms; has the incidence of early re-bleeding been over estimated. Journal of Neurology, Neurosurgery and Psychiatry 45: 774–779

Millikin C H 1975 Cerebral vasospasm and ruptured intracranial aneurysm. Archives of Neurology 32: 443–449

Mullan S, Hanlon K, Brown F 1978 Management of 136 consecutive supratentorial berry aneurysms. Journal of Neurosurgery 49: 794–805

Nishioka H 1966 Report on the Cooperative Study of intracranial aneurysms and subarachnoid haemorrhage Section VII, part I: Evaluation of conservative management of ruptured intracranial aneurysms. Journal of Neurosurgery 25: 574–592

Norlen G, Olivecrona H 1953 The treatment of aneurysms of the circle of Willis. Journal of neurosurgery 10: 404–415

Pakarinen S 1967 Incidence, aetiology and prognosis of primary subarachnoid haemorrhage. Acta Neurologica Scandinavica Suppl. 29: 1–128

Sahs A L, Nibbelink D W, Turner J C 1981 Aneurysmal subarachnoid haemorrhage. Report of the cooperative study. Urban & Schwargenberg, Baltimore

Sahs A L, Perret G E, Locksley H B 1969 Intracranial aneurysms and subarachnoid haemorrhage. A cooperative study. Lippencott, Philadelphia

Samson D S, Hodosh R M, Reid W R 1979 Risk of intracranial aneurysm surgery in the good grade patient: early versus late operation. Neurosurgery 5: 422–426

Sano K, Saito I 1978 Timing and indication of surgery for ruptured intracranial aneurysms with regard to subarachnoid vasospasm. Acta Neurchirugica 41: 49–60

Sano K, Saito I 1979 Cerebral aneurysms: advances in diagnosis and therapy. Springer Verlag, Berlin

Susuki K 1979 Cerebral aneurysms: advances in diagnosis and treatment. Springer Verlag, Berlin, p 413–418

Tappura M 1962 Prognosis of subarachnoid haemorrhage: study of 120 patients with unoperated intracranial arterial aneurysms and 267 patients without vascular lesions demonstrable in bilateral carotid angiograms. Acta Medica Scandinavica Suppl. 392: 1–75

Tovi D 1973 The use of antifibrinolytic drugs to prevent early recurrent aneurysmal subarachnoid haemorrhage. Acta Neurologica Scandinavica 49: 163–175

Weir B, Grace M, Hansen J, Rothberg C 1978 Time course of vasospasm in man. Journal of Neurosurgery 48: 173–178

Wilkins R H, Alexander J A, Odom G L 1968 Intracranial arterial spasm: a clinical analysis. Journal of Neurosurgery 29: 121–134

9. Does speech therapy influence the course of recovery from aphasia after stroke?

Anthony Hopkins

INTRODUCTION

Critchley (1970) records some of the testimonials of those who have recovered from aphasia, for the unimaginative few who cannot themselves foresee what it must be like to lose, at a stroke, the faculty of expressing and communicating their ideas, their wishes and their affections to family and to friends. Faced with such human tragedies, it is not surprising that others step in to help. Such individual, human, help for those suffering from disordered communication has become institutionalised over the last 50 years into a profession — the profession of speech therapy.

Criticism of work done by others is one of the less attractive aspects of human nature, however 'healthy' that criticism may be. However, the present competition for a share of limited resources for health care demands assessment of the worth of any therapy. Many of the older methods of management — consultation, reassurance, bed-rest, local heat, convalescence, physical rehabilitation — have yet to face the scrutiny of the 'controlled clinical trial' that is now demanded before the introduction of any new drug, and is, or should be, attempted at some stage in the assessment of new surgical therapies (e.g. European Coronary Surgery Study Group, 1982). The benefits of physiotherapy and speech therapy have not been so carefully assessed, with certain honourable exceptions (Sarno, Silverman & Sands, 1970; Darley, 1972; Basso, Capitani & Vignolo, 1979).

The crucial questions were put by Darley (1972): '1. Does language rehabilitation accomplish measurable gains in language function beyond what can be expected to occur as a result of spontaneous recovery? Or, stated differently, does therapy have a decisive influence on the course of recovery and the ultimate outcome? 2. Are the language gains attributable to therapy worth the necessary investment of time, effort and money?' Darley also put a third question: 'What are the relative degrees of effectiveness of various modes of treatment of aphasia?' — but it cannot be right to consider this question until an affirmative answer has been obtained to the first.

94

SPONTANEOUS RECOVERY FROM APHASIA

It is a clinical commonplace that some neurological recovery occurs after stroke, though the mechanisms of such recovery remain uncertain and, indeed, largely unexplored. It is against this background of spontaneous recovery that intervention must be measured.

The pattern of recovery of language after stroke has been placed on a more quantitative basis by Vignolo (1964), Culton (1969) and Sarno & Levita (1971). These last authors studied patients who received no treatment and measured changes in the Functional Communication Profile. Greater changes were seen in the first 3 months than in the next 3 months. Culton (1969) studied 11 patients recently rendered aphasic (9 after stroke) and they improved in all 8 measures studied — measures of auditory and visual decoding, and oral and graphic encoding. Spontaneous recovery of function was noted in the first month following the onset of aphasia and, although a further increase in mean scores was noted, significant improvement was not evident during the second month. The significance of these results is supported by studies on a further group of aphasic subjects who had been aphasic between 11 and 48 months. These subjects showed no significant change in performance of the eight tasks within the time limits of the study.

Kenin & Swisher (1972) did find that some elements of aphasia improved spontaneously more than others. Copying of writing showed the greatest improvement, followed by tests of comprehension. Expressive speech, involving description of the use of objects and sentence construction, showed the least spontaneous improvement.

ASSESSMENTS OF THE EFFICACY OF SPEECH THERAPY

Darley (1982) reviewed at length the previous efforts in this area. In many of the earlier studies there were gross weaknesses in the design of the assessment; although patients have dissimilar and unrevealed causes for their stroke, the various types of dysphasia are all treated as one, improvement is scaled on the basis of oral speech alone on a not improved, improved and much improved scale, the intensity and type of speech therapy is variable, and the performance in control subjects without therapy is not considered. Of the many individual case studies and trials of various quality reviewed by Darley, two are chosen for discussion here.

One attempt at a non-randomised but controlled trial is that of Sarno, Silverman & Sands (1970). These American workers assigned 31 severe receptive-expressive dysphasic subjects to one of three groups at least 3 months and up to 144 months after their stroke. The patients were scaled on Taylor's Functional Communication Profile, and all had overall values of less than 31%. For the most part such patients had no speech function and little understanding of speech. Sixteen of these patients had programmed therapy, 7 non-programmed therapy with defined goals, and 8 acted as controls. This assignment was non-random and depended on the location of patients and availability of therapists.

Treatment ranged from 4–36 weeks and the number of 30-minute sessions from 13–91. At retesting, there were small gains in some areas of the Functional Communication Profile, but these gains were seen in non-treated patients as well. The non-programmed therapy group did better than the controls in two tests of visual matching and recognition, but there was no significant improvement in either of the groups receiving therapy compared to the controls in tasks in the important areas involving imitation, writing-copying, auditory comprehension and expressive speech.

Sarno and her colleagues themselves stated that further studies involving larger groups of patients were required. Their report may be criticised on the following grounds:

1. Only patients with gross aphasia were studied. These patients are the most difficult to communicate with, and are acknowledged to have, at 3 or more months after the stroke, the worst prognosis.

2. There was no attempt to match the groups for site and size of lesion, for premorbid intelligence or linguistic competence. Although the mean ages and duration of symptoms were roughly comparable between the groups, the average figure conceals a very considerable scatter of ages and duration of symptoms. No information is given as to the numbers of patients, and their distribution in the groups, who received relatively few treatment sessions over a few weeks (range 4–36 weeks, mean 17.1) which many therapists would regard as inadequate treatment.

All this report may be said to have shown is that there are no striking benefits to be gained from speech therapy of severely dysphasic patients over a few weeks. In their last sentence Sarno and her colleagues state:

'. . . The speech pathologist might make more profitable use of his time attempting to refine the techniques for patient selection for speech therapy and improve methods of treatment for those more amenable to treatment.'

A more recent controlled trial is that of Basso, Capitani & Vignolo (1979). These workers from Milan studied 281 aphasic patients, all but 7 of whom were right-handed. The aphasia of the vast majority (85%) was caused by cerebrovascular disease. The time interval between onset and first examination was less than 2 months in 137 cases, from 2–6 months in 86 cases, and more than 6 months in 58 cases. Aphasia was assessed on oral expression (e.g. male patients were asked to describe how they shaved), visual naming, auditory comprehension of command, written description (e.g. about personal recent news or health), and reading. Points were allocated, and scores compounded. Only patients who received rehabilitative speech therapy by a 'stimulation approach' at a rate of at least three individual sessions per week for at least 5 months were considered 're-educated'. One hundred and sixty-two patients met these criteria. On the other hand, 119 patients were prevented from attending therapy by extraneous factors such as family or transportation problems. This was the non-randomised 'control' group. The second assessment of language was at least 6 months after the first, and was carried out by a therapist who had not treated the patient.

The results of this study are presented in complex tables, but fortunately the authors summarise their findings. Time since onset and overall severity of aphasia are both negatively correlated with improvement for both treated and untreated groups, confirming the clinical view, previously supported by Sarno, Silverman & Sands (1970) that the worse the aphasia at assessment, and the longer the interval between onset and assessment, the worse the prognosis for recovery. On the other hand, those who received speech therapy made significant gains in their ability to communicate through speaking, listening, writing and reading. Whether the dysphasia was fluent or non-fluent made no difference to outcome.

The authors themselves comment fairly on some biases in their study. The mean age of the control group was 53.4 years and of the treated group 47.8 years. Although neither the effect of age nor that of the interaction age-rehabilitation was significant, there was a weak inverse relation between age and improvement, which did not significantly interfere with the effects of rehabilitation. Nevertheless, the mean age of both groups of patients is surprisingly young, suggesting that the results might not apply at the older age at which usually strokes occur. The authors also consider that the 'family and transportation' problems might have biased the control group, but 'unsystematic information about these patients and their families suggests that objective difficulties rather than inadequate attitudes were the real obstacle in most cases'. As Benson (1979a) points out, 'although technical criticism may be made of this study . . . the number of patients studied is impressive and the results are striking . . .'

ALTERNATIVE METHODS OF COMMUNICATION AND NEW METHODS OF THERAPY

If one accepts the rather gloomy outlook for recovery of language for those with severe global aphasia revealed by clinical experience, and confirmed by Sarno, Silverman & Sands (1970), with or without speech therapy, then it is right to look around for other methods of communication. There may be a syllogism here, because communication must — unless one believes in the paranormal — require some emission of sign, symbol or scent from one body and the reception by another. It is reasonable to call the transmitted energy a 'language'. Indeed the phrase 'body language' has entered common parlance during the last decade. Non-verbal languages such as music are not really very different in their powers of communication of concepts and ideas from verbal languages, and this power could be increased if a common code of symbols were agreed, as in Morse. Critchley (1970) has reviewed the relevance of gesture to aphasia. Unfortunately many sign languages seem to demand as much linguistic competence as verbal language.

Some success has, however, been achieved with American Indian (Amerind) sign language (Skelly et al, 1974). These authors state:

'Sign is not a language. Signs do not represent discrete words, although even in explaining Sign we speak and act as if this were true. Signs are interpreted by the viewer in whatever language he uses . . . Since Sign is not a language, it has no grammatical structure but uses a logical associative order to the same purpose . . . There is no one correct Sign for an idea. Any Sign or group of Signs that conveys an idea adequately to a number of viewers reliably on different occasions is acceptable.'

The difference between Signs and, for example, deaf and dumb language using finger positions, is that Sign does not appear to have to be taught, although teaching obviously improves the efficacy of communication. In an earlier study Skelly and her colleagues had demonstrated that 'interested and motivated viewers could interpret the Sign at an 88% level of comprehension without any instruction'.

Skelly and her colleagues (1974) studied 6 patients with verbal apraxia where verbal scores on the Porch Index of Communicative Ability were exceeded by their gestural scores. All 6 patients mastered 50 Signs within the first 2 months. In an earlier study she had noted that varying degrees of oral movement and vocalisations accompanied Signing, so the patients were encouraged to focus on the therapist's articulatory movements while both were Signing. All 6 patients developed some spontaneous oral production synchronous with their Signing, suggesting that Sign may be a useful facilitator of verbalisation as well as providing an effective means of communication for aphasic subjects.

Such observations bring up the question of whether linguistic competence can be dissociated from 'natural language'. Baker et al (1975) wrote:

'A crucial test of the hypothesised dissociation between natural language and its cognitive pre-requisites is whether aphasic subjects can use arbitrarily designed symbols to represent elements of experience (events, properties, actions and so on); encode meaningful relationships in terms of the configurational properties, or syntax, of the symbol sequence; and have the capacity to encode such relationships in syntactic forms.'

These workers have used Visual Communication (VIC) non-verbal symbols carried on filing cards which are demonstrated to subjects and equated to an object, an action, or a person. The patient learns how to combine the symbols in a meaningful way. One patient proved to be an exceptionally rapid learner, and showed that he could 'understand and use the symbols in terms of normal categories of perceptual experience, could cope with novel messages, and was not bound by referentially constrained situations in his use of VIC'. The authors found no evidence of mapping of VIC symbols on to residual or recovering natural language functions, suggesting that there is indeed a dissociation between cognition and natural languages.

Further support for such dissociation comes from the work of Smith (1980), who designed inferential problems to be solved by aphasic and normal subjects which allowed selective consideration of logical as opposed to grammatical ability. Such constraints on reasoning that recurred were interpreted as resulting from defects in short-term memory rather than defects in logical ability. The dissociation between language and cognitive ability must not, however, be carried too far. The work of Drummond, Gallagher & Mills (1981) on aphasic word retrieval suggests that there is a dynamic interaction between linguistic and cognitive processes.

The possible practical importance of using both Sign and VIC symbols is that there appears to be a carry-over from improved facility with Sign or VIC into recovery of verbal language (Benson, 1979b). Such a carry-over, though presumably by different mechanisms, is also demonstrated by the use of Melodic Intonation Therapy (Sparks, Helm & Albert, 1974). These workers underscored the previously well recognised clinical point that well-articulated and linguistically accurate words are often produced by otherwise aphasic patients when they sing, and 'the dramatic contrast between non-propositional language of well memorised popular songs and the inefficient quality of propositional language which requires encoding of even the most basic thoughts.' Sparks and colleagues got their aphasic patients to sing propositional messages. They found that if 'sentences were adapted to already linguistally loaded melodies, the patient would revert to the lyrics associated with the song.' They therefore used limited pitch variations to 'compose' sentences so that inflection pattern, rhythm and stress were similar to the normal speech prosody of that sentence. Patient and therapist also initially tap out the rhythm as a phrase is intoned, but this tapping and stimulation by the therapist can be withdrawn and the patient himself can eventually continue the phrase without tapping. Useful recovery of function has been reported, especially for those with Broca's aphasia, but this method has not been assessed in a controlled trial.

Apart from the use of gesture or Sign, the aphasic patient has another weapon in his armoury to combat his aphasia — what Brookshire, quoted by Darley (1982), calls his 'knowledge of the world'. Messages delivered to him are likely to be meaningful in terms of his personal life and experience of what usually happens in less intimate real life situations.

THE APHASIC SUBJECT AT HOME

Introspective analysis of the quantity of verbal exchange with one's spouse, at, say, the end of a long car journey may suggest that one is becoming alarmingly taciturn! Personal observation of healthy elderly couples suggests that verbal exchanges become fewer at older ages, though I know of no 'fly on the wall' research to quantify this.

At home, non-verbal communication between spouses is likely to be enhanced by life-long experience of the significance of personal gesture. 'Moods' can be judged, and appropriate actions taken. The daily minutiae of their individual domestic lives is engrained by long habit. Spouses 'know what the other is thinking about'. Perhaps it is not surprising, therefore, that domestic life can continue with real enjoyment in spite of aphasia in many instances.

The observation by Helmick, Watamori & Palmer (1976) that spouses typically consider their aphasic husbands or wives to be less handicapped than they 'really' (sic) are, as judged by objective tests (Darley, 1982), begs the question as to who is to be the judge. The point about aphasia in real-life situations has already been made. It is true, as Darley points out, that 'a knowing look, a ready nod of the head, an automatic 'yes' may convey to the spouse an impression of complete understanding, when in reality understanding is incomplete or absent, but many families get by with reasonable facility and felicity.

This does not deny the very real problems faced by some spouses, and analysed by Malone (1969) and by Kinsella & Duffy (1979). Malone pointed out that, in addition to the obvious financial problems caused by the loss of the aphasic subject's job, expenses are usually sharply increased. The spouse, if still working, may be forced to neglect his or her job in order to care for the aphasic subject at home. The change in roles may sharply alter the family dynamics and children too are affected, either being involved in the caring, or taking the alternative route of staying away from home. Kinsella & Duffy (1979) confirm these distressing insights of Malone. They used rating scales to compare the psycho-social adjustment of patients after hemiplegia with and without aphasia, thereby isolating the effect of aphasia from that of locomotor disability. They showed that the spouses of aphasic patients were significantly more lonely and bored, and female spouses of aphasic hemiplegics showed a significantly higher incidence of minor psychiatric disorder.

It must be remembered, however, that the researches of Malone, and of Kinsella and Duffy, were carried out on populations of patients referred for rehabilitation of language. It is likely that such a population is likely to be biased in the direction of dissatisfaction, as such spouses are more likely to press for 'something to be done' and reach speech therapists. The place of patient satisfaction in illness behaviour has recently been explored in another context (Fitzpatrick & Hopkins, 1981).

THE ROLE OF VOLUNTEERS

Kinsella & Duffy (1979) relate the likelihood of psychiatric illness in the spouses of aphasic patients to 'the combination of coping with the severe crisis of the stroke whilst losing the protective function of an intimate relationship, or a supportive social network'. The last decade has seen, in the United Kingdom, the establishment of more than 100 Volunteer Stroke Schemes and 500 Stroke Clubs, affiliated to the Chest, Heart and Stroke Association. The importance of such a 'supportive social network' cannot, in my opinion, be over-estimated. Furthermore, there is evidence, reviewed below, which suggests that speech therapy given by untrained volunteers is as effective as that given by trained therapists.

Volunteer Stroke Schemes were begun by Miss Valerie Eaton Griffith, whose own efforts to help an aphasic neighbour have grown into the national network mentioned above. She has always stressed that, after early days, she has received help and guidance from trained therapists. Each of the 100 Volunteer Stroke Schemes has a paid part-time supervisor, and between 18 and 40 volunteers whose travel expenses are sometimes paid. Eaton Griffith's philosophy and first results were reported in the British Medical Journal in 1975. Some of what she writes is worth quoting verbatim:

'. . . Some families were better at coping with the patient than others; and, most important of all, the fighting spirit and determination of the patients varied greatly. Spontaneous improvement must also be taken into consideration. Nevertheless, at its lowest valuation, we feel that the Scheme has contributed to the confidence, happiness and general attitude to life in 30 of the 31 patients . . .

. . . Firstly, we offered help as neighbours and did not judge or comment on the disability; we accepted it. Secondly, because we did not know the patient before the stroke, he felt none of the shame with us which he felt with his family and friends who were so shocked by the change in him; he had no need to try to hide his inadequacies and would therefore make greater efforts to talk with us . . . Thirdly, during their visits the volunteers took time to encourage the patient's independence. They waited while he struggled to find the right word, pick up a pencil, or prepare a precarious cup of coffee. Over-protection by the family from the best motives was almost universal and could destroy whatever desire for independence remained . . .

. . . It became clear that however great the speech disability the resulting depression and apathy were an even greater handicap. Once these were overcome the patient could find a way to communicate.' (Eaton Griffith, 1975).

These observations were extended by Eaton Griffith & Miller (1980), and have been validated in two trials in which the outcome of therapy given by trained speech therapists and by untrained volunteers was compared (Meikle et al, 1979; David, Enderby & Bainton, 1982). The first of these lacked sufficient patients to give a clear answer, but the second recently published study seems irrefutable. One hundred and fifty-five patients entered the trial from 14 different hospitals in England and Scotland. No patient was entered unless he had achieved a score of less than 85% on the Functional Communication Profile (FCP) on two successive occasions 1 week apart, and at least 3 weeks had elapsed from the time of the stroke. Patients were randomly allocated to one of two groups. One group received individual treatment from a trained speech therapist who gave such treatment as she thought appropriate for 30 hours over 15–20 weeks. In the other group, volunteers were asked to devote 2 hours a week to their patients and were asked 'to encourage their patient to communicate as well as possible'. This 'encouragement' was given in the speech therapy department, not in the patients' homes. Assessments, always by trained therapists, were carried out at intervals; the assessing therapist was never the treating therapist.

The groups were comparable in all respects except for age. The authors advance statistical reasons for believing that the higher mean age in the speech therapy group (70 as opposed to 66 years) was not relevant in determining the outcome of the study, nor the number of drop-outs, which was approximately equal in the two groups.

Recovery in relation to the initial severity of the aphasia was investigated by dividing the patients into two groups according to whether their baseline FCP score was higher or lower than the median. Figure 9.1 is reproduced from the paper by David and her colleagues (1982). Both severely and less severely affected patients benefited from treatment, and there was no difference between the recovery curves of patients treated by volunteers or by trained therapists.

Although the shape of the curves in Figure 9.1 suggests that much of the improvement occurs in the first 8 weeks following treatment, not all patients entered the trial as soon as 3 weeks after the stroke. Figure 9.2, reproduced from

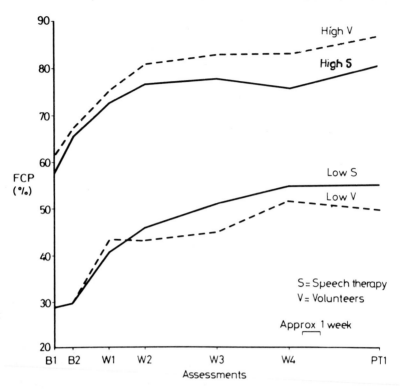

Fig. 9.1 Pattern of recovery of Functional Communication Profile (FCP) for aphasic patients treated by volunteers, and by speech therapy. High and low refers to the severity of the aphasia as judged by the baseline FCP score in relation to the median. (Reproduced by kind permission of Dr Rachel David and the Editor of the Journal of Neurology, Neurosurgery and Psychiatry.)

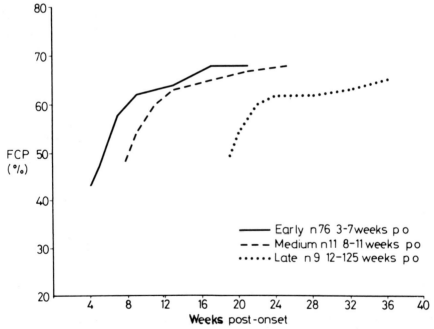

Fig. 9.2 Recovery pattern of FCP scores of patients referred at varying intervals post onset (p.o.) of their aphasia. (Reproduced by kind permission of Dr Rachel David and the Editor of the Journal of Neurology, Neurosurgery and Psychiatry.)

102

the same paper, shows that worthwhile improvement occurs even in the group entered late after onset, and the shapes of the recovery curves are surprisingly similar. The authors suggest that this indicates that 'treatment rather than spontaneous remission was responsible for most of the improvement shown by all the groups'. An alternative view is that 'interest, support and stimulation' can give worthwhile gains in functional communication without doing anything to the central core of language. That is to say, relief of social isolation and encouragement in coping should be the root of treatment, and it is not necessary to indulge in complex linguistic, semantic and contextual therapies to aid recovery.

FINANCIAL IMPLICATIONS OF SPEECH THERAPY

Eaton Griffith's work has important implications. There is the obvious humanitarian point that neighbourly help is kind and worthwhile, but it is just as well that the trial by David and her colleagues turned out the way it did. I have previously reviewed the alleged need for speech therapy after stroke in the United Kingdom (Hopkins, 1975). Tables 9.1 and 9.2 are reproduced from that publication. Even if bed-ridden aphasic survivors are subtracted from the figures shown, the tables indicate that there remain in the United Kingdom at least 26 000 aphasic survivors from stroke. This number is renewed annually by a further 5200 new aphasic subjects who survive at least 6 months. Given the recommended case load of 20 stroke patients per therapist (HMSO, 1972), more than the total number of therapists in post in the United Kingdom treating all kinds of disorders of speech and language are required to treat aphasia following stroke alone. Even so, the recommended case load would allow only $1\frac{1}{2}$ hours' speech therapy a week, making no allowance for record-keeping or travelling (Hopkins, 1975).

Table 9.1 Incidence and prevalence of stroke and stroke survivors. (Reproduced by kind permission from *Health Trends,* 1975, Volume 7, 58–60.)

	Column 1[1] Rates per 100 000	Column 2[2] Numbers in UK population
Annual incidence of stroke	164	90 000
Annual incidence of stroke survivors to 6 months	101	55 000
Annual incidence of dysphasic survivors at 6 months	9.4	5 200
Prevalence of stroke survivors	559	310 000
Prevalence of dysphasic survivors	52	29 000[3]

1 The figures in column 1 are based on a population study in Rochester, Minnesota, for the years 1955–1969 inclusive (Matsumoto et al, 1973. Data from their tables 2, 5 and 6). The figures per 100 000 are age-sex corrected to the USA white population of 1950.

2 The numbers in column 2 are rounded to two significant figures. They assume that the UK population of 55 million has the same age and sex distribution as that of the USA white population of 1950.

3 See text for explanation of this figure.

Table 9.2 Status of dysphasic survivors (Table 9.1) 6 months after a stroke. (Reproduced by kind permission from *Health Trends,* 1975, Volume 7, 58-60.)

Status	Column 1[1] Number of patients	Column 2[2] Prevalence rate/100 000	Column 3[3] Number in UK
Dysphasic only, not working	7	6.4	3 500
Dysphasic working	15	13.7	7 500
Dysphasic, not working, capable of self care	30	27.5	15 000
Dysphasic, bedridden	5	4.6	2 500
Total	57	52.2	29 000

1 The figures in column 1 are derived from Table 6 of Matsumoto et al, 1973.
2 The rate in column 2 are age-sex corrected to the USA white population of 1950.
3 The numbers in column 3 are rounded to two significant figures, and assume that the UK population of 55 million has the same age-sex distribution as that of the USA white population of 1950.

Clearly, speech therapy for stroke can never become widely available. The figures suggest that until now speech therapy has been given on the basis of availability and demand; observation suggests that the patients who obtain treatment reflect the ethnic and social class of the therapists themselves. It is as well that the work of Eaton Griffith and of David and her colleagues has come in time to prevent further resources being diverted to this field. This is not to deny the benefits to be obtained from an assessment by a trained therapist. Indeed, in the study by David and her colleagues it is acknowledged that the volunteer workers were given the results of the speech therapy assessments done on their patients. Nevertheless, I believe it would make more sense if there were a small national elite of highly trained speech therapists conducting research into language and modes of therapy. The role of advising the family and volunteers to cope with disabling situations like stroke could be taken on, I believe, by what might be termed generic rehabilitation workers. These would combine some of the knowledge and skills of social workers, physiotherapists, occupational therapists and speech therapists (Hopkins, 1975; Helander, 1978). Such workers could well be more effective than inadequate numbers of highly trained specialists in each of these fields of rehabilitative medicine.

REFERENCES

Baker E, Berry T, Gardner H, Zurif E, Davis L, Veroff A 1975 Can linguistic competence by dissociated from natural language functions? Nature 254: 509-510
Basso A, Capitani E, Vignolo L A 1979 Influence of rehabilitation on language skills in aphasic patients. A controlled study. Archives of Neurology 36: 190-196
Benson D F 1979a Aphasia rehabilitation. Archives of Neurology 36: 187-189
Benson D F 1979b Aphasia, alexia, and agraphia. Churchill Livingstone, New York, p 213
Broadbent D E 1964 Perceptual and response factors in the organisation of speech. In: de Reuck A V S, O'Conner M (eds) Disorders of language. Ciba Foundation Symposium. Churchill, London
Critchley M 1970 Aphasiology. Edward Arnold, London
Culton G L 1969 Spontaneous recovery from aphasia. Journal of Speech and Hearing Research 12: 825-832
Darley F L 1972 The efficacy of language rehabilitation in aphasia. Journal of Speech and Hearing Disorders 37: 3-21
Darley F L 1982 Aphasia. Saunders, Philadelphia, p 285

David R, Enderby P, Bainton D 1982 Treatment of acquired aphasia: speech therapists and volunteers compared. Journal of Neurology, Neurosurgery and Psychiatry

Drummond S S, Gallagher T M, Mills R H 1981 Word-retrieval in aphasia: an investigation of semantic complexity. Cortex 17: 63–82

Eaton Griffith V 1975 Volunteer scheme for dysphasia and allied problems in stroke patients. British Medical Journal 3: 633–635

Eaton Griffith V, Miller, C 1980 Volunteer stroke scheme for dysphasic patients with stroke. British Medical Journal 4: 1605–1608

Eisenson J 1973 Adult aphasia assessment and treatment. Appleton-Century-Crofts, New York, p 240 (see p 123)

Enderby P 1982 Unpublished paper submitted to the Chest, Heart and Stroke Association, London

European Coronary Surgery Study Group 1982 Long term results of prospective randomised study of coronary artery bypass surgery in stable angina pectoris. Lancet ii: 1173–1180

Fitzpatrick R, Hopkins A 1981 Referrals to neurologists for headache not due to structural disease. Journal of Neurology, Neurosurgery and Psychiatry 44: 1061–1067

Helander E 1978 Towards a multipurpose rehabilitation therapist. Rehabilitation 1: 26–29

Helmick J W, Watamori T S, Palmer J M 1976 Spouses' understanding of the communication abilities of aphasic patients. Journal of Speech and Hearing Disorders 41: 238–243

Hopkins A P 1975 The need for speech therapy for dysphasia following stroke. Health Trends 7: 58–60

HMSO 1972 Speech therapy services. Report of the Committee appointed by the Secretaries of State for Education and Science, for the Social Services, for Scotland and for Wales in July 1969

Kenin M, Swisher L P 1972 A study of pattern of recovery in aphasia. Cortex 8: 58–68

Kinsella G, Duffy F 1979 Psychosocial readjustment in the spouses of aphasic patients. A comparative survey of 79 subjects. Scandinavian Journal of Rehabilitation Medicine 11: 129–132

Malon R L 1969 Expressed attitudes of families of aphasics. Journal of Speech and Hearing Disorders 34: 146–151

Meikle M, Wechsler E, Tupper A, Benenson M 1979 Comparative trial of volunteer and professional treatments of dysphasia after stroke. British Medical Journal 1: 87–89

Sarno M T, Silverman M, Sands E 1970 Speech therapy and language recovery in severe aphasia. Journal of Speech and Hearing Research 13: 607–623

Sarno M T, Levita E 1971 Natural course of recovery in severe aphasia. Archives of Physical Medicine and Rehabilitation 52: 175–178

Skelly M, Schinsky L, Smith R W, Frust R S 1974 American Indian Sign (Amerind) as a facilitator of verbalisation for the oral verbal apraxic. Journal of Speech and Hearing Disorders 39: 445–456

Smith M D 1980 Memory and problem solving in aphasia. Cortex 16: 51–66

Sparks R, Helm N, Albert M 1974 Aphasia rehabilitation resulting from melodic intonation therapy. Cortex 10: 303–316

Vignolo L A 1964 Evolution of aphasia and language rehabilitation: a retrospective exploratory study. Cortex 1: 344–367

10. Does ergotamine work for migraine?

David Thrush

'Contumacious and Rebellious Disease . . .
Deaf to the Claims of Every Medicine'

Thomas Willis

There is no dearth of advice on how to treat and master migraine. There are regular national and international conferences, a proliferation of papers, articles appear frequently in the press proclaiming yet another cure (at present cervical manipulation and biofeedback are fashionable) and local radio phone-ins attempt to educate society.

Although headache is never the only symptom of a migraine attack, it is the patient's cardinal complaint and the one he most wants relieved. Ideally, treatment should be based on a knowledge of the pathogenesis of the attack and pain relieved or prevented by the alteration of physiological mechanisms. Unfortunately the doctor is at a considerable disadvantage. There is no satisfactory definition of migraine, the pathogenesis is poorly understood and the severity, frequency and type of migraine attacks vary enormously, some patients being able to continue work while others are totally incapacitated. Experimental animals do not suffer from migraine and vascular smooth muscle is far from uniform in its functional properties; not only do veins differ from arteries and arteries from arterioles, but vessels in different sites may also differ from one another in their functional activity (Robinson & Collier, 1979).

For more than 40 years ergotamine has been the traditional treatment for an acute attack of migraine, though its mechanism of action is not fully understood. The strong clinical support for its efficacy: 'There is no doubt, that ergotamine, ever since its introduction in therapeutics, still remains the drug of choice in acute attacks of migraine' (Saxena & de Vlaam-Schluter, 1974); 'Ergotamine is the drug of choice in the treatment of migraine attacks all over the world' (Tfelt-Hansen et al 1980); 'Ergotamine tartrate is the most consistently effective drug for the treatment of acute attacks' (Dalessio 1981), is not supported by clinical trials.

WHAT IS THE ACTION OF ERGOTAMINE?

There is a reference to 'a noxious pustule in the ear of grain' on an Assyrian tablet of 600 B.D. (Unger & Cristol, 1971) and epidemics of chronic ergotism ('Ignis

106

Sacer', or St Anthony's fire) caused by eating rye contaminated by the fungus Claviceps pupurea occurred throughout Europe in the Middle Ages. The fungus appears as black, slightly curved spurs in the head of grain and the name ergot is derived from the French word meaning a cockspur. Although it was thought in the 17th century that ergot was the cause of these epidemics, they continued into the 20th century, the last probably being in France in 1951 (Gabbai et al 1951).

The ergot alkaloids, among which are ergotamine, ergometrine, lysergic acid, bromocriptine and methysergide, possess a wide and divergent spectrum of pharmacological actions. Ergotamine was isolated by Stoll in 1918 but its chemical structure was not known until 1951 and it was finally synthesised by Hoffman, Frey and Ott in 1961 (Hoffman, 1978).

Ergotamine is an amino-acid ergot alkaloid and within the normal therapeutic range it has four basic properties (Fozard, 1975).

Vasoconstriction
Vasoconstriction results from the direct action of ergotamine on alpha adreno-receptors and it has been shown that there is a degree of selective vasoconstriction in the carotid circulation, at least in the dog (Saxena & de Vlaam-Schluter, 1974) and monkey (Mylecharane et al, 1978), though this may simply reflect differing amounts of the drug arriving at active sites caused by differences in regional blood flow and dilution. Aellig & Berde (1969) showed that the action of ergotamine was dependent on pre-existing vascular tone. If the tone was below 4 R.U. (1 R.U. = 1 resistance unit = 1 mm mercury per ml per min) vasoconstriction resulted, but at high vascular resistance vasodilatation occurred. This biphasic action may be an important factor in determining its effect on the cranial and extracranial circulations. In addition, the vasoconstrictor effect is enhanced by the synthesis of prostaglandin E which probably results from the potent vasoconstriction caused by ergotamine (Robinson & Collier, 1979).

Sensitisation of smooth muscle
In vitro experiments have demonstrated sensitisation of smooth muscle to sympathetic stimulation and stimulant drugs, possibly caused by inhibition of noradrenaline uptake, but this hypothesis remains controversial.

Antagonism of serotonin
Both in vitro and in vivo experiments have confirmed the inhibitory effect of ergotamine on the pressor responses caused by serotonin on vascular smooth muscle (Saxena & de Vlamm-Schluter, 1974) though much higher concentrations are required to inhibit the stimulant effect on extravascular smooth muscle, e.g. bronchi and intestine (Gaddum & Hameed, 1954).

Inhibition of reflex baroceptor vasodilatation
Intravenous noradrenaline, sufficient to raise systemic blood pressure, causes peripheral vasodilatation which results from reflex baroceptor activity inhibiting the vasomotor centre. Ergotamine tartrate inhibits this reflex, the site of inhibition being peripheral (Wellens, 1964).

At higher concentrations, ergotamine has an inhibitory effect on the carotid occlusion reflex, inhibits tryptamine-evoked pulmonary spasmogen release and monoamine uptake, becomes an alpha adreno-receptor blocking agent and inhibits autonomic neuronal transmitter release (Fozard, 1975).

WHERE COULD ERGOTAMINE ACT IN A MIGRAINE ATTACK?

Despite considerable research during the last decade, the pathogenesis of migraine remains ill-understood. Experimental findings are complex, difficult to evaluate and understand and often conflicting. The classical theory that constriction of intracranial vessels followed by dilatation of extracranial arteries, with constriction of scalp capillaries, remains, in simple terms, true. Studies using intracarotid Xenon 133 have confirmed the reduction of cerebral blood flow which may be global (Norris et al, 1975) or regional (Skinhøj, 1973) during the prodromal phase, and this appears to be caused by arteriolar and not arterial vasoconstriction. The cause of the vasoconstriction is a subject of considerable debate. Many biochemical abnormalities have been found, but most research has focussed on the roles of noradrenaline, serotonin and platelets. An eclectic theory can be summarised as follows. Patients with migraine have a genetically determined neurovascular instability. Various factors, (e.g. tyramine, hypoglycaemia) trigger the release of neural noradrenaline, which increases platelet aggregation and also acts on alpha-receptors causing vasoconstriction. The aggregation, possibly aided by a serotonin-releasing factor (e.g. fatty acids or tyramine), releases serotonin and adenosine diphosphate from platelets. Both serotonin and adenosine diphosphate cause further platelet aggregation, and in addition serotonin constricts extracranial arteries but probably dilates scalp capillaries. A number of studies have demonstrated a fall in plasma serotonin at the onset of a migrainous headache with a corresponding rise in urinary hydroxy-indole acetic acid. The fall in serotin appears to be specific for migraine and has not been found in patients with tension headaches, or vomiting, or under stress (Lance, 1978). In addition reserpine, a serotonin depletor, frequently precipitates migraine in susceptible patients, and the headache has been relieved by intravenous serotonin (Kimball et al, 1960). Further support for serotonin playing a major role in migraine comes from platelet behaviour studies. During headache-free periods migraine sufferers have a higher aggregation response to adenosine diphosphate than control patients; during the prodromal phase aggregation increases and then falls during the headache phase (Deshmukh & Meyer, 1977).

The cause of the headache is poorly understood. Both intracranial and extracranial blood flow are increased during the headache phase and may persist after ergotamine has relieved it. It has been postulated that a post-ischaemic lactic acidosis, confirmed by increased lactate and low bicarbonate levels in the cerebrospinal fluid, is responsible for cerebral hyperfusion (Skinhøj, 1973), but there appears to be little relationship between the duration and severity of the ischaemia and the severity of the headache. In addition, severe headache is not a common finding in patients who have cerebral anoxia resulting from other causes, for example transient cerebral ischaemic attacks. It is probable that other factors, possibly prostaglandins which are released by serotonin, play an important role. Vasodilatation per se is not responsible for the headache as this may occur for other reasons, e.g. after carbon dioxide inhalation, without causing headache. Most investigators support the hypothesis of a local sterile inflammatory response, the oedema resulting from the irritant effect of serotonin on the vessel wall and the associated release of other vasoactive and inflammatory substances, e.g. kinins, prostaglandins and histamine. Others have suggested a more central mechanism, pain resulting from a functional disorder of neurotransmitters in the nociceptive system caused by serotonin (Sicuteri, 1978).

No theory provides an adequate explanation of the pre-prodromal features, such as increasing tension, hunger, thirst, feeling of well-being, etc, for the selectivity of vasoconstriction, for the prodromal symptoms occurring sometimes during the headache, sometimes towards its end, or for the unilaterality of the headache.

Ergotamine has a wide spectrum of pharmacological activity but whatever effectiveness it has almost certainly results from its vasoconstrictor properties. Graham & Wolff (1939) showed that intravenous ergotamine reduced the amplitude of pulsation of the superficial temporal and occipital arteries by an average of 50%; the reduction usually began immediately, though maximum decrease was obtained after 35 minutes. As a consequence there was a decline in the intensity of the headache which tended to parallel the decrease in amplitude of pulsation. They also demonstrated, in one patient during craniotomy, that intravenous ergotamine resulted in a 20% reduction in the diameter of the middle meningeal artery whereas, in another patient, it had no significant effect on the middle cerebral artery or its branches. A subsequent study in 16 patients confirmed that intramuscular ergotamine does not alter cerebral blood flow (Hachinski et al, 1978). In contrast, a more recent study of patients during a migraine attack failed to show a significant asymmetry of temporal artery pulsation and from these and other studies using photoplethysmographic recordings during compression of the common carotid and superficial temporal arteries, the authors concluded that there was an intracranial contribution to the headache (Lance & Drummond, 1981).

Whether ergotamine's antagonism of serotonin has a meaningful role remains uncertain. Recent work on opiate receptors has shown that serotonin is necessary to inhibit afferent transmission of pain sensation. The ergotamine molecule has the same indole ring as serotonin; during the headache serotonin levels fall and it has been postulated that ergotamine may relieve headache by replacing serotonin and allowing endogenous opiates to inhibit afferent pain impulses (Orton, 1979).

THE ROLE OF ERGOTAMINE IN TREATMENT

Ergotamine was first used in the treatment of migraine by Eulenburg (1883) and Thomson (1894). The first systematic study, of 12 patients with favourable results in 8, was published by Tzank (1928) and was followed by a number of papers over the next decade which recorded the efficacy of ergotamine. Lennox (1934) reported the abrupt termination of headache in 90% of patients using subcutaneous or intravenous ergotamine and commented that 'the distracted physician to migraine patients has a new weapon in his armamentarium.'

O'Sullivan (1936) reported the abrupt termination of 1042 headaches in 89 patients using subcutaneous ergotamine: she stressed that it should be given as early as possible and calculated that her patients had been freed from 39 000 hours of suffering. Friedman & Merritt (1957) in a study of 2500 patients with migraine also stressed the importance of early and adequate administration. Oral or rectal administration did not influence the outcome, good results being achieved in 50% of patients, but when given parentally the success rate increased to 80%. A similar result was reported by Wilkinson (1971). In a recent study of effervescent ergotamine, Blowers et al (1981) reported that 40.2% of attacks were successfully treated and moderate relief was obtained in a further 37.9%, though the authors did not define success.

The reader, like the author, may now begin to wonder why he sees so many patients with migraine.

More recent trials have not supported these early claims. Sublingual ergotamine was found to be no more effective than placebo (Crooks et al, 1964), and it was later demonstrated that therapeutic amounts of ergotamine cannot be absorbed through the buccal mucosa (Sutherland et al, 1974). In a double-blind cross-over trial of 88 patients, oral ergotamine was no more effective than placebo (Waters, 1970). In contrast, a study of 20 patients showed oral ergotamine to be more effective than placebo but no more effective than Tolfenamic acid (a potent inhibitor of prostaglandin biosynthesis) in reducing the duration and intensity of attacks (Hakkarainen et al, 1979). Studies comparing ergotamine with other drugs have shown that it is less effective than Midrid, a drug containing isometheptene, paracetamol and dichloralphenazone (Yuill et al, 1972), and as effective as Migraleve (General Practitioner Clinical Research Group, 1973) — though few would agree that the mean duration of headache following treatment with ergotamine (13.5 hours) and following treatment with Migraleve (18.8 hours) showed that either was effective. Both ergotamine and dextropropoxyphene compound (dextropropoxyphene napsylate 100 mg, acetylsalicylic acid 350 mg and phenazone 150 mg) were equally effective and superior to acetylsalicylic acid in reducing the frequency and severity of attacks (Hakkarainen et al, 1980); and in a more recent trial comparing ergotamine with metoclopramide and a combination of the two drugs, both were equally efficient and the combination was more effective in reducing the duration of attacks (Hakkarainen & Allonen, 1982). In all these trials the side-effects with ergotamine have been significantly greater than with other drugs.

The results of these trials are variable and they are in marked contrast to statements supporting the efficacy of ergotamine in textbooks and review articles on migraine. Is there an explanation?

Drug trials in the treatment of migraine are notoriously difficult for three reasons. The frequency, severity and type of migraine attack vary enormously, and I suspect that when local doctors are informed about a migraine trial it is the chronic patients, whose symptoms are often tied up with considerable psychopathology, who are referred. Secondly, there are many problems in designing a trial; each patient has to be treated by a standardised regime and not by a dose which has been tailored to his requirements; despite careful instructions, patients may fail to take their tablets as soon as the attack starts, compliance may be variable, and until recently plasma ergotamine levels could not be estimated. In most trials the number of patients has been small and the cross-over period too short, in one trial a fortnight only (Stieg, 1977), so statistical conclusions are difficult to evaluate. Finally, it is only in recent years that we have begun to learn a little about the pharmacokinetics of ergotamine and studies have shown that its bioavailability varies enormously.

Ergotamine is poorly and irregularly absorbed from the gastrointestinal tract, metabolised in the liver and excreted in the bile (Nimmerfall & Rosenthaler, 1976). Using tritium labelled ergotamine, Meier & Schreier, (1976) predicted a peak dose of 3 ng/ml at 3 hours after taking 4 mg ergotamine with caffeine. Orton (1978), using a radioimmunoassay method, found ergotamine in the plasma within an hour in three normal subjects who had taken 1 mg effervescent ergotamine orally after fasting overnight, the mean level showing a peak of 2 ng/ml at 45 minutes; the level fell to below the limit of accuracy of the method within $2\frac{1}{2}$ hours. One subject, given 0.25 mg ergotamine intramuscularly, showed a maximum level at 15 minutes but no ergotamine was detected up to 4 hours later in a patient who took 0.36 mg of ergotamine by Medihaler though he had used the Medihaler with success in treating his migrainous neuralgia. Using high performance liquid chromatography with fluoroscein detection, no ergotamine was detected in the plasma of 9 men taking regular ergotamine despite clinical improvement occurring in several. Similarly, no ergotamine was detected in 3 migrainous patients after taking 2 mg ergotamine orally (Ekbom et al, 1981).

Using a radioimmunoassay technique Ala-Hurula (1979) measured the rate of absorption of ergotamine taken orally, rectally, and by intramuscular injection in 33 volunteers. Blood levels were highest at 30 minutes following intramuscular injection, 60 minutes after rectal administration, and 2 hours after oral administration, though there was considerable variation between subjects, even when ergotamine was given by intramuscular injection. A surprising finding was a secondary increase in levels between 24 and 48 hours but it has recently been shown that the vasoconstrictor effect of ergotamine lasts for over 24 hours (Tfelt-Hansen et al, 1982). The pharmacokinetics of effervescent ergotamine are similar to those of the oral and rectal preparations though absorption is faster (Ala-Hurula, 1982). Factors which influence the marked variation in bioavailability are gastric motility, which is reduced during a migraine attack (Volans 1975), the presence of food in the stomach and the dissolution rate of solid tablets.

CONCLUSION

Ergotamine is no wonder drug. It has been over-prescribed and abused and bioavailability studies and trials show that enteral ergotamine has little, if any, role in the treatment of the acute attack of migraine. It should never be used in prophylaxis, except in migrainous neuralgia when rectal ergotamine may be of value. Parenteral ergotamine is inconvenient for the patient, many recoil from the thought of having to inject themselves and I know of no trial comparing it to other medication or placebo.

Migraine continues to be surrounded by magic and mythology. It shows an amazing ability to respond to placebo medication and provided a doctor is empathetic and prescribes with confidence, whatever he gives will improve many patients' attacks. Too many patients, however, are 'looked at, investigated, drugged and charged' (Sachs, 1973). It is not always necessary to prescribe: many patients need only reassurance and an explanation of symptoms.

If treatment is necessary, I try simple analgesics first, usually with metoclopramide (though I have yet to be convinced that its addition makes a significant difference), and stress that the tablets should be taken as soon as the attack starts. If they fail, I try Migraleve or Midrid and if there is still no improvement I suggest parenteral ergotamine, the patient being taught to give it by subcutaneous or intramuscular injection. To those who are unwilling to inject themselves and if all other treatment has failed, I offer oral ergotamine, usually as Migril, in a single dose of 2–4 mg with metoclopramide, but I ask the patient not to repeat the dose if the headache continues. If ergotamine fails after the treatment of three attacks it should be abandoned.

I doubt that there will ever be one way of treating migraine and treatment will remain both an art and a science. The art lies in forging a satisfactory doctor–patient relationship by spending time listening and talking to the patient thereby establishing authority and confidence, and by treating the patient (and sometimes the family) as well as the disease. The science is making the correct diagnosis and giving the right drug in the right dosage to the right patient at the right time.

'The wisest physician is he who knows the uselessness of most medicines.' (Anon.)

REFERENCES

Aellig W H, Berde B 1969 Studies of the effect of natural and synthetic polypeptide type ergot compounds on peripheral vascular bed. British Journal of Pharmacology 36: 561–570
Ala-Hurula V 1982 Bioavailability and antimigraine efficacy of effervescent ergotamine. Headache 22: 167–170
Ala-Hurula V, Myllyla V V, Arvela P, Heikkilä J, Kärki N, Hokkanen E 1979 Systemic availability of ergotamine tartrate after oral, rectal and intramuscular administration. European Journal of Clinical Pharmacology 15: 51–55
Blowers A J, Cameron E G, Lawrence E R 1981 Effervescent ergotamine tartrate (Effergot) in the treatment of the acute migraine attack. British Journal of Clinical Practice 35: 188–190
Crooks J, Stephen S A, Brass W 1964 Clinical trial of inhaled ergotamine tartrate in migraine. British Medical Journal 1: 221–224
Dalessio D J 1981 Use of ergot preparations in acute migraine attacks (editorial). Headache 21: 75
Deshmukh S V, Meyer J S 1977 Cyclic changes in platelet dynamics and the pathogenesis and prophylaxis of migraine. Headache 17: 101–108
Ekbom K, Paalgow L, Waldenlind E 1981 Low biological availability of ergotamine tartrate after oral dosing in cluster headache. Cephalagia 1: 203–207
Eulenberg A 1883 Subcutane injectionen von ergotism — (tanret): Ergotinum citricum solutum (Gehre). Deutsche mediszinische Wochenschrift 9: 637
Fozard J R 1975 The animal pharmacology of drugs used in the treatment of migraine. Journal of Pharmacy and Pharmacology 27: 297–321
Friedman A P, Merritt H H 1957 Treatment of headache. Journal of the American Association 163: 1111–1117
Gabbai A, Lisbonne P, Pourquier J 1951 Ergot poisoning at Pont St Esprit. British Medical Journal 2: 650–651
Gaddum J H, Hameed E A 1954 Drugs which antagonise 5-hydroxytryptamine. British Journal of Pharmacology 9: 240–248
General Practitioner Clinical Group 1973 Migraine treated with an antihistamine-analgesic combination. Practitioner 211: 357–361

Graham J R, Wolff H G 1979 Mechanism of migraine headache and action of ergotamine tartrate. Archives of Neurology and Psychiatry 39: 737-763

Hachinski V, Norris J W, Edmeads J, Cooper P W 1978 Ergotamine and cerebral blood flow. Stroke 9: 594-596

Hakkarainen H, Allonen H 1982 Ergotamine vs metoclopramide vs their combination in acute migraine attacks. Headache 22: 10-12

Hakkarainen H, Quiding H, Stockman P 1980 Mild analgesics as an alternative to ergotamine in migraine. A comparative trial with acetylsalicylic acid, ergotamine tartrate, and a dextropropoxyphene compound. Journal of Clinical Pharmacology 20: 590-595

Hakkarainen H, Vapaatalo H, Gothoni G, Parantainan J 1979 Tolfenamic acid is as effective as ergotamine during migraine attacks. Lancet 2: 326-328

Hoffman A 1978 Historical view on ergot alkaloids. In: Spano P F, Trabucchi M (eds) Pharmacology supp 1. International Workshop on Ergot Alkaloids, p 1-11

Kimball R W, Friedman A P, Vallejo E 1960 Effects of serotonin in migrainous patients. Neurology 10: 107-111

Lance J W 1978 Migraine. In: Matthews W B, Glaser G H (eds) Recent advances in clinical neurology. Churchill Livingstone, Edinburgh, ch 8, p 145-162

Lance J W, Drummond P D 1981 the extracranial vascular change of headache. In Abstracts 12th World Congress of Neurology, Kyoto, Japan. Excepta Medica, Amsterdam, No 160

Lennox W G 1934 The use of ergotamine tartrate in migraine. New England Journal of Medicine 210: 1061-1065

Meier J, Schreier E 1976 Human plasma levels of some anti-migraine drugs. Headache 16: 96-104

Mylecharane E J, Spira P J, Misbach J, Duckworth J W, Lance J W 1978 Effects of methysergide, pizotifen and ergotamine in the monkey cranial circulation. European Journal of Pharmacology 48: 1-9

Nimmerfall F, Rosenthaler J 1976 Ergot alkaloids: hepatic distribution and estimation of absorption by measurement of total radioactivity in bile and urine. Journal of Pharmacokinetics and Biopharmaceutics 4: 57-66

Norris J W, Hachinski V C, Cooper P W 1975 Changes in cerebral blood flow during a migraine attack. British Medical Journal 3: 676-677

Orton D 1978 Ergotamine tartrate levels using radioimmunoassay. In: Greene R (ed) Current concepts in migraine research. Raven Press, New York, p 73-75

Orton D 1979 Migraine: can simple analgesics take the place of ergotamine. Modern Medicine (September), p 37-41

O'Sullivan M E 1936 Termination of 1000 attacks of migraine with ergotamine tartrate. Journal of the American Medical Association 107: 1208-1212

Robinson B F, Collier J G 1979 Vascular smooth muscle. Correlations between basic properties and responses of human blood vessels. British Medical Bulletin 35: 305-312

Sachs O 1973 Migraine. Evolution of a common disorder. Faber and Faber, London

Saxena P R, de Vlaam-Schluter 1974 Role of some biogenic substances in migraine and relevant mechanism in antimigraine action of ergotamine — studies in an experimental model for migraine. Headache 14: 142-163

Skinhøj E 1973 Haemodynamic studies within the brain during migraine attacks. Archives of Neurology 29: 95-98

Sicuteri F 1978 Endorphins, opiate receptors and migraine headache. Headache 17: 253-257

Stieg R L 1977 Double blind study of belladonna-ergotamine phenobarbital for interval treatment of recurrent throbbing headache. Headache 17: 120-124

Sutherland J M, Hooper W D, Eadie M J, Tyrer J H 1974 Buccal absorption of ergotamine. Journal of Neurology, Neurosurgery and Psychiatry 37: 1116-1120

Tfelt-Hansen P, Eickhoff J H, Olesen J 1980 The effect of single dose ergotamine tartrate on peripheral arteries in migraine patients: methodological aspects and time effect curve. Acta Pharmacologica et Toxicologica 47: 151-156

Tfelt-Hansen P, Eickhoff J H, Olesen J 1982 Duration on the . biological effect of ergotamine tartrate. In: Critchley M (ed) Advances in neurology. Raven Press, New York 33: 315-319

Thomson W H 1894 Ergot in treatment of periodic neuralgias. Journal of Nervous and Mental Disorders 21: 124

Tzank A 1928 Le traitement des migraines par le tartrate d'ergotamine. Bull et mém Soc méd de hôpital de Paris 52: 1057-1061

Unger L, Cristol J L 1971 Migraine — a series of 38 patients treated with ergotamine tablets. Medical Times 99: 97-102

Volans G N 1975 The treatment of migraine. In: Turner P (ed) Proceedings of a conference held at the Royal College of Physicians. Pitman Medical, London, p 156-172

Waters W E 1970 Controlled clinical trial of ergotamine tartrate. British Medical Journal 2: 325–327

Wellens D 1964 Inhibition of norepinephrine — induced reflex vasodilatation in dog hind limb. Archives Internationales de Pharmacodymie et de Therapie 151: 281–285

Wilkinson 1971 Migraine — treatment of acute attack. British Medical Journal 2: 754–755

Yuill G M, Swinburn W R, Liversedge L A 1972 A double trial of isometheptene mucate compound and ergotamine in migraine. British Journal of Clinical Practice 26: 76–79

11. Is L-dopa harmful?

A. J. Lees

Since its introduction into clinical practice 13 years ago, the aromatic amino acid, L-dihydroxyphenylalanine (L-dopa) has firmly established itself as the treatment of choice for patients with idiopathic Parkinson's disease. Such is its universal acceptance that debate regarding its administration is now centred more around when treatment should be started and at what dosage, rather than whether it should be used at all. The pioneer trials in the late nineteen sixties using large doses (2–8 g per 24 h) achieved an average 50% reduction of functional disabilities and a considerable improvement in all the cardinal features of the disease. The subsequent incorporation of a peripheral dopa decarboxylase inhibitor led to a more rapid therapeutic response and reduced the number of gastrointestinal and cardiovascular adverse reactions thereby permitting the large majority of patients to derive worthwhile benefit. In milder cases of the disease all symptoms and signs were temporarily abolished and some severely crippled patients were able to discard their wheelchairs and fend once more for themselves. Indeed, the early results were so spectacular that it was hoped that L-dopa might actually be curative. A further testimony to its striking success was the virtual disappearance of stereotactic surgical approaches to management within a year or two of the drug's introduction. However, despite its indisputable efficacy L-dopa continued to be looked upon as a difficult and dangerous drug to use and was appreciably underprescribed for several years. Concern existed from the beginning about its long-term safety; sensationalised media coverage of its idiosyncratic aphrodisiac effects and reports of fractures and angina also contributed to an unwarranted therapeutic nihilism on the part of many practitioners.

Experience with the drug over the next few years allayed many of these fears and, provided early side-effects could be surmounted, unwanted complications were rare in the first year or two of sustained treatment. Nevertheless, it was soon apparent that after a honeymoon period, former disabilities re-appeared in many patients and a constellation of perplexing and increasingly disabling drug-induced disturbances also slowly emerged. These included violent adventitious hyperkinesias, capricious diurnal swings in disease severity and visual hallucinations. The duration of benefit derived from each dosage also steadily dwindled so that improvement was only noticeable in short time periods. After 6 years of continuous treatment most patients returned to their pre-treatment level of disability and about one-quarter were exhibiting some degree of intellectual deterioration.

In spite of these challenging problems L-dopa improves the quality of life for patients with Parkinson's disease and apart from the newer synthetic dopamine receptor agonists is at least twice as potent as any other currently available medicine. Unlike stereotactic surgery and the anticholinergic drugs it is effective against the most disabling symptom, bradykinesia and, in contrast to amantidine, rapid tachyphylaxis does not occur.

There is also evidence to suggest that L-dopa might have a beneficial effect on the natural history of Parkinson's disease. Hoehn & Yahr (1967) analysed the case records of 602 patients treated with anticholinergic medication and followed in New York City between 1949 and 1964. They reported a mean duration of disease from diagnosis to death of 9 years, a mean age at death of 67 years and an excess mortality ratio of 2.9. A higher mortality ratio occurred inexplicably in women, and a benign tremulous variety of the disease was distinguishable. A quarter of the patients died or were severely disabled within 5 years of the onset of the disease, two-thirds by 9 years and 80% by 10 years or more. A similar mortality ratio of 3:1 in patients who had not received L-dopa was found by Diamond & Markham (1976) in a retrospective study. Kurland (1958), however, found a mortality ratio of only 1.4:1 in 44 untreated patients followed from 1940–1954 and other reports have shown that even before L-dopa was available as many as one-quarter of patients may be alive and active as long as 18 years after the onset of the disease (Pollock & Hornabrook, 1966). The mortality ratios in the best documented long-term L-dopa studies are shown in the Table 11.1. It can be seen that, with the exception of the poor results obtained by Barbeau (1976) in severely handicapped akinetic patients, an average mortality ratio of 1.5:1 occurs. Many of these early studies included severely disabled patients with

Table 11.1 Mortality ratio figures for L-dopa treated patients.

Investigator	No. of patients	Duration of therapy (y)	Mortality ratio
Diamond et al (1976)[a] UCLA, USA	93	6	0.96:1
Barbeau (1976)[a] Montreal, Canada	70	6	2.4:1
Diamond & Markham (1979)[c] UCLA, USA	327	6	1.45:1
McDowell & Sweet (1979)[b] New York, USA	100	10	1.54:1
Yahr (1976)[a] New York, USA	597	5–7	1.46:1
Joseph et al (1978)[a] US Multicentre	1625	6	1.03:1
Rinnie et al (1980)[b] Finland	349	9	1.59:1
Shaw et al (1980)[b] UCH, England	178	6	1.45:1

a L-dpa alone
b L-dopa alone then peripheral dopa decarboxylase inhibitor addition
c L-dopa plus a peripheral dopa decarboxylase inhibitor from the outset

a long duration of disease and were conducted with neat L-dopa rather than combination therapy. Even better figures, therefore, might be obtained with currently available medication and the additional opportunity to treat more patients early in the course of the illness. Improved life-expectancy, if indeed it occurs, is probably due to increased mobility preventing early deaths from hypostatic pneumonia rather than any intrinsic ameliorative effects on the underlying disease process.

It is on this background of incontrovertible success that the case against L-dopa must be brought. Although there are substantial theoretical arguments that can be marshalled against L-dopa therapy much of the currently available evidence is speculative, anecdotal or contentious and it is virtually impossible to disentangle the effects of inexorable disease progression from the possible toxic effects of the drug. Nevertheless, there is a growing view that chronic L-dopa administration may lead to irreversible detrimental changes in the brain and, for this reason, most physicians do not prescribe the drug in the very early stages of Parkinson's disease.

THE SELF-LIMITING NATURE OF L-DOPA THERAPY

Compensatory mechanisms within the basal ganglia prevent the appearance of Parkinson's disease until there has been a severe reduction in the number of pigmented nigral neurones. Increased dopamine turnover within the few surviving cells and hypersensitivity of postsynaptic striatal dopamine receptors enables neuronal function to be tenuously maintained for a considerable length of time.

The precise mode of action of L-dopa therapy is not known. One notion is that its effectiveness relies on the preservation of a minimum number of presynaptic dopaminergic terminals into which L-dopa is incorporated thus assisting in the greater release of dopamine per unit of time. Alternatively it may be converted to dopamine outside the catecholamine-rich neurones and function as a neuromodulator tonically bathing striatal neurones.

Sustained treatment returns cerebral dopamine levels towards normal and probably also evokes intermittent dopaminergic overactivity. As a result the compensatory mechanisms which have developed in the surviving neuronal apparatus may be shut-off. This could lead to changes in receptor sensitivity and also affect the physiological properties and even survival of the remaining dopaminergic neurones. This line of reasoning has been used to explain the apparent finite period of usefulness of L-dopa treatment.

THE DECLINE IN THERAPEUTIC EFFICACY

Progression of the underlying disease process is probably responsible for much of the deterioration observed in the course of long-term therapy. Markham & Diamond (1981) found that disability scores were similar in patients matched for duration of disease irrespective of the duration of L-dopa therapy, and in those patients able to tolerate long-term treatment life-expectancy was normal. These data support the rationale of giving L-dopa early, and implies that the current widely advocated policy of witholding treatment is wrong.

However, there are a few observations which suggest that the pharma-codynamic properties of L-dopa itself may also contribute to the waning response. For instance, uniform decline in benefit appears to occur after 2 or 3 years stable improvement. This occurs independently of the patients' initial level of therapeutic response or pretreatment level of disability (Fig. 11.1). Long-term metabolic effects of L-dopa seem a more likely explanation for this finding than a steady rate of cell death throughout the course of Parkinson's disease.

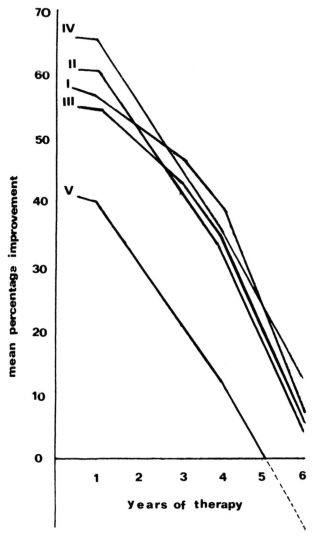

Fig. 11.1 The long-term response to L-dopa therapy with respect to pre-treatment disease severity using the Hoehn and Yahr classification of disease severity (personal data).

In a cross-sectional retrospective analysis using 22 pairs of patients matched for duration of disease Fahn's group in New York found that those patients who had received L-dopa for between 4–8 years had worse disability scores than those who had received treatment for 1–3 years (Lesser et al, 1979). It is possible, however, because of the retrospective nature of this study, that the pretreatment disease severity of those patients who began treatment at an earlier stage may have been greater than the group with a short duration of L-dopa exposure.

Fahn & Barrett (1979) have reported five patients who improved appreciably on modest dosages of L-dopa but then deteriorated when the dose was increased. Of particular interest here was the observation that two of these patients lost their peak-dose choreoathetosis as the signs of Parkinson's disease increased. Subsensitisation of receptors has been invoked as a possible explanation for this phenomenon and some support for this is now available from receptor binding studies in post-mortem brains (Rinne, 1982). Drug holidays are based on this sort of rationale but in my hands have proved ineffective and potentially dangerous.

THE LONG-TERM L-DOPA SYNDROME

Drug-induced abnormal involuntary movements occur in virtually all patients treated with maximum tolerated doses of L-dopa. They are dose-related, increase in severity as treatment continues and are readily reversible on discontinuing medication. The commonest variety consists of choreoathetosis occurring at the height of each interdose period when plasma dopa levels are at their highest and Parkinsonian disabilities at their least. These 'peak-dose' dyskinesias are generally assumed to arise as a result of dopaminergic overactivity in the corpus striatum. However, studies with the dopamine receptor agonist bromocriptine in previously untreated patients have revealed that in a small number of individuals therapeutic effects comparable to those achieved with L-dopa may be obtained with a greatly reduced frequency of dyskinesias (Lees & Stern, 1981). What is even more intriguing is that in patients in whom L-dopa has been discontinued dyskinesias occur frequently when bromocriptine is introduced. Furthermore, patients who have derived sustained benefit from bromocriptine therapy alone for several years without experiencing dyskinesias may develop them rapidly following L-dopa substitution. These findings suggest that the mechanism underlying the therapeutic effects of dopaminergic drugs in Parkinson's disease are quite distinct from those provoking dyskinesias. They also raise the possibility that L-dopa may actually irreversibly alter the metabolism of neurones in such a way as to lower the threshold for these abnormal movements.

The absence of oscillations in performance in patients receiving long-term bromocriptine as the only therapy also points to the likelihood of this complication being partly related to the pharmacokinetic and pharmacodynamic properties of L-dopa (Lees & Stern, 1981) and studies being carried out in the Department of Neurology at University College Hospital, London have also demonstrated that a constant intravenous infusion of L-dopa may smooth out, but not totally eradicate, fluctuations in performance in patients with the long-term L-dopa syndrome.

POST-MORTEM DATA

A comparison of the causes of death in patients dying with Parkinson's disease before and during the L-dopa era reveals no appreciable differences. Hypostatic pneumonia as a result of immobility and delirium remains the commonest cause of death and there is no suggestion of an increased incidence of neoplasia or vascular disease. Examination of the brain using conventional histological techniques and light microscopy has revealed no structural alterations (Yahr et al, 1972) although nigral cell counts and detailed electron microscopic studies have not yet been carried out.

Striatal dopamine levels are much higher in L-dopa treated patients than untreated controls and high concentrations are found in other parts of the brain after prolonged therapy. In addition, many patients who have received chronic treatment have a low or normal dopamine receptor binding affinity in the corpus striatum whereas in untreated patients hypersensitivity is usual (Lee et al, 1978). Whether these marked chemical changes resulting from treatment can lead to irreversible neuronal damage is unknown.

NEUROENDOCRINE EFFECTS

The acute administration of L-dopa causes a rise in serum growth hormone levels, suppression of prolactin release and a decreased glucose tolerance with a delayed and exaggerated insulin response (Boyd, Lebovitz & Pfeiffer, 1970). Similar changes in growth hormone and carbohydrate tolerance after 1 years treatment led to anxiety about the possible development of acromegaly and diabetes mellitus (Sirtori, Bolme & Azarnoff, 1972). Other studies, however, failed to show an increase in mean 24 hour growth hormone concentrations compared with age-matched controls (Malarkey, Cyrus & Paulson, 1974) and no increased incidence of either of these conditions has been found in practice. It has been suggested that periodic growth hormone surges induced by L-dopa might influence the long-term clinical response to the drug (Cotzias, Papavasiliou & Ginos, 1976). Subsequent studies have failed to substantiate any effects of endogenous growth hormone release (Galea-Debono et al, 1977) or exogenous human somatotropin administration (Papavasiliou et al, 1979) on the long-term side-effects of L-dopa and it seems probable that the powerful neuroendocrine effects are quite independent from the anti-Parkinsonian effects.

L-DOPA AND DEMENTIA

There is a marked discrepancy between the frequency of intellectual impairment reported in recent studies and the two most carefully conducted trials in the pre-L-dopa period. Mjones (1949) reported a prevalence of definite dementia of only 3.2% in a cross-sectional study carried out in Sweden and a similar study in New Zealand obtained the only slightly higher figure of 8% (Pollock & Hornabrook, 1966). In contrast most of the investigations in the last 10 years have reported prevalence figures for dementia of 20–40% (Celesia & Wanamaker, 1972; Lieberman et al, 1979; Shaw, Lees & Stern, 1980). It is uncertain whether improved life-expectancy, a deleterious effect of L-dopa or simply greater awareness on the part of clinicians is responsible for this change. L-dopa has been reported to improve intellectual function in Parkinson's disease (Loranger et al, 1972) although this effect is rarely prolonged. Botez & Barbeau (1973) noted clear-cut cognitive deficits in patients on dopaminergic therapy when compared with patients receiving only anticholinergics. It is also known that the administration of L-dopa to Parkinsonian patients with dementia may provoke states of excitement, catatonia, impulsions, perseverations and somnolence. Complete disintegration of higher mental functions may then ensue to be followed after withdrawal of the drug by exacerbated Parkinsonism and an irreversible aggravation of dementia (Sacks et al, 1972). However, discontinuation of L-dopa therapy in patients who develop a progressive dementing illness in the course of therapy rarely leads to any slowing in the insidious decline of mental faculties. A primary disorder of the isodendritic core with clinical overlap between Parkinson's disease and Alzheimer's disease and a mesocorticolimbic dementia due to degeneration of the ascending cortical dopamine pathways have been postulated as possible causes of dementia in Parkinsonism and it is conceivable that L-dopa therapy might accelerate either of these two processes.

L-DOPA AND MELANOMA

There are at least three convincing case reports of recurrence of melanomata within 1–12 months of starting L-dopa therapy (Lieberman & Shupack, 1974). The most likely mechanism for this acceleration of neoplastic change is the incorporation of the drug into the tumour stimulating its growth directly.

POSSIBLE NEUROTOXIC MECHANISMS

Formation of toxic metabolites

Many mammalian species possess large concentrations of catecholamines within the basal ganglia but it is only in the primates and particularly man that neuromelanin accumulates to any appreciable degree. Marsden (1965) has hypothesised that this may be due to lower catecholamine requirements in the phylogenetically ancient brain stem nuclei as their function is taken over by the development of higher cortical centres. Consequently the metabolism of typrosine is diverted away from catecholamine synthesis and towards the formation of neuromelanin.

The biosynthesis of neuromelanin is still poorly understood. Unlike cutaneous melanin its formation does not appear to be mediated by tyrosinase since albinos possess normal amounts of brain pigment. Non-enzymatic auto-oxidation of catechols is probably of primary importance leading to o-quinone formation, leukochromes and finally by a series of polymerisation steps neuromelanin is formed. This process causes a univalent reduction of oxygen with the formation of hydrogen peroxide by the transfer of two electrons. Recent attention has also been focussed on the one electron transfer product superoxide. Both hydrogen peroxide and superoxide destroy cells but the superoxide radical may initiate lipid peroxidation and is particularly lethal. Fortunately most mammalian tissues possess an enzyme, superoxide dismutase, which detoxifies superoxide to molecular oxygen and hydrogen peroxide which in turn is then catabolised by peroxidase and catalase. However, the simultaneous formation of superoxide and hydrogen peroxide may, through a bimolecular reaction, form the hydroxyl radical which is known to cause alterations in nuclear DNA and be responsible for several forms of radiation damage. The quinones per se may also have toxic effects being sulphydryl agents capable of inhibiting DNA and RNA polymerase and certain steps in energy metabolism. Normally the cells' content of reduced glutathione, ascorbic acid and superoxide dismutase offers protection against these potentially damaging effects.

It has been suggested that Parkinson's disease may be caused by a primary defect in the storage (Cohen et al, 1976) transport, or degradation (Graham, 1979) of catecholamines resulting in a life-long increase in the formation of cytotoxic by-products which act as free radicals and alter redox potentials in nerve cells. A reduced level of peroxidase and catalase has been found in one study in patients with Parkinson's disease although the authors acknowledge that this may simply be a secondary effect consequent upon the degeneration of nigrostriatal neurones (Ambani, VanWoert & Murphy, 1975). No reduction in superoxide dismutase concentrations have been found in Parkinson's disease and monoamine oxidase, another source of hydrogen peroxide, is also normal. Although L-dopa is a potent scavenger of the superoxide radical, administration of large doses might lead to excessive oxidative stress on the surviving neurones and accelerate cell death.

It has been known for some time that 6-hydroxydopamine is a powerful selective neurotoxin with a predilection for catecholamine-containing neurones. Indeed use of this property has been made in laboratory animals to produce selective lesions in the ascending dopamine pathways. It is likely that its cytotoxic effects occur as a result of its rapid auto-oxidation to hydroxyl radicals, superoxide and hydrogen peroxide. Sandler (1970) has suggested that the formation of small amounts of 6-hydroxydopamine endogenously might cause Parkinson's disease and a partial deficiency of superoxide dismutase might be the predisposing factor for cell damage. Sandler has also shown that when L-dopa and a peripheral dopa decarboxylase are given together, transamination metabolic pathways assume a greater significance and trihydroxyphenylacetic acid has been found in the urine of L-dopa treated patients. This substance is structurally related to 6-hydroxydopamine and if concentrated in the brain could cause neuronal death (Sandler et al, 1974).

Excessive trapping of methyl groups by large doses of L-dopa with a profound albeit transient reduction in s-adenosylmethionine also has potentially dangerous consequences. For example it might induce methionine or choline deficiency, impair synthesis of RNA or by chronic depletion of methyl groups cause liver damage (Wurtman & Romero, 1972).

Excessive neuromelanin formation
Neuromelanin is a naturally occurring pigment related to lipofuscin which accumulates as a waste product in catecholamine-rich neurones within the brain. It first appears in the human substantia nigra at about 18 months of age and then increases linearly up to about 60 years after which mean pigment levels slowly decline (Mann & Yates, 1974). This decrease has been attributed to a selective loss of those neurones with the highest neuromelanin content. Cytoplasmic RNA is also slowly lost and by the age of 90 years a 20% reduction in nucleolar volume has occurred in the surviving nigral neurones (Mann, Yates & Barton, 1977). This reduction in the protein synthesising capacities of the cell may be regarded as a harbinger to subsequent cell death. Excessive pigment accumulation may cause

damage to the neurones' endoplasmic reticulum through mechanical disruption or displacement of membranes.

In Parkinson's disease Mann & Yates (1981) have reported a reduction of 22% in melanin in the surviving neurones compared with age-matched controls which they believe to be due to a further-reduction in the number of highly pigmented neurones. If these observations are confirmed it follows that L-dopa therapy might be disadvantageous in the long-term. Although initial benefit occurs with an increase in striatal dopamine levels towards normal, a simultaneous increase in pigment formation in the surviving neurones could occur leading to further damage and premature cell death.

CONCLUSION

Although there are compelling hypothetical arguments to suggest that chronic amino acid administration in high dosages could be harmful, there is no hard proof that L-dopa exerts lasting deleterious effects on the brain. It is also debatable whether L-dopa in fact has a finite period of usefulness as has been suggested. In my experience even the most severely debilitated patients who have steadily lost ground on sustained therapy usually deteriorate further if the drug is withdrawn. Long-term adverse side-effects are however a major challenge, and hopefully greater understanding of the pharmacokinetic effects of L-dopa will lead to improved methods of administration. The recent long-term studies with dopamine receptor agonists and the discovery of dopaminergic antagonists with selective effects further suggest that more powerful and less noxious dopaminergic drugs may soon be developed.

CURRENT PRESCRIBING POLICY

I now start treatment with small doses of L-dopa in combination with a peripheral dopa decarboxylase inhibitor (up to 400 mg a day in divided doses). As treatment continues small incremental doses (6–12 administrations per 24 h) may be required but I endeavour to keep the total daily dose below 800 mg. I no longer give amantidine and am prescribing anticholinergics less and less particularly in the elderly. While accepting that anticholinergics have a synergistic effect with L-dopa and are often useful as an adjuvant in suppressing tremor and drooling, in the majority of patients these benefits are outweighed by the problems of polypharmacy, psychotoxicity and possible long-term irreversible effects on cognition and memory. In the few patients with idiopathic Parkinson's disease unable to tolerate L-dopa, and in postencephalitic Parkinson's disease anticholinergics still have a role to play. In neuroleptic-induced Parkinsonism the offending drug should wherever possible be withdrawn following which disappearance of symptoms almost invariably occurs in weeks or months, but occasionally after periods as long as 1 year. If medication must be continued thioridazine is probably the drug with the lowest incidence of reversible extrapyramidal side-effects. Occasionally both anticholinergics and L-dopa may be temporarily needed in patients who have been rendered severely akinetic by depot phenothiazines.

FUTURE RESEARCH

One way of ascertaining whether L-dopa is harmful would be to set up a controlled prospective long-term study comparing the therapeutic effects of L-dopa with those obtained with maximum tolerated doses of a dopamine receptor agonist drug, such as bromocriptine. The problem, however, is that present evidence suggests that far fewer patients are able to tolerate and derive comparable benefit from bromocriptine inevitably leading to a high early drop-out rate in one arm of the trial. An alternative approach might be to compare the long-term response to maximum tolerated doses of L-dopa with that obtained with small doses of L-dopa supplemented if necessary with a dopamine receptor agonist or the selective monoamine oxidase inhibitor (-) deprenyl. A study of this sort has in fact just been started at University College Hospital but because of the problems in obtaining a sufficiently large number of previously untreated patients it is likely to take some years to reach fruition.

REFERENCES

Ambani L M, Van Woert M H, Murphy S 1975 Brain peroxidase and catalase in Parkinson's disease. Archives of Neurology 32: 114–117
Barbeau A 1976 Six years of high-level levodopa therapy in severely akinetic parkinsonian patients. Archives of Neurology 33: 333–338
Botez M I, Barbeau A 1973 Long-term mental changes in levodopa treated patients. Lancet 2: 1028–1029
Boyd A E, Lebovitz H E, Pfeiffer J B 1970 Stimulation of growth hormone by L-dopa. New England Journal of Medicine 283: 1425–1429
Celesia G G, Wanamaker W M 1972 Psychiatric disturbances in Parkinson's disease. Diseases of the Nervous System 3: 557–583
Cohen G, Dembiec D, Mytilineou C, Heikkila R E 1976 Oxygen radicals and the integrity of the nigrostriatal tract In: Birkmayer W, Hornykiewicz O (ed) Advances in Parkinsonism. Roche, Basle, p 251–257
Cotzias G C, Papavasiliou P S, Ginos J Z 1976 Therapeutic approaches in Parkinson's disease: possible roles of growth hormone and somatostatin. In: Yahr M D (ed) The basal ganglia. Raven Press, New York, p 305–316
Diamond S G, Markham C H 1976 Present mortality in Parkinson's disease: the ratio of observed to expected deaths with a method to calculate expected deaths. Journal of Neural Transmission 38: 259–269
Diamond S G, Markham C H, Treciokas L J 1976 Long-term experience with L-dopa; efficacy progression and mortality. In: Birkmayer W, Hornykiewicz O (eds) Advances in Parkonsinism. Roche, Basle, p 444–455
Diamond S G, Markham C H 1979 Mortality of Parkinson patients treated with Sinemet. In: Poirier L J, Sourkes T L, Bédard P J (eds) Advances in neurology, vol. 24. Raven Press, New York, p 489–497
Fahn S, Barrett R E 1979 Increase of Parkinsonian symptoms as a manifestation of levodopa toxicity. In: Poirier L J, Sourkes T L, Bédard P J (eds) Advances in neurology, vol. 24. Raven Press, New York, p 451–460
Galea-Debono A, Jenner P, Marsden C D 1977 Plasma dopa levels and growth hormone response to levodopa in Parkinsonism. Journal of Neurology, Neurosurgery and Psychiatry 40: 162–167
Graham D G 1979 On the origin and significance of neuromelanin. Archives of Pathology and Laboratory Medicine 103: 359–362
Hoehn M M, Yahr M D 1967 Parkinsonism: onset, progression and mortality. Neurology 17: 427–442
Joseph C, Chassan J B, Koch M-L 1978 Levodopa in Parkinson's disease. Annals of Neurology 3: 116–118
Kurland L J 1958 Epidemiology: incidence, geographic distribution and genetic considerations. In: Field W S (ed) Pathogenesis and treatment of Parkinsonism. Thomas, Springfield, Illinois, p 5–43
Lee T, Seeman P, Rajput A, Farley I J, Hornykiewicz O 1978 Receptor basis for dopaminergic supersensitivity in Parkinson's disease. Nature 273: 59–61

Lees A J, Stern G M 1981 Sustained bromocriptine therapy in previously untreated patients with Parkinson's disease. Journal of Neurology, Neurosurgery and Psychiatry 44: 1020-1023

Lesser R P, Fahn S, Snider S R, Cote L J, Isgreen W P, Barrett R E 1979 Analysis of the clinical problems in Parkinsonism and the complications of long-term levodopa therapy. Neurology 29: 1253-1260

Lieberman A N, Shupack J L 1974 Levodopa and melanoma. Neurology 24: 340-343

Lieberman A, Dziatolowski M, Kupersmith M, Serby M, Goodgold A, Korein J, Goldstein M 1979 Dementia in Parkinson's disease. Annals of Neurology 6: 353-359

Loranger A W, Goodell H, McDowell F H, Lee J E, Sweet R D 1972 Intellectual impairment in Parkinson's disease. Brain 95: 405-412

McDowell F H, Sweet R 1979 Ten year follow up study of levodopa treated patients with Parkinson's disease. In: Poirier L J, Sourkes T L, Bedard P J (eds) Advances in neurology, vol. 24. Raven Press, New York, p 475-497

Malarkey W B, Cyrus J, Paulson G W 1974 Dissociation of growth hormone and prolactin secretion in Parkinson's disease following chronic L-dopa therapy. Journal of Clinical Endocrinology and Metabolism 39: 229-235

Mann D M A, Yates P O 1974 Lipoprotein pigments — their relationship to ageing in the human nervous system. II, The melanin content of pigmented nerve cells. Brain 97: 481-488

Mann D M A, Yates P O, Barton C M 1977 Neuromelanin and RNA in cells of substantia nigra. Journal of Neuropathology and Experimental Neurology 36: 379-383

Mann D M A, Yates P O 1974 Levodopa: long-term impact on Parkinson's disease. British Medical Journal 282: 985-986

Markham C H, Diamond S G 1981 Evidence to support early levodopa therapy in Parkinson's disease. Neurology 31: 125-131

Marsden C D 1965 Brain pigment and its relation to brain catecholamines. Lancet 1: 475-476

Mjones H 1949 Paralysis agitans, a clinical and genetic study. Acta Psychiatrica et Neurologica Scandinavica Suppl. 54: 1-195

Papavasiliou P S, McDowell F H, Rosal V, Miller S T 1979 Administration of human somatotropin in levodopa-treated patients with Parkinsonism. Archives of Neurology 36: 624-627

Pollock M, Hornabrook R W 1966 The prevalence, natural history and dementia of Parkinson's disease. Brain 89: 429-448

Rinne U K 1982 Brain neurotransmitter receptors in Parkinson's disease. In: Marsden C D, Fahn S (eds) Movement disorders. Butterworth Scientific, London, p 59-74

Rinne U K, Sonninen V, Siirtola T, Marttila R 1980 Long-term responses of Parkinson's disease to levodopa therapy. Journal of Neural Transmission Suppl. 16: 149-156

Sacks O W, Kohl M S, Messeloff C R, Schwartz W F 1972 Effect of levodopa in Parkinsonian patients with dementia. Neurology 22: 516-519

Sandler M 1970 The role of minor pathways of dopa metabolism. In: Barbeau A, McDowell F H (eds) L-Dopa and Parkinsonism. F A Davis, Philadelphia, p 72-75

Sandler M, Johnson R D, Ruthven C R J, Reid J L, Calne D B 1974 Transamination is a major pathway of L-dopa metabolism following peripheral decarboxylase inhibition. Nature 247: 364-366

Shaw K M, Lees A J, Stern G M 1980 The impact of treatment with Levodopa on Parkinson's disease. Quarterly Journal of Medicine 49: 284-293

Sirtori C R, Bolme P, Azarnoff D L 1972 Metabolic responses to acute and chronic L-dopa administration in patients with Parkinsonism. New England Journal of Medicine 287: 729-733

Wurtman R J, Romero J A 1972 Effects of levodopa on nondopaminergic brain neurons. Neurology 22: Suppl. 511: 72-81

Yahr M D 1976 Evaluation of long-term therapy in Parkinson's disease mortality and therapeutic efficacy. In: Birkmayer W, Hornykiewicz O (eds) Advances in Parkinsonism. Roche, Basle, p 435-443

Yahr M D, Wolf A, Antunes J-L, Miyoshi K, Duffy P 1972 Autopsy findings in Parkinsonism following treatment with levodopa. Neurology 22: Suppl. 511: 56-65

12. Should surgery be the first resort for involuntary movement disorders?

D. L. McLellan

With the sole exception of facial nerve decompression for hemifacial spasm, no treatment provides more than symptomatic alleviation of involuntary movements. Successful surgery has many attractions for the patient. Once the discomfort of his operation is past, the involuntary movement has gone and he can carry on normally without having to take tablets. Most patients taking drugs for involuntary movements have to put up with side-effects. The movements recur as soon as a dose is missed, and so the tablets are not only irksome but become, in the minds of many patients, a symbol of continuing illness. With such advantages, why is surgery so often postponed until the patient has been stupefied by medication or has reached the last stages of neurological dissolution? Is this another example of the legendary conservatism of neurologists, or should surgery indeed be regarded as a humane way of nudging the terminal patient through to the other side?

Part of the answer to this question is that the benefits and risks of the surgery of involuntary movements have never been subjected to a prospective controlled clinical trial. In three recent world symposia on advances in stereotactic and functional neurosurgery (Siegfried et al, 1978; Gildenberg, 1980; Gillingham et al, 1980) encompassing 28 reports on the use of surgical procedures for involuntary movements and spasticity, only one controlled trial (a very small one) was reported. So the conservatism of neurologists is counterbalanced by intuitive optimism among neurosurgeons, whose operations graduate into the surgical repertoire on the basis of optional self-assessment.

To state this antithesis so baldly is not in any way to impugn the motives or skills of those who have pioneered the treatment of these intractable and distressing conditions. But the reason for divergencies in opinion and practice is a serious lack of information upon which the effects of medical and surgical treatments over the patient's lifetime can be compared with each other, and with the natural history of the disease. It is much easier, of course, to study the effects of tablets of standard potency than to assess surgery undertaken by practitioners with different degrees of skill. Another factor that decides the result of an operation is chance — indeed, but for serendipitous mistakes, new targets for stereotactic attack would have taken much longer to identify. There is an intuitive element in the conduct of stereotactic operations, the precise location of lesions tending to be decided by the particular clinical features of the individual patient;

126

many surgeons have evolved personal and independent strategies for some of these conditions. Similar difficulties have been overcome by surgeons in other fields and there is no overwhelming reason why the treatments of involuntary movements should have a more controversial basis. Surveying the range of medical opinion, a pragmatist would be forgiven for concluding that there can be very little to choose between the treatments that are available and the vicissitudes of the untreated disease. Nonetheless, there are many reports of operations which have dramatically improved an individual patient's condition and so it is extremely important for each patient that the correct decision is made in his particular case.

In this chapter a personal viewpoint will be presented, with a few general references to guide the reader to the relevant literature. Some of these questions have been well discussed at length in a recent review by Marsden & Fahn (1982).

Parkinsonism

Stereotactic thalamotomy for Parkinsonism is the best established surgical treatment for involuntary movement but since the advent of more effective drug treatment it is rarely performed. Unilateral tremor that causes marked distress or disability, and which has not responded to drugs while under the supervision of a neurologist, remains a good indication for surgery. Thalamotomy does not improve uncomplicated bradykinesia. Before the advent of levodopa, its effect was to remove tremor rather than to restore function but this is not to deny that the abolition of moderate or severe tremor does restore some function to a bradykinetic hand. Levodopa treatment has greatly improved the outlook for bradykinesia. Thus a patient who remains incapacitated by severe tremor in the upper limbs despite a good response to levodopa (evidenced, for example, by improved gait and balance) can expect even greater gains in function from thalamotomy than in the days before levodopa was introduced.

The risk of death or serious disability as a result of surgery is approximately 1-3%, being greater in the elderly and in the presence of arterial hypertension or dementia. It is perfectly reasonable to perform a unilateral procedure on a patient with a bilateral tremor, because restoring good function to one hand enables the patient to achieve most daily living activities. Bilateral surgery, even when separated by a gap of 3 months, carries a 20-30% risk of dysarthia and dysphagia, and a smaller risk of impaired voluntary movement of the limbs. Bilateral surgery is not therefore indicated for tremor except in exceptional circumstances.

The second indication for thalamotomy is for the patient whose dopaminergic therapy affords mobility only at the expense of gross chorea and athetosis, especially when these involuntary movements are unilateral (Siegfried 1980). By restricting the dose that a patient can tolerate, chorea can reduce the effectiveness of drug treatment. Controlateral thalamotomy abolishes or greatly reduces the drug-induced involuntary movements, allowing the patient to increase the dose to a level at which mobility improves. It is possible that these dyskinesias might be avoided by starting treatment, in the newly diagnosed patient, with bromocriptine rather than with levodopa. In patients who already show dyskinesia, drug combinations of levodopa and decarboxylase inhibitors in staggered regimens, or concurrently with a dopamine agonist or a monoaminoxidase-B inhibitor, will usually avoid this particular indication for surgery.

Idiopathic tremor

Idiopathic tremor is a variable condition. It most commonly resembles either an accentuated physiological tremor at about 12 Hz or a rather slower postural (action) tremor at about 8 Hz. Some sporadic cases and some familial cases are characterised by a tremor at rest indistinguishable from the tremor of Parkinsonism; others have an intention tremor and may show associated abnormalities such as titubation of the head or fragments of torticollis which throw the precise nosology of their complaint into some doubt. Some authorities have sought to categorise idiopathic tremor on the basis of synchronous rather than alternating bursts of activity in antagonistic muscle groups, a criterion that would exclude many cases with this clinical diagnosis. These features are mentioned here only in order to draw attention to the likelihood that idiopathic tremor is a syndrome with different pathological and physiological causes. Despite this, few trials of treatment have systematically analysed the influence of these features in determining the natural history of the condition or its response to treatment.

When drug treatment for idiopathic tremor is effective it has to be taken for the rest of the patient's life, usually at the cost of side-effects such as dry mouth or sedation. Some cases show a remarkable response to alcohol, a slippery slope with very obvious drawbacks. Mild cases are often well controlled by intermittent drug treatment at times of stress but moderate or severe tremor usually requires stereotactic surgery.

The effect of thalamotomy for these tremors depends to some extent upon where the lesion is made. Using precise physiological recording techniques, Narabayashi (1982) can place a 3 mm lesion in the ventral intermediate (Vim) nucleus of the thalamus which abolishes tremor for at least 1 year in 98% of cases. This compares with success rates of 71% for a 7 mmm lesion in the globus pallidus and 92% for a lesion in or just below the ventrolateral (anterior) nucleus of the thalamus. The older operation of pallidotomy would suppress idiopathic tremor for up to 20 years and there is reasonable agreement that ventrolateral thalamotomy can satisfactorily suppress tremor in 85% of patients with Parkinsonism for the lifetime of the patient (about 15 years).

How much use is a unilateral thalamotomy for bilateral tremor? Most activities of daily living can be achieved with one good hand and one 'simple gripping' hand and thus the prime indication for surgery is loss of function because of tremor. The cosmetic effects of unilateral surgery are less than half successful and in particular titubation of the head is unlikely to be improved.

Intention tremor

Isolated intention tremor occurring as a form of idiopathic tremor can often be suppressed by stereotactic surgery but intention tremor occurring in the context of more generalised disease, such as multiple sclerosis, is much more difficult to treat. In addition, the risks of surgery are much greater, presumably because of the presence of other lesions in the brain and the risk that the surgery can provoke a relapse of the disease. Multiple sclerosis is a progressive disease and the relief of disability for a limited period of several years is therefore a reasonable goal. Unilateral thalamotomy is not suitable for mild or only moderately disabled patients but surgery must not, on the other hand, be postponed until the patient is so dysarthric and grossly disabled that the risks of surgery have become unacceptable.

Generalised torsion dystonia (dystonia musculorum deformans)

This condition is usually progressive, running its most rapid course in patients who are young at the onset of symptoms (especially in the first decade of life) and whose signs appear in the lower limbs. The mildest cases have little disability over a lifetime but more often the disability is progressive, with severe painful deformities and prostration within a few years in severe cases.

There is considerable disagreement about the best way of treating this disease. Cooper (1969, 1976) pioneered the surgical treatment and over the years his group has evolved a strategy involving multiple bilateral thalamic lesions in stages. The first stage may involve a lesion in the Vim of the thalamus contralateral to the most severe symptoms, followed a week later by a lesion of the pulvinar on the opposite side. This is a much less risky procedure than bilateral thalamotomies. After delay of several months, further lesions may be made depending upon the patient's symptoms. Targets include the posterior sensory nucleus and centrum medianum of the thalamus. The immediate effect of these lesions upon dystonia differs in a most important respect from the effects of thalamotomy on the tremor of Parkinsonism. In Parkinsonism, the tremor is immediately abolished but in dystonia there may be less obvious immediate change at the time the lesion is made. Over the next 3–6 months the dystonia may show progressive improvement. This time course, not unlike the appearance of spasticity after a stroke, appears to represent a progressive adaptation to the effects of thalamotomy.

Several points about Cooper's approach need to be emphasised. First, the use of a cryogenic probe enables the temporary effects of cooling to be observed before a permanent lesion is made. Second, the precise size of the initial lesion is determined in practice by the immediate effects of cooling. Third, several lesions may be necessary to improve symptoms in a particular patient and the timing, size and location of these is determined by the patient's signs, response to each successive lesion and the manner in which the disease is progressing. When one considers the difference between this type of therapy and the administration of tablets from a single bottle the difficulties of controlling stereotactic surgery for the purposes of objective evaluation become all too apparent.

Cooper's view is that stereotactic thalamotomy not only relieves the symptoms but prevents the progression of the disease, so that the only reasons for withholding surgery are: (1) that the symptoms are too mild to warrant it; (2) that there is good chance of spontaneous remission or very slow progression of symptoms (suggested by family history) or (3) the patient is too young to cope psychologically with the surgery. Drugs such as clonazepam and carbamazapine help some patients, especially those with mild symptoms that fluctuate in response to stress. Dopaminergic drugs are, in Cooper's view, dangerous as his impression has been that they can cause non-reversible acceleration of torsion dystonia. It is doubtful that any other department can match Cooper's experience of several hundred cases of this rare disease but the lack of controlled observations makes it very difficult for other clinicians to gauge the effect that such treatment would be likely to have on their own patients, or to evaluate the relative efficacy of the different lesion locations that have been tried. If Cooper's results had been confirmed by other surgeons in the field there is no doubt that stereotactic surgery would be the treatment of first choice for progressive torsion dystonia.

Why is there a discrepancy between the results of different neurosurgeons? Placebo effects and observer bias must be assumed to account for some of the reported improvement. The other difficulty, differences in surgical technique, has been alluded to above and this is particularly important when trying to compare results from different surgical centres. Now that the precise site and volume of lesions can be assessed with CT scanning, the time is ripe for detailed study of the precise anatomical location and size of the lesions that have actually been made.

Chronic electrical stimulation of the spinal cord
There have been a number of reports that chronic electrical stimulation of the upper cervical cord by electrodes implanted posteriorly over the dura can improve many of the features of torsion dystonia. This treatment is much easier to standardise but, needless to say, no prospective trials have been done. Spinal stimulation carries a smaller operative risk than stereotactic surgery and is a simpler procedure that can be performed under general anaesthesia. However, long-term effects upon the tissues in the cervical spinal canal are unknown and in children and adolescents who are still growing, surgical rearrangement of the lead wires or the electrodes may be necessary.

Conclusion
My personal approach to torsion dystonia is as follows. Patients whose disease is mild and not rapidly progressive are treated conservatively. If medication is well tolerated and effective then it can be continued, otherwise there is no virtue in it. Clonazepam, carbamazepine and anticholinergic drugs may be helpful but long-term phenothiazines and dopaminergic drugs are to be avoided.

Patients who are young and whose dystonia is steadily progressive, and especially those whose dystonia started in the lower limbs, are referred to a neurosurgeon experienced in the stereotactic surgery of torsion dystonia. Those in whom stereotactic surgery would carry greater than usual risks, or who are unable to cope psychologically with the considerable demands of stereotactic surgery, can be treated on a trial basis with high cervical cord stimulation using an implanted electrode. This needs to be done in a unit that has the technical resources to calibrate the implanted equipment and subsequently to monitor its function; preferably the surgery should be done as part of an organised prospective study. Unless a satisfactory result has been obtained within 4 months, the stimulating apparatus including the electrodes should be removed.

Spasmodic torticollis

This is the most intractable of all movement disorders to treat. Stereotactic thalamotomy is very much a last resort because the bilateral anteriorly placed lesions that are needed pose grave risks to speech, swallowing and mobility without promising more than a 30% chance of a good result. Multiple denervation of the cervical muscles also has unpleasant side-effects which are postponed for a year or two, but are nevertheless disabling — severe, painful spondylosis with root compression and myelopathy and dysphagia. The involuntary movements persist in the few remaining muscles in at least half the cases. Drug treatment with clonazepam, anticholinergic drugs and carbamazepine is worth trying but usually ineffective. At the time of writing, this gloomy outlook is enlivened by several reports of good responses in up to 70% of cases by chronic electrical stimulation of the upper cervical spinal cord (Waltz, 1982). Whether this will turn out to be a mirage like the other treatments remains to be seen. Stimulation is certainly safer than the other surgical treatments and can be given a trial as described above if the disorder is severe. Finally, mild cases of torticollis are said to respond well to careful training in relaxation of the neck muscles, supplemented by augmented sensory feedback using electromyographic signals on the overactive muscles.

Surgery is very much a last resort for spasmodic torticollis. My personal approach is to use relaxation training supplemented, in the few cases where it works, by drug treatment. In patients whose life is becoming disrupted, chronic cervical cord stimulation can be tried, preferably under the conditions described above.

Hemifacial spasm and blepharospasm

These rare conditions are usually tolerated by the patient in preference to the small but definite risks of surgery. The frequency of the movements and the patient's concern about them can usually be alleviated with tranquillising drugs for stressful occasions. Decompression of the facial nerve often relieves hemifacial spasm. If blepharospasm is sufficiently severe to occlude vision, peripheral resection of the relevant muscles relieves it at the cost of impaired movements of the upper part of the face.

Chorea and athetosis

Chorea and athetosis rarely need treating but tetrabenazine is reasonably effective. Surgery is indicated only in exceptional cases of levodopa-induced dyskinesias, as described above.

Conclusion

Many patients tolerate their involuntary movements and do not wish to run the risks of surgical treatment or to put up with the side-effects of drugs. However, they are probably less innately cautious and conservative than neurologists. In my view we do not use surgery often enough in movement disorders, partly because we are never quite sure where the surgeon is going to make his lesion and partly because we favour the temporary drug side-effects in comparison with the permanent complications of surgery. But to the patients, a successful ablative operation for tremor or dystonia can provide a period of freedom from medical attention lasting many years. The recently introduced techniques of chronic electrical stimulation of the cervical cord are probably safer than thalamotomy but they tend to produce an unpleasant tingling around the shoulders and the upper limbs, and they also require constant surgical and medical surveillance. These and other stimulation treatments are still in the research phase and it may well be that other targets in the brain and spinal cord will give better results in the future. There is no hope of a consensus view on these matters until neurologists and neurosurgeons sink their differences and conduct objective prospective trials of different treatments over the natural lifetime of their patients.

REFERENCES

Cooper I S, 1969 Dystonia. Involuntary, movement disorders. Hoebner, Harper and Row, New York, ch 4, D 131–292
Cooper I S 1976 Tewnty year follow up of study of the neurosurgical treatment of dystonia muscular deformans. Advances in Neurology 14: 423–452
Gildenberg P L (ed) 1980 Proceedings of the meeting of the American Society for stereotactic and functional neurosurgery. Applied Neurophysiology 43: 89–266
Gillingham F J et al (eds) 1980 Advances in stereotactic and functional neurosurgery 4 (Proceedings of 4th meeting of the European Society for stereotactic and functional neurosurgery). Acta Neurochirurgica Suppl. 30
Marsden C D, Fahn S (eds) 1982 Movement disorders. Butterworths, London
Narabayashi H 1982 Surgical approach to tremor. In: Marsden C D, Fahn S (eds) Movement disorders. Butterworths, London, p 292–299
Siegfried J 1980 Neurosurgical treatment of Parkinson's disease. Present indications and value. In: Rinne U K et at (eds) Parkinson's disease: current progress, problems and management. Elsevier/North-Holland, ch 23, p 369–383.
Siegfried J et al (eds) 1978 Neural prostheses and neurostimulation. Proceedings of 8th meeting of World Society for stereotactic and functional neurosurgery. Applied Neurophysiology 45: 1–208
Waltz J M 1982 Surgical approach to dystonia. In: Marsden C D, Fahn S (eds) Movement disorders. Butterworths, London, p 300–307

13. When can anticonvulsant drugs be stopped?

David Chadwick

'The effect of a convulsion on the nerve centres is such as to render the occurrence of another more easy, to intensify the predisposition that already exists. Thus every fit may be said to be, in part, the result of those which had preceded it, the cause of those which follow it.'

William Gowers (1881)

The converse of Gowers dictum has also gained wide clinical acceptance; that is, if seizures are completely controlled over a prolonged period of 3 or more years then anticonvulsant withdrawal may be attempted with some hope of success. It is the aim of this article to review the evidence upon which this clinical practice is based.

THE PROGNOSIS OF EPILEPSY

Whilst control of seizures is only one of many factors which contribute to the overall morbidity and handicap of patients with epilepsy, it is germane to consider the probability that patients will achieve a remission in seizures after starting therapy.

Table 13.1 summarises remission rates in those studies reviewed by Rodin (1968) and in some important subsequent studies. Many problems exist in the interpretation of these data, not least the varying minimum period required as a definition of remission, Bridge (1949) having emphasised that success in control of seizures is inversely proportional to the length of follow-up. The majority of studies are hospital based, which undoubtedly has an adverse effect on the outcome, patients with more severe and refractory epilepsy being more likely to be referred to specialist centres. In this respect the study of Annegers et al (1979) is of particular importance; 457 patients were followed for at least 5 years, and 141 for 20 years. The probability of being in a remission lasting for 5 years or more was 61% at 10 years, and as high as 70% at 20 years. These figures are considerably higher than other studies, reflecting the community basis of the study. The majority of other studies are striking in that remission rates are consistent at between 20 and 30% despite the fact that they include periods before the advent of modern anticonvulsant therapy. Turner recorded a 2 year remission

Table 13.1 Prognosis for remission.

Author	No. of patients	Min. duration Remission (years)	% remitted
Habermas (1901)	937	2	10
Turner (1907)	212	2	33
Grosz (1930)	91	10	11
Kirstein (1942)	174	3	22
Alstroem (1958)	897	5	22
Kiørboe (1958)	130	4	22
Strobos (1959)	228	1	38
Probst (1960)	83	2	31
Trolle (1961)	799	2	37
Juul-Jensen (1963)	969	2	32
Lorge (1964)	177	2	34
Rodin (1968)	90	2	32
Annegers et al (1979)	457	5	70
Sofijanov (1982)	512	2	50
Jap. study (1981)	1868	3	58

rate in 1907, identical to that reported by Rodin in 1968! This suggests that remission in epilepsy largely reflects the natural history of the disease rather than the influence of anticonvulsant medication, a suggestion which receives some support from Annegers et al (1979) who were unable to show major changes in remission rates in patients diagnosed with epilepsy between the years of 1935 and 1959 and those diagnosed between 1960 and 1974. Whether the introduction of serum anticonvulsant monitoring will have a substantial impact on remission rates has yet to be proved.

Two more recent studies demand comment as they show higher remission rates than earlier studies. The group for the study of prognosis of epilepsy in Japan (1981), from a hospital based population, reported an overall 3 year remission rate of 58% in 1868 patients. There are reservations about this study in that this population represented only 42% of those originally seen between the years of 1975 and 1977. Sofijanov (1982), studying a population of 512 epileptic children, found a terminal remission of 2 years or more in 50% of the patients studied. This probably reflects the more benign aspects of some childhood epileptic syndromes, e.g. petit mal and benign focal epilepsy of childhood. Similarly high remission rates of between 40% and 60% have previously been reported in children (Livingstone, 1961; Breg & Yannet, 1962).

A number of factors are of importance in the prognosis for remission of seizures. The age of onset of epilepsy is perhaps one of the most important, although some controversy exists on this point. Rodin (1968) quoted several authors to suggest that seizure disorders starting in childhood remit less frequently than those starting later in life. Where this problem has been examined in some detail a rather different picture emerges. Within the group of epilepsies commencing in childhood there is general agreement that the commencement of seizures within the first year of life (when it is usually symptomatic of cerebral pathology), carries an adverse prognosis (Kiørboe, 1961; Hedenstroem & Schorsch, 1963; Strobos, 1959; Sofijanov, 1982). The group for the study of the prognosis of epilepsy in Japan (1981) emphasised the poor prognosis for seizures beginning before the age of 1 compared with those commencing between the ages of 1 and 10. They comment that childhood epilepsy is more likely to remit than adult onset epilepsy. Annegers et al (1979) found that both partial and generalised epilepsies had a better prognosis should they start before the age of 20.

Whatever the age of onset, the duration of the epilepsy prior to treatment is an important prognostic factor. Gowers (1881) stated that 83% of patients would have their seizures arrested if treated within 1 year. Annegers et al (1979) showed that most patients who achieve remission do so early during the course of treatment. With continuing seizures and the passage of time it becomes progressively less likely that an individual patient will enter remission. Thus there is a plateau in the number of patients in remission 15–20 years after the onset of epilepsy. Similar findings have been reported with shorter term follow-up in children (Sofijanov, 1982) and in adults (Shorvon & Reynolds, 1982). Rodin (1968) also emphasised that the fewer and the less frequent the seizures, the better the prognosis for remission.

Seizure type is of major importance. Remission rates range from approximately 60% for patients with only tonic clonic seizures to between 20 and 40% in patients with complex partial seizures (Yahr et al, 1952; Trolle, 1961; Juul-Jensen, 1963; Reynolds et al, 1981). The combination of complex partial seizures with secondary generalised tonic-clonic seizures seems to have a particularly adverse prognosis (Rodin, 1968; the group for study of prognosis of epilepsy in Japan 1981) and in such patients it is common to find that whilst tonic-clonic seizures come under increasingly good control with anticonvulsant therapy, partial seizures remain resistant to drug therapy (Rodin, 1968; Reynolds et al, 1981; Turnbull et al, 1982). Other generalised epilepsies of childhood carry varying prognoses. Between 70 and 80% of patients with simple absences (petit mal) are likely to enter remission (the group for the study of prognosis of epilepsy in Japan 1981, Sofijanov, 1982). Complex absences show a lesser remission rate (33–65%), and in patients with the West or Lennox-Gastaut syndromes remission rates may be as low as 35–50%.

Epilepsy of unknown aetiology has a better prognosis than symptomatic epilepsy (Juul-Jensen 1963, the group for the study of prognosis of epilepsy in Japan 1981; Annegers et al, 1979). In keeping with this, epilepsy complicated by an associated neuropsychiatric deficit carries an adverse prognosis (Sofijanov, 1982; Shorvon & Reynolds, 1982).

Rodin (1968) drew attention to the adverse prognosis associated with the occurrence of injuries during seizures, and the clustering of attacks in close temporal association.

There is a considerable volume of literature on the EEG and its prognostic value. Those interested should refer once again to Rodin (1968). He did not feel that prognostic statements could be made on the basis of the EEG alone, but what evidence there was suggested that a more important prognostic factor was normalisation of the EEG during the course of treatment.

WHY WITHDRAW ANTICONVULSANTS?

Patients with epilepsy are in many ways unique in that they often receive drug therapy over many decades. Anti-epileptic drugs have been associated with acute idiosyncratic and dose related adverse reactions, and with increasingly well documented chronic toxic effects. Such effects are often subtle, and their recognition has usually lagged 20 or 30 years behind the introduction of the responsible drugs (Reynolds, 1975). Whilst we remain ignorant of the possible long-term effects of therapy with newer anti-epileptic drugs such as carbamazepine and valproate, the ability of hydantoin and barbiturate anticonvulsants to effect skin, connective tissue, haemapoietic and lymphoreticular systems, and hepatic metabolism are now well recognised (Reynolds, 1975), and constitute a major argument in favour of a policy of anticonvulsant withdrawal in patients with epilepsy who enter remission.

More potent arguments for anticonvulsant drug withdrawal may be the increasing evidence of effects of anti-epileptic drugs on the central nervous system. The adverse behavioural effects of phenobarbitone have long been recognised in children (Ounsted, 1955), as has the unusual pseudodementia seen in patients with chronic phenytoin intoxication (Logan & Freeman, 1969). However, recent studies have suggested that many anticonvulsant drugs, even in therapeutic dosage, may have adverse effects on both behaviour and cognitive function. These may be of considerable importance in the development and education of children with epilepsy.

The administration of phenobarbitone (Tchicaloff & Gaillard, 1970), phenytoin (Rosen, 1968; Stores, 1975) and primidone (Rodin et al, 1976) may all result in impaired performance on a variety of psychometric tests. Carbamazepine appears somewhat less harmful (Rodin et al, 1976; Dodrill & Troupin, 1977). The effects of these drugs on psychometric testing appear related to serum level, the most severe disturbances being seen in patients with greater than optimal serum levels. Changes may also occur, however, with serum levels within the optimal range (Reynolds & Travers, 1974). It seems that patients with lower IQ or brain damage are most susceptible to adverse behavioural and cognitive disturbances produced by anticonvulsants (Trimble, 1979), and anticonvulsant withdrawal if possible may be particularly beneficial for behaviour and learning in this group of patients (Davis et al, 1981).

STUDIES OF ANTI-EPILEPTIC DRUG WITHDRAWAL

Few studies have been undertaken to determine the success of anticonvulsant withdrawal, and the factors which identify patients likely to remain seizure free. Table 13.2 summarises the outcome reported in these studies.

Comparison of these studies presents considerable difficulties, because there is often a sparsity of information about the patients studied, a lack of uniformity in the length of remission before anticonvulsant withdrawal, and an absence of information about the period of time over which anticonvulsant withdrawal was undertaken, and for how long the patients were followed up. Perhaps the most useful and well organised study of anticonvulsant withdrawal has been that of Juul Jensen (1964, 1968), who undertook a prospective study of a series of 200 patients who had been seizure free for 2 or more years. Withdrawal was accomplished over a period of 2 to 3 months although 34 disregarded advice and

Table 13.2 Relapse after anticonvulsant withdrawal.

Authors	No.	Age	Period in remission before withdrawal (years)	Period of withdrawal	Follow-up (years)	Total	Relapse rate during drug reduction	after cessation
Holowach et al (1972)	148	Children	>4	NS	5–12	36 (24%)	18	18
Zenker et al (1957)	117	Children	0.5–9	NS	NS	24 (21%)	—	—
Emerson et al (1981)	68	Children	>4	2–3 mth	0.5–6	18 (26%)	—	—
Yahr et al (1952)	26	NS	>2	NS	NS	12 (46%)	—	—
Juul-Jensen (1968)	200	NS	>2	2–3/12	5	79 (39%)	20	59
Strobos (1959)	41	NS	>2	NS	NS	19 (46%)	—	—
Merrit (1958)	89	NS	>3	NS	NS	39 (44%)	30	9
Janz & Sommer-Burkhardt (1976)	253	NS	>2	NS	<5	124 (49%)	92	32
Oller-Daurella et al (1976)[a]	317	NS	>5	Years	0.5–27	55 (17%)	26	29

a In this series there was a 13% relapse rate in 39 patients on unchanged medication.
NS = not stated.

discontinued their therapy abruptly. By 2 years 70 patients had suffered a relapse, and in half of these relapse occurred during reduction or discontinuation of their anticonvulsants. During the third to fifth year a further 9 patients had suffered relapse (giving a final relapse rate of 40%). This figure is in good agreement with the majority of studies which have included adult onset epilepsy (see Table 13.2). A lower rate of relapse is seen in studies restricted to patients with the onset of epilepsy in childhood (Zenker et al, 1957; Holowach et al, 1972; Emerson et al, 1981).

Oller-Daurella et al (1976) reported results in 356 patients who had been seizure free for 5 or more years. Of 317 patients who commenced anticonvulsant withdrawal this was completed in 138. Whilst 26 patients (8%) relapsed during anticonvulsant reduction, 29 (9%) relapsed following withdrawal of drug therapy. One hundred and fifty-three patients were still gradually withdrawing therapy at the time of this report. It is of interest that 39 patients remained on unchanged anticonvulsant medication. Whilst this does not represent a control group relapses occurred in 5 (13.8%) of these patients, compared with 55 (17%) relapses in patients who reduced or withdrew medication. This study is interestingly at variance with many of the other studies in showing such a low total relapse rate. The possibility that this is due to slow anticonvulsant withdrawal after prolonged periods of remission (up to 22 years) demands consideration. As in other studies (Juul-Jensen, 1964; Janz & Sommer-Burkhardt, 1976), approximately 60% of relapses occurred within 6 months of discontinuation of therapy. Relapses later than 5 years after drug withdrawal are uncommon (Thurston et al, 1982).

Several groups have examined factors associated with a good prognosis on withdrawal of anticonvulsant drugs. These show a striking similarity to those influencing remission during anticonvulsant therapy (see above). There is general agreement that the onset of epilepsy in childhood is associated with a low risk of relapse. Holowach et al (1972) found that a particularly qood prognosis was associated with epilepsy commencing before the age of 3 and where anticonvulsants could be withdrawn by the age of 8, although this finding was less striking when the group of patients were followed for 15–23 years (Thurston et al, 1982). This is at variance with Emerson et al's (1981) finding of a 47% relapse rate in patients with the onset of epilepsy before 3 years, compared with 25% relapse rate in those with epilepsy commencing between 2–7 years, and only 6% relapse rate in children whose epilepsy began after 7 years. In a more adult population Juul-Jensen (1964) found that epilepsy with onset before the age of 30, carried a better prognosis for anticonvulsant withdrawal than that commencing later in life. Janz & Sommer-Burkhardt (1976) agreed that patients with an onset of epilepsy before the age of 10 were less likely to relapse than patients with later onset. The duration of the patients' epilepsy also seemcd important, shorter durations carrying a better prognosis. Thurston et al (1982) found that only 24% of 116 children whose epilepsy was of less than 6 years duration relapsed, compared with 89% of 9 children whose epilepsy was of longer duration.

There is agreement that the severity of epilepsy, as judged by the number and frequency of seizures prior to remission, is directly related to the likelihood of relapse (Juul-Jensen, 1964; Janz & Sommer-Burkhardt, 1976; Oller-Daurella et al, 1976). Little evidence is available from these studies on the importance of the duration of control and the likelihood of subsequent relapse. Only Oller-Daurella et al (1976) comment that the likelihood of relapse seems to be least in patients who have been seizure free for many years (in this study as many as 27 years).

The type of epilepsy has important consequences. Yahr et al (1952), and Merritt (1958) commented on the rarity of relapse in patients with petit mal epilepsy, a finding borne out in larger, later series (Holowach et al, 1972; Janz & Sommer–Burkhardt, 1976; Oller-Daurella et al, 1976). The combination of petit mal absence, with myoclonic jerks and grand mal attacks significantly increases the risk of relapse (Janz & Sommer–Burkhardt, 1976). Surprisingly Oller-Daurella et al (1976) reported that up to 75% of patients with secondary generalised epilepsy (e.g. West and Lennox-Gastaut syndromes) avoid relapse which is a surprising finding in view of the generally poor prognosis for these conditions (Rodin, 1968). Patients suffering only grand mal attacks of apparent primary origin also have a relatively good prognosis with relapse rates of between 8 and 33%. Partial seizures are more likely to relapse and it may be that complex partial and simple motor seizures carry a particularly high risk, as does the combination of differing seizure types in an individual patient (Oller-Daurella et al, 1976; Thurston et al, 1982).

Holowach et al (1972) found that the presence of associated neuropsychiatric deficit carried a high risk of relapse following anticonvulsant withdrawal. Similarly the presence of known cerebral pathology increased the rate of relapse in the study of Juul-Jensen (1964).

The EEG may be a prognostic aid. In a series of children, EEG's were recorded at the time of withdrawal. It was shown that 16% of patients with normal recordings relapsed. The rate of relapse was greater in patients whose pre-withdrawal record showed some kind of paroxysmal activity but overall the relapse rate was still only 27% (Holowach et al, 1972). Emerson et al (1981) produced similar but more clear-cut findings, again in children. Only 12% of patients with a normal EEG (immediately prior to drug withdrawal) relapsed, compared to 57% of those with a 'definitely abnormal' EEG. Juul-Jensen (1964) found that a degree of abnormality in the initial EEG did not correlate well with prognosis following drug withdrawal. However, normal or slightly abnormal EEG's taken immediately before withdrawal were associated with relapse rates of 31 and 38% respectively. The presence of delta wave foci, or bilateral paroxysmal activity were associated with a relapse rate of 100%, and 75% respectively. Janz & Sommer-Burkhardt (1976) however found that normality or otherwise of the EEG did not help with prognosis. Strobos (1959) reported that patients with bilateral paroxysmal discharges on the EEG which disappeared with drug therapy were less likely to relapse on anticonvulsant withdrawal than patients whose EEG continued to be abnormal. This was not the case for patients with focal EEG abnormalities.

Emerson et al (1981) have assessed the relative contribution of these several factors indicative of successful drug withdrawal. They found that a normal EEG prior to withdrawal, and a history of only a few tonic-clonic seizures were of greatest importance. Thurston et al (1982) undertook a multivariate analysis of prognostic factors, and found the duration of epilepsy to be the most important, but focal motor seizures, combinations of seizure types and neurological deficit also played important roles.

Thus, in summary there is agreement that up to 50% of patients who become seizure free for periods of 2 or more years will relapse when medication is reduced or withdrawn. The risks of relapse decrease rapidly with the passage of time after withdrawal. Patients with the onset of epilepsy between the ages of 1 and 16, who have suffered a small number of primary generalised seizures, who have no associated neurological or psychiatric handicap and whose EEG is normal at the end of their period of drug therapy, have a high expectation of remission which will be maintained following anticonvulsant withdrawal.

AREAS OF UNCERTAINTY

There are, however, many unanswered questions. There is no available information to compare relapse in patients randomly allocated to continuance or withdrawal of therapy, although there is some evidence to suggest that withdrawal is associated with a higher risk of relapse (Oller-Daurella et al, 1976; Annegers et al, 1979). No study has addressed the question of whether increasingly long seizure free periods while on anticonvulsants carry a better prognosis, although this was suggested from the retrospective data of Oller-Daurella et al (1976). Certainly there is no specific information on whether anticonvulsant withdrawal is best considered after 2, or 3, of 5 or more years of remission. A further problem arises with the growing number of patients who are started on anticonvulsants as a prophylactic measure following head injury or supratentorial craniotomy. The rationale of such a policy is open to question (Janz, 1982), but in those instances where it is undertaken, when is it safe to withdraw drugs if seizures do not occur?

There is no data which allows one to assess the importance of relative speed of anticonvulsant reduction. All clinicians are aware of the dangers of sudden discontinuation of therapy and abrupt withdrawal of anti-epileptic drugs probably represents the most common cause of status epilepticus. It is striking that all authors agree that most relapses occur during or shortly after reduction or cessation of therapy and Oller-Daurella et al (1976) suggested that slow withdrawal of anticonvulsants lessened the risk of relapse. This raises the question of how we should regard seizures arising in close association with anticonvulsant withdrawal. Do they simply reflect a relapse in the underlying epileptic tendency or are they a withdrawal phenomenon, similar to that seen with shorter acting sedative drugs which as alcohol, barbiturates and benzodiazepines (Victor, 1970; Wikler & Essig, 1970)? Whilst the latter are always generalised tonic-clonic seizures, and those precipitated by anti-epileptic drug withdrawal in epileptic patients are usually identical to those occurring naturally in the individual patient (Spencer et al, 1981), the question is at present impossible to answer, but has profound implications for the management of seizures occurring in association with anticonvulsant withdrawal after prolonged remission.

If complete withdrawal of anticonvulsants carries a high risk, should partial withdrawal be considered? Schmidt & Janz (1977) found that 15 patients who had recently commenced therapy, and whose seizures continued after the initiation of therapy, allowing determination of both sub-therapeutic and therapeutic plasma concentrations, had markedly higher therapeutic serum concentrations of phenytoin and phenobarbitone than a group of 32 patients who had been seizure free for long periods of time. Whilst these results may be explained by those patients who had been seizure free for prolonged periods having less severe epilepsy, the possibility that the minimum therapeutic level of anticonvulsant drugs declines with increasing periods of seizure control demands consideration. If correct this observation may prompt consideration of a policy of relative rather than absolute drug withdrawal in some patients.

All these unanswered questions demand further investigation, and any future study should be prospective, and should involve randomisation to differing rates of anticonvulsant withdrawal, and should compare relapse rates in patients who have been seizure free for 2, 3, or 5 years, with that in a control group of patients continuing therapy. Any such study must include large numbers of well documented patients, in order to add further information on the prognostic factors associated with relapse and to provide an assessment of an individual patient's risk similar to that produced by Jennet (1975) for the risk of developing post-traumatic epilepsy.

CURRENT POLICY

In the meantime clinicians are faced with the problem of advising patients who have been seizure free for long periods whether or not they should attempt anticonvulsant withdrawal. Inevitably the patient must be the final arbiter of this decision as the recurrence of seizures may jeopardise his or her work, social life, and driving. In the United Kingdom the Department of Transport suggest that patients with driving licences gained after a period during which they have been seizure free, and who wish to withdraw their anticonvulsants, should discontinue driving for at least 6 months. Should they experience further seizures they will be banned from driving for a further statutory period (presently 2 years). This provision, whether or not one agrees with it, will in itself often be sufficient to discourage patients with epilepsy from discontinuing their therapy. It is therefore of the greatest importance to explain to patients considering the withdrawal of anticonvulsants the risks which are involved.

REFERENCES

Alstroem C H 1950 A study of epilepsy in its clinical, social, and genetic aspects. Munksgaard, Copenhagen
Annegers J F, Hauser W A, Elverback L R 1979 Remission of seizures and relapse in patients with epilepsy. Epilepsia 20: 729–737
Breg W R, Yannet H 1962 The child in a convulsion. Paediatric Clinics of North America 9: 101–112
Bridge E M 1949 Epilepsy and convulsive disorders in children. Mcgraw-Hill, New York
Davis V J, Poling A D, Wysocki T, Breuning S É 1981 Effects of phenytoin withdrawal on matching to sample and workshop performance of mentally retarded persons. Journal of Nervous and Mental Disease 169: 718–725

Dodrill C B, Troupin A S 1977 Psychotropic effects of carbamazepine in epilepsy: a double blind comparison with phenytoin. Neurology 27: 1023–1028

Emerson R, D'Souza B J, Vining E P, Holden K R, Mellits E D, Freeman J M 1981 Stopping medication in children with epilepsy. New England Journal of Medicine 304: 1125–1129

Gowers W R 1881 Epilepsy and other chronic convulsive diseases. Churchill, London

Grosz W 1930 Ueber den Ausang der genuinen Epilepsie: (auf Grund katamnestischer Erhebungen). Archiv fur Psychiatrie und Nervenkrankheiten 90: 765–776

Group for the study of the prognosis of epilepsy in Japan 1981. Natural history and prognosis of epilepsy: report of a multi-institutional study in Japan. Epilepsia 22: 35–53

Habermaas 1901 Ueber die Prognose der Epilepsie Allgermeine. Zeitschrift fur Psychiatrie 58: 243–253

Hedenstroem I, Schorsch G 1963 Ueber thereapierestente Epileptiker. Archiv fur Psychiatrie und Nervenkrankheiten 204: 579–588

Holowach J, Thurston D L, O'Leary J 1972 Prognosis of childhood epilepsy. New England Journal of Medicine 286: 169–174

Janz D 1982 Prognosis and prophylaxis of traumatic epilepsy. In: Clifford-Rose F (ed) Research progress in epilepsy. Pitman, London, p161–175

Janz D, Sommer-Burkhardt E-M 1976 Discontinuation of antiepileptic drugs in patients with epilepsy who have been seizure-free for more than two years. In: Janz D (ed) Epileptology. Thieme-Verlag, Stuttgart, p 228–234

Jennet B 1975 Epilepsy after non-missile head injuries. Heinemann, London

Juul-Jensen P 1963 Epilepsy, a clinical and social analysis of 1020 adult patients with epileptic seizures. Munksgaard, Copenhagen

Juul-Jensen P 1964 Frequency of recurrence after discontinuance of anticonvulsant therapy in patients with epileptic seizures. Epilepsia 5: 352–363

Juul-Jensen P 1968 Frequency of recurrence after discontinuance of anticonvulsant therapy in patients with epileptic seizures. A new follow-up study after 5 years. Epilepsia 9: 11–16

Kiørboe E 1961 The prognosis of epilepsy. Acta Psychiatrica Scandinavica 36 (suppl. 150): 166–178

Kirstein L 1942 A contribution to the knowledge of the prognosis of epilepsy. Acta Medica Scandinavica 112: 515–523

Livingstone S 1961 Living with epileptic seizures. Journal of Paediatrics 59: 128–137

Logan W J, Freeman J M 1969 Pseudodegenerative disease due to diphelylhydantoin intoxication. Archives of Neurology 21: 631–637

Lorge M 1964 Epilepsie und Lebensschicksal: Ergebnisse katamnestischer Untersuchungen. Psychiatrica et Neurologica (Basel) 147: 360–381

Merritt 1958 Medical treatment in epilepsy. British Medical Journal 1: 666–669

Oller-Daurella L, Pamies R, Oller L 1976 Reduction or discontinuance of antiepileptic drugs in patients seizure-free for more than 5 years. In: Janz D (ed) Epileptology. Thieme-Verlag, Stuttgart, p 218–227

Ounsted C 1955 The hyperkinetic syndrome in epileptic children. Lancet 2: 303–311

Probst C 1960 Ueber den Verlauf von hirnelektrisch strummen Epilepsien. Schweizer Archives fur Neurologie, Neurochirugie und Psychiatrie 85: 357–400

Reynolds E H 1975 Chronic antiepileptic toxicity: a review. Epilepsia 16: 319–352

Reynolds E H, Travers R D 1974 Serum anticonvulsant concentrations in epileptic patients with mental symptoms. British Journal of Psychiatry 124: 440–445

Reynolds E H, Shorvon S D, Galbraith A W, Chadwick D, Dellaportas C I, Vydelingum L 1981 Phenytoin monotherapy for epilepsy: a long-term prospective study, assisted by serum level monitoring, in previously untreated patients. Epilepsia 22: 475–488

Rodin E A 1968 The prognosis of patients with epilepsy. Thomas, Springfield, Illinois

Rodin E A, Kitano H, Lewis R, Rennick P M 1976 A comparison of the effectiveness of primidone versus carbamazepine in epileptic outpatients. Journal of Nervous and Mental Disease 163: 41–46

Rosen J A 1968 Dilantin dementia. Transactions of the American Neurological Association 93: 273

Schmidt D, Janz D 1977 Therapeutic plasma concentrations of phenytoin and phenobarbitone. In: Gardener-Thorpe C, Janz D, Meinardi H, Pippenger C E (eds) Antiepileptic drug monitoring. Pitman, Tunbridge Wells, p 214–225

Shorvon S D, Reynolds E H 1982 The early prognosis of epilepsy. British Medical Journal 285: 1699–1701

Sofijanov N G 1982 Clinical evolution and prognosis of childhood epilepsies. Epilepsia 23: 61–69

142

Spencer S S, Spencer D D, Williamson P D, Mattson R H 1981 Ictal effects of anticonvulsant medication withdrawal in epileptic patients. Epilepsia 22: 297-307

Stores G 1975 Behavioural effects of anticonvulsant drugs. Developmental Medicine and Child Neurology 17: 647-658

Strobos R R J 1959 Prognosis in convulsive disorders. Archives of Neurology 1: 216-225

Tchicaloff M, Gaillard F 1970 Quelques effects indesirables antiepileptiques sur les rendements intellectuels, Revue de Neuropsychiatrie Infantile et d'Hygiene Mentale de l'Enfance. 18: 599-602

Thurston J H, Thurston D L, Hixon B B, Keller A J 1982 Prognosis in childhood epilepsy. New England Journal of Medicine 306: 831-836

Trimble M 1979 The effects of anticonvulsant drugs on cognitive abilities. Pharmacology and Therapeutics 4: 677-685

Trolle E 1961 Drug therapy in epilepsy. Acta Psychiatrica Scandinavica (suppl. 150) 36: 187-199

Turnbull D M, Rawlins M D, Weightman D, Chadwick D W 1982 A comparison of phenytoin and valproate in previously untreated epileptic patients. Journal of Neurology, Neurosurgery and Psychiatry 45: 55-59

Turner W A 1907 Epilepsy, a study of the idiopathic disease. Macmillan, London

Victor M 1970 The role of alcohol in the production of seizures. In: Modern problems in pharmacopsychiatry: epilepsy. Karger, Basel, p 185-199

Wikler A, Essig C F 1970 Withdrawal seizures following chronic intoxication with barbiturates and other sedative drugs. In: Modern problems in pharmacopsychiatry: epilepsy. Karger, Basel, p 170-184

Yahr M D, Sciarra D, Carter S, Merritt H H 1952 Evaluation of standard anticonvulsant therapy in three hundred nineteen patients' Journal of American Medical Association 150: 663-667

Zenker C, Groh C, Roth G 1957 Problems und Erfahrungen beim Abentzen anticonvulsiver Therapie. Neue Osterrich Zeitschrift fur Kinderheilkunde 2: 152-163

14. What is postlumbar puncture headache and is it avoidable?

D. Hilton-Jones

INTRODUCTION

Soon after Quincke introduced the technique of lumbar puncture (LP) in 1891 it was obvious that headache following the procedure was common. Despite the numerous contradictions in the extraordinarily vast literature, with regard to cause and prevention, there is at least general agreement as to the character of postpuncture headache. Usually it starts within 24 hours of puncture, but the onset may be delayed for several days; for example, bed-rest for 24 hours after puncture delays the onset of headache but does not prevent it (Carbaat & Van Crevel, 1981). The symptoms gradually resolve in a few days but occasionally persist for several weeks. Headache and other symptoms lasting up to 1 year have been reported but it is uncertain whether they can be attributed directly to the initial LP (Vandam & Dripps, 1956). Frontal headache is about twice as common as generalised or occipital headache, and pain in other sites occurs in under 10% (Noon, 1949). Associated neck stiffness is not uncommon. The pain is usually a dull ache, but may be throbbing. Although virtually any type of headache occurs there are certain common characteristics of postpuncture headache; most strikingly, the pain is almost invariably eased partially or completely by lying down and it is exacerbated by head shaking and jugular vein compression. Nausea may occur with the headache and occasionally even in its absence. Vomiting is much less common. A few patients complain of unsteadiness when walking, and vertigo may occur. Ocular and auditory disturbances in association with headache are well recorded but, fortunately, uncommon (Vandam & Dripps, 1956).

THE INCIDENCE OF POSTLUMBAR PUNCTURE HEADACHE

In their extensive review of the literature from 1891 onwards, Tourtellotte et al (1964) found the incidence of headache following *diagnostic* LP to vary between 3 and 60% with an average of 32%, assuming no special measures were taken to prevent headache. Following LP for spinal anaesthesia the incidence was lower; between 0 and 40%, with averages of 18% and 13% for the obstetric and non-

144

obstetric sub-groups respectively. The differing incidence between the three groups is important. Firstly, it suggests that something other than simply dural puncture is involved in the pathogenesis of headache and, secondly, that comparison of studies between rather than within the three groups must be made with considerable caution.

The lower incidence of headache after spinal anaesthesia is probably related to several factors:

1. Fluid is introduced rather than removed
2. The fluid introduced is an anaesthetic
3. There is a tendency to use smaller needles than for diagnostic LP
4. Postoperative patients may have prolonged bed-rest
5. The absence of neurological disease in most patients undergoing spinal anaesthesia.

We are concerned, primarily, with headache following diagnostic LP, though many comments also apply to spinal anaesthesia and certain techniques are hardly mentioned outside the anaesthetic literature. Indeed, there is a great divide between the literature dealing with diagnostic LP and that concerned with spinal anaesthesia. In part, this is due to the appalling lack of randomised controlled trials of the preventive techniques under discussion, resulting in each camp quoting anecdotes at the other. In part, it is a failure to understand the specific circumstances of each group of patients, the limitation of staff trained in certain techniques, and the differing requirements of dural puncture in each of the groups.

It is often stated that patients with dementia, syphilis and a variety of psychiatric conditions, particularly schizophrenia, have a lower incidence of postpuncture headache (Tourtellotte et al, 1964; Fuller Torrey, 1979; Ballenger et al, 1979). Conclusive proof is lacking but this has not inhibited several suggestions to explain the difference. Possibly, these patients do not mobilise as rapidly after LP, or undertake the same degree of physical activity. Their diseases may interfere with the patients' ability to report symptoms or the doctors' willingness to believe them. Gowdy (1979) believes that the low incidence in schizophrenic patients is due to insensitivity to pain and suggests that there may be an underlying metabolic defect. Daniels & Sallie (1981) do not agree that schizophrenics have altered pain perception, and conclude that suggestion is a major factor in influencing the development of headache.

THEORIES OF CAUSATION

There have been almost as many theories to explain the development of postpuncture headache as there have been years since the first lumbar puncture. Fortunately, the vast majority can be rapidly discounted for lack of any proof. There is now general agreement that the prime cause of postpuncture headache is continued cerebrospinal fluid (c.s.f.) leakage through the dural hole made at the time of lumbar puncture (Wolff, 1972). This leads to loss of the brain's normal supportive cushion of c.s.f with subsequent stretching of pain sensitive structures, and to dilatation of intracranial veins. If this theory is correct, then:

1. It should be possible to demonstrate continued c.s.f. leakage
2. Headache should correlate with a state of c.s.f. hypotension
3. The development of headache should be favourably influenced by methods that counteract or prevent c.s.f. leakage.

C.s.f. leakage

Continued c.s.f. leakage through the dural hole was first suggested by Sicard (1902) and was demonstrated in man at autopsy by Ingvar (1923). Six days after LP, Mixter (1932) noted persistence of the dural hole at laminectomy. Pool (1942), when performing myeloscopy on patients 2–4 days after LP, frequently found large collections of epidural fluid. Persisting leakage has even been noted at laminectomy several months after LP on one occasion (Brown & Jones, 1962). Radioisotopes have also been used to demonstrate persistent leakage (Gass et al, 1971; Kadrie et al, 1976). Indirect evidence comes from studies of patients subjected to dural puncture without removal of c.s.f. For example, Sciarra & Carter (1952) performed a normal LP on 62 patients and removed 10–12 ml of c.s.f. A second group of 45 patients underwent dural puncture without c.s.f. removal. There was no significant difference in the incidence of headache, being 46% and 38% respectively. That the development of headache is independent of the volume of c.s.f. removed, within certain limits, had previously been suggested by Alpers (1925) who found no difference in removing volumes between 10 and 25 ml. The volume of c.s.f. lost by leakage often exceeds, probably to a large extent, the volume of c.s.f. removed for diagnostic purposes.

C.s.f. hypotension

Jacobaeus & Frumerie (1923) repeated LP on 2 patients with postpuncture symptoms and recorded extremely low c.s.f. pressures. Both patients had headache and in both cases intrathecal injection of saline was accompanied by a rise in c.s.f. pressure and resolution of headache. Nelson (1930) also found very low c.s.f pressure on repeat puncture in 3 patients with typical postpuncture headache. In a further 7 such patients Pickering (1948) found, on repeat puncture, pressures around atmospheric in 6 cases and a pressure at the lower limit of normal in the seventh. Intrathecal injection of saline sufficient to increase the c.s.f. pressure to the normal or upper normal range abolished the headache. Marshall (1950) performed repeat LP on 43 patients irrespective of the development of headache. Of 5 patients with typical postpuncture headache 3 had low c.s.f. pressures and 2 had normal pressures. Of those patients without headache 4 had pressures below 50 mm of c.s.f. He concluded that the association between low c.s.f. pressures and headache was not invariable, and that other factors must play a part.

The lack of a simple direct relationship between low c.s.f. pressure and headache does not detract from the theory that loss of c.s.f. volume is in large part responsible for the development of headache. In an elegant study of experimental c.s.f. drainage headache, Kunkle et al (1943), emphasising the very close similarity with postpuncture headache, demonstrated that headache does not correlate directly with lowered c.s.f. pressure, but is closely associated with a change in the normal pressure differential between the inside and outside of the intracranial veins, resulting in venous dilatation. Such venous dilatation following c.s.f. removal has been demonstrated in cats (Forbes & Nason, 1935). The dilatation, together with traction on the veins, produces pain. Jugular compression causes further venous dilatation and an increase in severity of the headache, despite tending to reverse the state of c.s.f. hypotension.

Reduction of leakage

Despite the very many techniques that have been described to prevent postpuncture headache, only the use of a small calibre needle and epidural blood patching are of proven value, and these have in common the mechanism of reducing the amount of c.s.f. leakage. The successful and unsuccessful methods will be considered in more detail later.

Brown & Jones (1962) described a patient with a prolapsed lumbar intervertebral disc who developed typical postpuncture headache after myelography. After 2 months his headache and sciatica persisted and repeat LP demonstrated no measurable spinal fluid pressure. Five months after myelography, with headache still persisting, laminectomy and discectomy were performed for his sciatica. At operation a continuous flow of c.s.f. was seen coming from a dural rent at the site of the first LP. No evidence of the second dural puncture was found. The c.s.f. leak was arrested by applying dural clips and he had no further posture related headache. Persistent c.s.f. leakage occurs because the lumbar c.s.f. pressure exceeds the pressure in the epidural space, and indeed this differential may contribute to the continuing patency of the hole itself and is increased by standing. In the erect position the c.s.f. pressure at the level of the cisterna magna is approximately zero (Kunkle et al, 1943), suggesting that puncture at this level would not result in persistent c.s.f. leakage. Controlled trials are lacking, but it appears that cisternal puncture is associated with a lower incidence of headache than lumbar puncture (Kulchar, 1940).

Perkel (1925) noted a lower incidence of postpuncture headache in patients with an abnormal c.s.f. Associated meningeal inflammatory changes may be relevant by causing more rapid closure of the dural hole, but confirmation is lacking. Alternatively, these patients may, in general, be less well than those with normal fluid, and thus be more confined in their activities immediately following LP (Wolff, 1972).

There is, therefore, considerable evidence that postpuncture headache is in large part caused by continued c.s.f. leakage through the dural hole left after LP. Many other theories have been proposed but none have found scientific support and few, if any, have been tested in adequate experimental studies. Alteration in the rate of c.s.f. production, both increase and decrease, has been suggested, as has the vague concept of autonomic instability. Some earlier authors favoured asthenia or migraine, and suggestions that the development of headache is related to local climatic circumstances or the wearing of glasses have found little support. A variety of technical difficulties have been incriminated, and certainly, multiple dural puncture may result in a greater leakage of c.s.f.. Tourtellotte et al (1964) reviewed these and other theories, and concluded that c.s.f. leakage was the most important factor.

Psychogenic factors

There is still considerable discussion surrounding the role of psychogenic factors in the development of postpuncture headache (Hilton-Jones, 1981), some authors believing them to be of major importance (Paulley, 1980; Daniels & Sallie, 1981), others discounting them (Crawford, 1981). This discrepancy of opinion can, in part, be attributed to the relative lack of controlled trials studying these aspects of the problem and most of what has been written is anecdotal. Redlich et al (1946) studied a group of psychiatric inpatients and tried to evaluate the contribution of physical and psychogenic factors to the development of postpuncture symptoms. They concluded that continued c.s.f. leakage was the major factor with only a small, statistically insignificant contribution from anxiety, hypochondriasis and other emotional elements. However, they were studying a highly selected group of patients and caution must be taken in extrapolating their results. Although they found no difference in the frequency of postpuncture headache between the sexes many reports indicate a higher frequency of headache amongst females, though rarely reaching statistical significance, and there are no reports showing a higher frequency amongst males. In a recent study on healthy volunteers, Tourtellotte et al (1972) found headache and several other complaints to be significantly more frequent amongst females. This sex difference has been used by several authors to support the view that functional factors significantly contribute to the development of postpuncture headache (Tourtellotte et al, 1964).

Kaplan (1967) performed an interesting study on 100 healthy 'volunteers' from a convict population. Lumbar puncture was performed normally on 50 subjects, followed by bed-rest for 4 hours. The other 50 subjects underwent an identical procedure but without dural puncture, the needle only entering as far as the ligamentum flavum or into a paravertebral muscle. There was no significant difference in the incidence of headache between the two groups, being 28% and 22% respectively. Before the procedure was performed, 15 of the subjects in the sham puncture group expressed concern about the development of headache. The incidence of headache in this sub-group was 47%, which was significantly higher than the incidence of 11% in those subjects who expressed no such fears. Kaplan concluded that psychogenic factors were of primary importance in the development of postpuncture headache. This study is not beyond criticism even if the unusual choice of subjects is discounted. It was double-blind in that assessment of headache was made by an independent physician, but unfortunately he did not record sufficient detail to determine adequately the nature of the headache in each of the two groups. This emphasises an important point. To evaluate the success of methods designed to reduce the incidence of headache it is obviously necessary to be certain that headaches reported after LP are typical postpuncture headaches as described earlier, and not some form of non-specific headache related to tension, stress or anxiety. Kaplan's study would have been more valuable if this distinction had been made.

Conclusion

Continued c.s.f. leakage after LP is the major factor in the development of postpuncture headache. Psychogenic factors probably contribute to an extent not adequately determined at the present time. Sometimes the headache following LP may be a form of stress or tension headache and not directly related to the dural puncture. Inadequate characterisation of the type of headache makes the results of some studies difficult to interpret.

PREVENTION

Tourtellotte et al (1964) reviewed more than 40 methods reported to lower the incidence of postpuncture headache. Mostly the results were inconclusive, due in large part to poor trial design, lack of randomised control groups, small numbers of subjects, and inadequate patient information. They concluded that the use of small calibre needles was a major factor in reducing the incidence of headache, and it was conceivable that recumbency after LP was of some importance. With regard to multiple dural punctures and state of hydration after LP the evidence was inconclusive. They considered the use of fibrinogen injected epidurally to form a clot over the dural hole, but rejected it at that time because of the risk of hepatitis. They did not consider epidural blood patching, which had been introduced some 4 years earlier. Of the numerous drugs that have been recommended for prophylaxis against, and treatment for postpuncture headache, all except one were of unproven value. The exception, dimenhydrinate, was shown to reduce the incidence of headache following spinal analgesia for vaginal delivery, but this has not been confirmed. Since 1964 vasopressin and its synthetic analogue DDAVP have been studied with a suggestion that the severity but not incidence of headache may be slightly reduced (Aziz et al, 1968: Cowan et al, 1980).

Intrathecal instillation of fluid may abolish established postpuncture headache, and several authors have suggested routinely instilling normal saline before removing the needle. The epidural instillation of fluid may decrease leakage by increasing the pressure in the epidural space, but the effect of a single injection is short lived. The continuous infusion of fluid into the epidural space for 24 hours after LP has been found, in an uncontrolled study, to lessen the frequency and severity of headache (Crawford, 1972) and other authors have suggested the instillation of a bolus of saline into the epidural space at the time of dural puncture, and again 24 hours later, as being effective prophylaxis (Craft et al, 1973). Both studies reported only small numbers of patients, and both were concerned with the selected sub-group of patients who inadvertently had the dura punctured during attempted epidural anaesthesia during labour. Epidural fluid was instilled through a catheter, and such a technique is inappropriate following diagnostic LP, which is usually performed by staff inexperienced in such techniques.

On theoretical grounds it has been argued that increasing the patients' state of hydration may lead to increased rate of c.s.f. secretion, thereby counteracting continued leakage. The oral intake of large quantities of fluid in the 24 hours after LP is frequently recommended (Birkahan & Heifetz, 1969), though its beneficial effect has not been adequately assessed. Similarly, the value of intravenous isotonic and hypotonic fluids is unproven although there is a transient increase in c.s.f. pressure, largely due to increased c.s.f production, and this may be accompanied by relief of postpuncture headache (Thorsén, 1947). The effect of a single infusion probably lasts no more than a few hours (Thorsén, 1947; Noon, 1949) and some authors have not found any relief of headache (Marx & Hershey, 1952). A more prolonged infusion may confer lasting benefit, but this has not been adequately studied. Such a technique is likely to restrict the patients' mobility, which may be a complicating factor in analysis. Possibly these methods of increasing hydration, unless continued for unacceptably long periods, simply delay the onset of headache.

Posture

The role of posture immediately following LP is the subject of considerable discussion. Sicard (1902) was the first to suggest the importance of 24 hours bed-rest following LP but this has only very recently been studied in an adequate trial. Carbaat & Van Crevel (1981) compared the effects of 24 hours bed-rest with immediate mobilisation, and found that the frequency of headache was not significantly affected. What 24 hours bed-rest did was delay the onset of headache by a similar period of time. Unfortunately the patients were not randomly allocated to each of the study groups, but this is the only major criticism of their study.

Apart from duration of bed-rest after LP, the position assumed by the patient during and after LP has been considered important. The few studies comparing the incidence of headache following LP performed in either the lying or sitting position suggest little if any difference between the methods (Tourtellotte et al, 1964). Nor does the degree of back flexion during the procedure influence the occurrence of headache (Miller & Crocker, 1964). Brocker (1958) reported that the incidence of postpuncture headache could be reduced to less than 1% if patients lay prone for 3 hours after LP. However, there were several deficiencies in the design of the trial, and such dramatic but unlikely results have not been substantiated by other workers. Easton (1979) suggested, without giving actual figures, that elevating the foot of the bed after LP reduced the incidence of headache. Further study by Smith et al (1980) failed to show any statistically significant benefit from bed tilting although there was a trend towards lower frequency of headache. In the light of these reports Handler et al (1982) studied the effect of 4 hours prone bed-rest against 30 degrees head down tilt for 30 minutes followed by supine bed-rest for $3\frac{1}{2}$ hours. Five hours after LP there was a lower incidence of headache in the prone group, but the difference did not reach statistical significance. At the end of 1 week there was no difference in the incidence of headache between the two groups. Our own recent study did not show any significant benefit from head down tilting and/or the prone position (Hilton-Jones et al, 1982). Indeed, the lowest frequency of headache occurred in patients who assumed the supine position without bed tilting, although this did not achieve statistical significance. However, the figures did suggest that even in a very much larger trial it would be unlikely that bed tilting and the prone posture could ever be shown to confer any significant benefit.

The posture assumed after LP and the period of bed-rest, at least if it is within 24 hours, make no significant contribution, beneficial or otherwise, to the

150

development of headache, though it is clear that lying down relieves established headache. These findings are probably not surprising. If postural manoeuvres prevent headache, either they decrease the size, or increase the speed of repair, of the dural hole. If this does not occur, headache will develop at much the same frequency as it does without these special measures, though delayed in onset until the patient stands up. A very long period of bed-rest may allow repair of the hole so that headache does not occur on mobilisation, but is not likely to be practical.

Small calibre needles

Even without special precautions not all patients develop headache, and this is thought to be because they have less c.s.f. leakage due to more rapid and/or complete closure of the dural hole. It seems likely that early closure of the hole is related to local mechanical factors rather than to specific repair mechanisms. In the position required for LP dura and arachnoid membranes may slide over each other. When the patient resumes a more normal position the membranes move and the degree of overlap of the holes in each membrane will dictate the amount of c.s.f. leakage. Any residual leakage will eventually be sealed off by a fibrinous plug (Jones, 1974). Thus, the smaller the initial dural hole, the less c.s.f. leakage there is likely to be, resulting in a lower incidence of headache. I am aware of only one publication that has adequately tackled the effect of needle size. Tourtellotte et al (1972), in a randomised double-blind trial, found the incidence of headache to be significantly lower when using a 26 SWG needle, compared with a 22 SWG needle. Furthermore, severe headache and a variety of miscellaneous complaints were significantly less frequent in the former group. Overall the frequency of headache was reduced from 1 in 3 to 1 in 9 patients. The incidence of headache in the 26 SWG needle group was 9% and 19% for males and females respectively. Thus a significant number of patients still get headache, and these figures are higher than those reported in many other series which were without randomised controls and almost certainly biased. For example, Gerner (1980) found an incidence of headache of less than 1% when using a 26 SWG needle. It seems likely that the figures from Tourtellotte et al, with their more critical evaluation, more closely reflect the true value of using a small needle.

Not only may the size of the needle be important, but also its direction of insertion. Autopsy studies have shown, not surprisingly, that larger needles leave larger holes, but also that if the needle bevel is introduced at right angles to the longitudinally running dural fibres a larger hole results (Greene, 1923; Franksson & Gordh, 1946). Hatfalvi (1977) noted no cases of postpuncture headache in a personal series of 600 spinal anaesthetics, and attributed this to his preferred technique of introducing the spinal needle from a lateral approach. In an experimental study on isolated meninges he demonstrated no leakage after tangential insertion of a 20 SWG needle, but leakage occurred if this or a smaller needle was inserted perpendicularly. Furthermore, he showed in cadavers that a 20 SWG needle inserted in the mid-line entered the dura at right angles, whereas a 25 SWG needle, although inserted in the mid-line, becomes deviated by structures between the skin and dura, and actually enters the dura tangentially. He concluded that the angled approach resulted in less overlap of the dura and arachnoid holes after LP, with subsequent reduction in c.s.f. leakage. Thus a small needle may be effective in reducing headache not only because of its smaller diameter, but also because of its inherent flexibility.

Unfortunately there are disadvantages in using fine calibre needles. Their flexibility necessitates the use of an introducer, which may conveniently be an ordinary blood-letting needle of slightly larger diameter, although special introducers are manufactured. Such a method requires a little more practice but is perhaps not suited for staff performing LP infrequently. Static pressure measurements may be made, but dynamic recordings require a transducer. The needle tip is easily occluded by nerve roots and manipulation to avoid this can be difficult. Rate of fluid flow is so slow that syringe aspiration is required. In view of these limitations it is not surprising that the greatest advocates of the use of small needles are anaesthetists. They have much more opportunity to use and become experienced in the method than most junior medical staff who nowadays perform relatively few lumbar punctures, and furthermore they are concerned with the introduction rather than removal of fluid.

Epidural blood patching
If continued c.s.f. leakage is the main cause of postpuncture headache, then mechanical blockage of the dural hole should alleviate or prevent headache. Nelson (1930) tried blocking the hole with catgut, and although he showed some improvement in the frequency of headache the results were inconclusive. A few further studies failed to show any significant benefit, and the technique was frequently complicated by low back pain and pain in the legs. In passing, Nelson commented on the possible effect of bleeding induced by the needle rupturing a blood vessel, resulting in a bloody tap. He suggested that such bleeding may help to plug the dural hole. Gormley (1960) noted a low incidence of postpuncture headache following bloody taps and was inspired to try the effect of the epidural injection of autologous blood in patients with established headache. In his initial report all six patients had immediate and permanent cure of their headache. Numerous reports have appeared since then and the success rate is in the order of 90% (DiGiovnai et al, 1972; Abouleish et al, 1975). The technique has been used prophylactically, injecting blood as the spinal needle is withdrawn through the epidural space. Using this method Ozdil & Powell (1965) reported no headache in a series of 100 patients following spinal anaesthesia and Gutterman & Bezier (1978) found a significant reduction in the number of headaches following myelography. The technique has been used successfully up to 11 weeks after onset of headache (Cass & Edelist, 1974).

I am not aware of any report, dealing with reasonable numbers of patients, on the treatment or prophylaxis of headache with epidural blood patching following *diagnostic* LP, though it seems reasonable to conclude that similar results may be found. The technique should not be difficult to master but, requires practice. The most important factors are strict asepsis when taking the patients' blood, and accurate placement of the blood in the epidural space which may be made difficult by a pool of c.s.f. if there has been considerable leakage. Anaesthetists are more expert than most in finding the epidural space, which perhaps explains why they are the main proponents of the technique.

In expert hands the technique is relatively safe, though several complications have been reported. By far the commonest is back pain at the site of injection which occurs in up to 35% of patients, this figure being similar to the number of patients likely to develop headache, and although usually transient it may be persistent and troublesome (Abouleish et al, 1975). Radicular pain and paraesthesiae have been reported (Nicholson, 1973; Cornwall & Dolan, 1975), and lumbosacral meningismus probably due to subarachnoid injection of blood has been described (Wilkinson, 1980). Many authors have been concerned with the possibility of the introduction of infection, but fortunately this has not yet been reported. Local sepsis of the back or septicaemia are absolute contraindications to the procedure.

Conclusion

No single technique is invariably effective in preventing postpuncture headache. Small needles decrease the incidence of headache, but the benefit is not as dramatic as is sometimes claimed. Epidural blood patching may be very effective, but is perhaps best reserved for the treatment of intractable postpuncture headache rather than for prophylaxis. Both these techniques require some practice and it is probable that their widespread use by inexperienced staff, performing LP only infrequently, would lead to more rather than fewer complications. The epidural infusion of fluid for 24 hours after dural puncture may be beneficial, but has no practical role following diagnostic LP. The value of increasing hydration with oral or intravenous fluids is still uncertain, but at least the former is unlikely to have any major side-effects. We and others have been unable to show any beneficial effect from postural manoeuvres after LP, including 24 hours bed-rest.

It must be remembered that postpuncture headache is usually a benign self-limiting problem, and only a few patients develop severe or persisting symptoms. It is, therefore, imperative that any method of prophylaxis or treatment does not have more side-effects than the symptoms being treated. Excessive therapeutic enthusiasm must be carefully guarded against. If patients with intracranial mass lesions are excluded, serious sequelae of lumbar puncture are extremely rare and some of these, such as isolated cranial nerve palsies, are only transient. Newrick & Read (1982) have recently reviewed the literature on intracranial subdural haematoma after spinal puncture. They found 12 cases and added a further 2. It is pertinent to note that in all 14 cases dural puncture was performed either for spinal anaesthesia or inadvertently during attempted epidural anaesthesia, and I am not aware of any reports of this complication following diagnostic LP. It is probable that predisposing factors apart from dural puncture were present in some of the patients. Nine of the 14 cases recovered completely. Considering how frequently lumbar puncture is performed subdural haematoma must be an extremely unusual complication but despite this it has been suggested that epidural blood patching or epidural infusion is mandatory for the treatment of postpuncture headache in order to prevent such an outcome (Garrett & Bolsin, 1982). Such an extreme view would only be tenable if these manoeuvres carried no significant complications, but this is manifestly not the case.

CURRENT PRACTICE

Prior to performing LP the patient is told the purpose of the procedure and what it entails. I usually tell them that it is little different in terms of discomfort from venepuncture. Generally patients are not forewarned of headache, although patients going home the same day are told that should they develop headache it is self-limiting and will be relieved by lying down. The procedure is performed at the bedside. The elaborate ritual of transferring the patient to a clinical room, donning gloves, mask, hat and gown is not only unnecessary, but daunting for the patient. I use the left lateral position from personal preference. After skin cleansing a small skin bleb is raised with 2% lignocaine over the chosen interspace. I use a 20 or 22 SWG disposable spinal needle as this allows pressure measurement and the collection of enough c.s.f. (approximately 10 ml) in a reasonable period of time without the need for syringe aspiration. After the procedure the patient is allowed to get up and the nursing staff encourage oral fluid intake. If headache develops the patient is instructed to lie down, and in most cases this is adequate treatment. Simple analgesics are given if headache persists despite lying down. I have found severe headache to be very uncommon, and following several hundred LPs in the Oxford neurology department in the last 2 years only 2 patients have had their discharge from hospital delayed because of headache. In both cases headache resolved within 5 days with simple supportive measures. I would consider epidural blood patching if headache proved to be intractable but as yet have had no cause to use this technique.

FURTHER RESEARCH

There are several unanswered questions with regard to factors that may predispose to the development of headache or favourably influence recovery of established headache. Bearing in mind the thousands of patients having an LP every year, it should be a simple matter to put these to the test. As has been emphasised, trial design is of major importance, particularly with respect to adequate numbers of patients and suitable control groups. Postpuncture headache is a specific entity and care should be taken to exclude or at least separately analyse non-specific headache not directly related to c.s.f. hydrodynamic disturbances.

It would be of interest to know whether forewarning the patient of the possible development of headache influences its occurrence, and if it does so in a deleterious manner whether the headache is a typical postpuncture headache. Posture during LP appears to be irrelevant, but there are no good trials comparing lying against sitting. The volume of c.s.f. seems unimportant, at least within certain limits, but as there is now a trend to remove larger quantities of c.s.f. for sophisticated immunological assays it may be worth comparing the effect of removing volumes between 5 and 20 ml. Oral hydration after LP has theoretical backing but has not been formally assessed.

CONCLUSION

Postpuncture headache is usually a benign self-limiting condition. Persistent c.s.f. leakage is the major factor in its development, though other factors may play a part. Despite numerous and mostly useless reports, the only two methods known which will definitely prevent headache are the use of a small calibre needle and epidural blood patching, the latter also being effective in treating established headache. Both techniques have their problems, which limit their routine use for diagnostic LP. The vast literature is confused by inadequate trials, anecdote and excessive therapeutic enthusiasm. It is extraordinary that such a simple and common procedure as LP is surrounded by so much folklore, to the extent that in many hospitals money is wasted by admitting patients so that they can lie on their backs doing nothing for 24 hours.

REFERENCES

Abouleish E, de la Vega S, Blendinger I, Tio T 1975 Long-term follow up of epidural blood patch. Anesthesia and Analgesia 54: 459–463
Alpers B J 1925 Lumbar puncture headache. Archives of Neurology and Psychiatry 14: 806–812
Aziz H, Pearce J, Miller E 1968 Vasopressin in prevention of lumbar puncture headache. British Medical Journal 4: 677–678
Ballenger J C, Post R M, Sternberg D E, van Kammen D P, Cowdry R W, Goodwin F K 1979 Headaches after lumbar puncture and insensitivity to pain in psychiatric patients. New England Journal of Medicine 301: 110
Birkahan J H, Heifetz M 1969 Lumbar puncture headache. British Medical Journal 1: 782
Brocker R J 1958 Technique to avoid spinal-tap headache. Journal of the American Medical Association 168: 261–263
Brown B A, Jones O W 1962 Prolonged headache following spinal puncture. Journal of Neurosurgery 19: 349–350
Carbaat P A T, van Crevel H 1981 Lumbar puncture headache: controlled study on the preventive effect of 24 hours' bed rest. Lancet 2: 1133–1135
Cass W, Edelist G 1974 Postspinal headache. Journal of the American Medical Association 227: 786–787
Cornwall R D, Dolan W M 1975 Radicular back pain following lumbar epidural blood patch. Anesthesiology 43(6): 692–693
Cowan J M A, Durward W F, Harrington H, Johnston J H, Donovan B 1980 DDAVP in the prevention of headache after lumbar puncture. British Medical Journal 280: 224
Craft J B, Epstein B S, Coakley C S 1973 Prophylaxis of dural-puncture headache with epidural saline. Anesthesia and Analgesia 52(2): 228–231
Crawford J S 1972 The prevention of headache consequent upon dural puncture. British Journal of Anaesthesia 44: 598–600
Crawford J S 1981 Headache after Lumbar Puncture. Lancet 2: 418
Daniels A M, Sallie R 1981 Headache, lumbar puncture, and expectation. Lancet 1: 1003
Digiovanni A J, Galbert M W, Wahle W M 1972 Epidural injection of autologous blood for postlumbar-puncture headache. Anesthesia and Analgesia 51(2): 226–232
Easton J D 1979 Headache after lumbar puncture. Lancet 1: 974–5
Forbes H S, Nason G I 1935 The cerebral circulation. Archives of Neurology and Psychiatry 34: 533–547
Franksson C, Gordh T 1946 Headache after spinal anesthesia and a technique for lessening its frequency. Acta Chirurgica Scandinavica 94: 443–54
Fuller Torrey E 1979 Headaches after lumbar puncture and insensitivity to pain in psychiatric patients. New England Journal of Medicine 301: 110
Garrett C P O, Bolsin S N 1982 Subdural haematoma as a complicaton of spinal anaesthetic. British Medical Journal 285: 1047
Gass H, Goldstein A S, Ruskin R, Leopold N A 1971 Chronic postmyelogram headache. Archives of Neurolgoy 25: 168–170
Gerner R H 1980 Posture and headache after lumbar puncture. Lancet 2: 33

Gormley J B 1960 Treatment of postspinal headache. Anesthesiology 21: 565–6

Gowdy J M 1979 Headaches after lumbar puncture and insensitivity to pain in psychiatric patients. New England Journal of Medicine 301: 110–1

Greene H M 1923 A technique to reduce the incidence of headache following LP in ambulatory patients. Northwest Medicine 22: 240

Gutterman P, Bezier H S 1978 Prophylaxis of postmyelogram headaches. Journal of Neurosurgery 49: 869–871

Handler C E, Perkin G D, Smith F R, Rose F C 1982 Posture and lumbar puncture headache: a controlled trial in 50 patients. Journal of the Royal Society of Medicine 75: 404–7

Hatfalvi B I 1977 The dynamics of post-spinal headache. Headache 17(2): 64–66

Hilton-Jones D 1981 Headache after lumbar puncture. Lancet 2: 253–4

Hilton-Jones D, Harrad R A, Gill M W, Warlow C P 1982 Failure of postural manoeuvres to prevent lumbar puncture headache. Journal of Neurology, Neurosurgery and Psychiatry 45: 743–746

Ingvar S 1923 On the danger of leakage of the cerebrospinal fluid after lumbar puncture. Acta Medica Scandinavica 58: 67–101

Jacobaeus H C, Frumerie K 1923 About the leakage of the spinal fluid after lumbar puncture and its treatment. Acta Medica Scandinavica 58: 102–108

Jones R J 1974 The role of recumbency in the prevention and treatment of postspinal headache. Anesthesia and Analgesia 53: 788–96

Kadrie H, Driedger A A, McInnis W 1976 Persistent dural Cerebrospinal fluid leak shown by retrograde radionuclide myelography. Journal of Nuclear Medicine 17: 797–799

Kaplan G 1967 The psychogenic etiology of headache post lumbar puncture. Psychosomatic Medicine 29: 376–379

Kulchar G V 1940 Cisternal puncture. American Journal of Syphilis, Gonorrhea and Veneral Diseases 24: 643–650

Kunkle E C, Ray B S, Wolff H G 1943 Experimental studies on headache. Archives of Neurology and Psychiatry 49: 323–58

Marshall J 1950 Lumbar-puncture headache. Journal of Neurology, Neurosurgery and Psychiatry 13: 71–4

Marx G F, Hershey S G 1952 Prophylaxis of postspinal analgesia headache following vaginal delivery. New York State Journal of Medicine 52: 1906–1908

Miller E V, Crocker J S 1964 The flexed back and post-lumbar puncture headache. Anesthesiology 25: 80–81

Mixter W J 1932 Conclusion in: Fremont-Smith F, Merritt H, Lennox W G (eds) The relationship between water balance, spinal fluid pressure and epileptic convulsions. Archives of Neurology and Psychiatry 28: 956–959

Nelson M O 1930 Postpuncture headaches. Archives of Dermatology and Syphilology 21: 615–27

Newrick P, Read D 1982 Subdural haematoma as a complication of spinal anaesthetic. British Medical Journal 285: 341–342

Nicholson M J 1973 Comment on: Complications following Epidural blood patch for postlumbar-puncture headache. Anesthesia and Analgesia 52: 67–71

Noon Z B 1949 Postspinal puncture headache. Arizona Medicine 6: 19–23

Ozdil T, Powell W F 1965 Post lumbar puncture headache. Anesthesia and Analgesia 44: 542–545

Paulley J W 1980 Posture and headache after lumbar puncture. Lancet 2: 33

Perkel J D 1925 Contribution a l'étude des accidents secondaires qui suivent la ponction lombaire. La Presse Medicale 33: 1320–1322

Pickering G W 1948 Lumbar-puncture headache. Brain 71: 274–280

Pool J L 1942 Myeloscopy: intraspinal endoscopy. Surgery 11: 169–182

Quincke H 1891 Die Lumbarpunktion des Hydrocephalus. Klinisches Wochenschrift 28: 929–933, 965–968

Redlich F C, Moore B E, Kimbell I 1946 Lumbar puncture reactions: relative importance of physiological and psychological factors. Psychosomatic Medicine 8: 386–398 Sciaara D, Carter S 1952 Lumbar puncture headache. Journal of the American Medical Association 148: 841–842

Sicard J A 1902 Le Liquide Céphalo-Rachidien. Masson, Paris

Smith F R, Perkin G D, Rose F C 1980 Posture and headache after lumber puncture. Lancet 1: 1245

Thorsén G 1947 Neurological complications after spinal anesthesia and results from 2493 follow-up cases. Acta Chirurgica Scandinavica 95(suppl 121)

Tourtellotte W W, Haerer A F, Heller G L, Somers J E 1964 Post-lumbar puncture headaches. Thomas, Illinois

Tourtellotte W W, Henderson W G, Tucker R P, Gilland O, Walker J E, Kokman E 1972 A randomized double-blind clinical trial comparing the 22 versus 26 gauge needle in the production of the post-lumbar puncture syndrome in normal individuals. Headache 12: 73–78

Vandam L D, Dripps R D 1956 Long-term follow-up of patients who received 10 098 spinal anaesthetics. Journal of the American Medical Association 161: 586–591

Wilkinson H A 1980 Lumbosacral meningismus complicating subdural injection of blood patch. Journal of Neurosurgery 52: 849–51

Wolff H G 1972 Headache and other head pain, 3rd edn. Oxford University Press, New York

15. Does biopsy or any surgery influence the outcome in patients with supratentorial malignant gliomas?

Jonathan Punt

INTRODUCTION

Considering the accepted role of surgical excision in the majority of solid tumours, it is interesting to be questioning the value of any surgery for a specific tumour nearly 100 years after the first technically successful removal of a glioma by Bennett and Godlee in 1884 (Bennett & Godlee, 1885): the 25-year-old patient complained only of focal motor seizures with brachial monoparesis and was dead from meningitis 4 weeks after the operation. Despite this inauspicious start the neurological establishment of the day enthused and in the ensuing discussion (Ferrier et al, 1885) all agreed that further cases should be referred. At Guy's Hospital, White (1886) was more sanguine suggesting that only 4 out of 24 patients with gliomas would have benefited from surgical treatment. Thereafter, the physicians and surgeons of successive generations notably Cushing (1932), Cairns (1935), McKenzie (1936), Pennybacker et al (1950), Bender & Elizan (1962), Hitchcock & Sato (1964), Garfield & Dayan (1973) and Northfield (1973) have continued to remind us of the very modest achievements of surgery in this inevitably fatal disease. In the last decade most workers have pursued various aspects of radiotherapy and chemotherapy, the benefits of excisional surgery — as well as the shortcomings — being assumed. A reappraisal is therefore timely. Although rarely expressed publicly, it is clear that many British physicians and surgeons continue to have grave reservations about submitting patients with gliomas to operation and the writer suspects that many are highly selective in their practice.

DEFINITION OF INFLUENCE

In this article, only supratentorial tumours in adults will be considered and the term malignant brain glioma will be used to cover all those tumours variably described as glioblastoma multiforme, anaplastic glioma and malignant astrocytoma.

How to define influence? If one's desire is purely to palliate then clearly any manoeuvre that alleviates the burden on the patient and his family has influence.

158

Alternatively, if the aim is 'cure' a more objective measure is required. The yardsticks used by the Brain Tumour Group of the European Organisation for Research into Treatment of Cancer (EORTC) and the American Brain Tumour Study Group are those of symptom free interval or median time to progression, and survival time from operation. These parameters have the advantage of ready and accurate measurability, but do they really indicate any true influence of treatments under trial on the biological behaviour of the disease? As Saloman (1980) has shown, the exponential shape of survival curves for patients with malignant brain gliomas resembles that of a disseminated, slowly growing tumour, the characteristics of which have been defined by Shackney et al (1978). Response to treatment for this type of tumour is typically not durable. I would suggest that our treatments for malignant brain gliomas are usually only applied towards the end of the natural history of the disease and the value of median survival time in such slowly growing tumours is therefore questionable (Saloman, 1980). In effect, one is only measuring palliation. If one seeks evidence of any real influence of treatments on the behaviour of the tumour, then the time from first symptom to either progression or death may be a better parameter, though less accurately obtained. Both these interpretations of 'influence' are valid, the 'palliative' and the 'curative', and both will be considered in their place. However, the major concern of this article will be with the latter.

THE INFLUENCE OF BIOPSY

Is biopsy really necessary, or is it reasonable to prognosticate and plan further management without histological confirmation of the diagnosis of malignant brain glioma? Following his innovative introduction of 'arterial encephalography' in July of 1927, Moniz (1931) stated that the technique could demonstrate a characteristic pattern for each type of cerebral tumour and Lorenz (1940) confirmed this assertion. Subsequent experience led neurosurgeons to question the infallibility of arteriography although the occasional physician has based non-operative treatment of supposedly malignant brain tumours upon angiographic appearance alone (Bender & Elizan, 1962). The advent of computer assisted tomographic (CT) scanning produced similar claims and again experience has shown that even the most thorough clinical evaluation combined with a good quality CT scan does not provide the same diagnostic accuracy as histological examination of an operative specimen: metastatic tumour, meningioma, abscess, infarct and herpes simplex encephalitis can all mimic glioma. Future generations of CT scanner, possibly complimented by other investigative tools such as nuclear magnetic resonance and more specific radionuclide brain imaging, may be honed fine enough to render tissue diagnosis obsolete but until that time, it is my view that the majority of patients with mass lesions of the cerebral hemispheres should be offered biopsy as the basis of their management, especially if this includes measures that are time consuming, unpleasant or hazardous.

Tissue may be obtained simply and cheaply by burrhole biopsy under local anaesthesia, the disadvantages of this technique being failure to obtain adequate or representative tissue and abrupt deterioration in the patient's condition from uncontrolled intracerebral haemorrhage. The latter risk has probably been overstated because burrhole biopsy has frequently been reserved for moribund patients and the high mortality is hardly surprising. For example, in a retrospective series in which 58% of the patients were subjected to burrhole biopsy, Hitchcock & Sato (1964) reported an operative mortality of 27% for burrhole biopsy compared to 4% when extirpation was performed. As their policy had been to manage the older and more disabled patients with more extensive disease with burrhole biopsy this observation is hardly surprising. Reduction of intracranial pressure by steroids prior to biopsy is probably the most important factor, apart from operative technique, in reducing mortality and morbidity from burrhole biopsy and in this respect it is relevant that Hitchcock & Sato (1964) found the mortality to be 32% in the presence of raised intracranial pressure compared to 4% if this feature was absent.

Marshall et al (1974) reported their experience of 60 patients, suspected on clinical and radiological grounds of harbouring malignant brain gliomas, who were subjected to standard burrhole biopsy under local anesthetic coupled with immediate histological examinaton of the tissue obtained. All patients received steroids pre and postoperatively. Mortality and morbidity were low: 2 patients, both moribund preoperatively, died and a further 1 suffered a transient hemiparesis. Accuracy was high being positive for malignant glioma in 53 out of 60 cases. One biopsy was erroneously reported as meningioma and in 6 cases, diagnostic tissue was not obtained; all proved to be malignant gliomas at subsequent craniotomies. That 90% of patients were spared major open surgery for an incurable disease outweighs the 10% failure rate. Shetter et al (1977) reported the results of freehand and stereotactic biopsy performed in 54 cases of suspected malignant brain tumours all of whom received preoperative steroids. A definite histological diagnosis was obtained in 49 cases, 46 being malignant tumours, and 3 infarcts. The single death was from haemorrhage in a patient with multiple metastases. Morbidity was higher than in the study of Marshall et al (1974), 7 patients experiencing an increase in neurological deficit, permanently so in 2 cases of malignant glioma. The rate of positive diagnosis was 95% with freehand biopsy compared to 82% with the stereotactic method though the latter was free of permanent aggravation of neurological deficit. Although it is my practice to reserve burrhole biopsy for patients who are unsuitable for excisional surgery either because of advanced and crippling neurological disability, or because of the site of the tumour, the experience of Marshall et al (1974) and Shetter et al (1977) provides justification for the more widespread application of this technique to patients in better neurological condition. Having obtained a tissue diagnosis such patients are still eligible for radiotherapy, chemotherapy or other treatments but have been spared major intracranial surgery. In addition, the occasional patient with a large cystic tumour will benefit from the reduction in intracranial pressure afforded by drainage at the time of burrhole biopsy.

In patients with minimal disability and accessible tumours, I favour open biopsy at a craniotomy in order to be certain of obtaining diagnostic tissue at minimum risk. Most of these patients have either very diffuse lesions with little focal enhancement on CT scan or have presented with epilepsy alone. Many physicians feel that such patients should not be operated upon at all at this stage, but merely treated for their epilepsy until such time as the glioma progresses. As the number of patients with gliomas suffering only from epilepsy increases, through more active investigation with CT scanning, the opportunity for treating gliomas earlier arises. As discussed by Saloman (1980) early diagnosis may give therapies the optimal chance of success. It is in this respect that biopsy has the greatest, and as yet unrealised, potential to influence the outcome in malignant brain glioma. For the majority of patients who presently receive biopsy alone, the procedure provides the necessary factual basis for their management and for the fortunate minority an alternative, less malignant, condition is disclosed.

THE INFLUENCE OF EXCISIONAL SURGERY

Despite the demonstration by Scherer (1940) that malignant brain gliomas are not localised or encapsulated tumours, the description by Maxwell (1946) of the frequency of interhemispheric extension, the fact that longevity following surgery is so unusual as to occasion reports in the literature (Netsky et al, 1950), neurosurgeons — myself included — continue to perform excisional surgery in patients who are neither moribund nor severely disabled. The rationale for such operations is based upon the following tenets: the patient, the family and the referring physician feel that definitive action is being taken; histological diagnosis is established more safely than by burrhole biopsy; internal decompression by relieving raised intracranial pressure and reducing neurological deficit improves the quality of survival; reduction of the volume of tumour renders the residuum more sensitive to adjuvant oncolytic therapy. The first of these is probably true, though as some neurologists rarely refer their patients with gliomas to a neurosurgeon, the need to feel that something is being done is certainly not universal. The second, although widely believed, is no longer tenable in patients adequately prepared with steroids and operated upon with fastidious technique, as demonstrated by Marshall et al (1974) and Shetter et al (1977) and already discussed above. The other possible advantages to accrue from excisional surgery will be discussed at length.

Excision of gliomas prolongs life?
Writing in 1958, Frankel & German bemoaned the paucity of articles concerning malignant brain glioma and indeed the basis for the belief that extirpation influences the outcome of the disease stems from a handful of reports. In considering these, it must be remembered that many span more than a decade during which time surgical practices concerning the general care of the patient may have changed considerably (Goldsmith & Carter, 1974). In addition, although it seems usual to distinguish between subtotal and gross total excision, I have reservations regarding the reality of this distinction especially when based upon retrospective reviews of other surgeons operation notes. Indeed, any estimate of the extent of radical excision not supported by cavity biopsies and postoperative CT scanning must be suspect. As none of the published series included the former and all preceded the latter, there is clearly room to question the actual proportion of tumour removed.

161

Davis et al (1949) reported a series of 211 cases of verified malignant brain glioma 187 of which were operated upon with a mortality (death within 1 month of operation) of 30.2%. Of the surviving 110, 18% of those receiving only an open biopsy, 21% of those having a subtotal resection and 26% of those in whom a gross total resection was achieved were still alive more than one year from operation. These figures do not take into account radiotherapy, re-operation, or the neurological state of the surviving patients and the small differences in survival rates between the groups suggests that excision had little influence on the outcome.

Frankel & German (1958) described 183 patients operated upon by many different surgeons between 1924 and 1952 with a surgical mortality (death within 1 week of operation) of 18.5%, an average survival of 3 months and 1 year survival of 13%. Two interesting findings emerge from this study; first, although those receiving 'total' resection survived longer than those having partial resection (22% of 50 cases alive at 1 year from operation compared with 8% of 105 cases), by 18 months there was little difference between the two groups. Furthermore, of 32 patients having a lobectomy, 40% were alive at 9 months from operation compared with 17% of 149 cases not receiving a lobectomy, but by 1 year, there was no difference between the two groups. This would strongly suggest that the principal influence of excision was merely the creation of an internal decompression rather than any fundamental effect on the tumour. Secondly, when survival from the onset of symptoms was compared between 178 operated cases and 30 unoperated cases, the median survival time was 9 months for the former and 5 months for the latter; percentage survival for the two groups was roughly the same by 12 months suggesting that the benefits of surgery only occur in the first year from operation and only modify the outcome for 3–6 months. This strongly supports the view of Saloman (1980), which I share, that median time to progression is more a measure of the palliative effect of surgery than of its biological influence.

In a retrospective study of 495 patients seen between 1928 and 1953, Roth & Elvidge (1960) found survival time from operation ranged from 11.5 months for incomplete removal to 18.4 months for 'complete' removal: if the effect of radiotherapy was eliminated there was little difference between the two groups except at 6 months from operation when the percentage surviving was 20.4% for imcomplete and 34.4% for 'complete' removal.

Hitchcock & Sato (1964), noting that encouraging results were more often due to selection than to treatment, reported 225 cases treated at Oxford between 1950 and 1960 with a median survival rate for the untreated (including the 58% with burrhole biopsy only) of less than 1 month compared to 3–6 months for those undergoing excisional surgery with or without radiotherapy. Although this implies a modest achievement for excision, there was interestingly no difference between external decompression and extirpation when both were followed by radiotherapy, the median survival for both groups being 9–12 months; this provides further evidence that any influence of excisional surgery is occasioned by the simple mechanical effect of creating space. Taveras et al (1962) also found only a slight difference between biopsy and excision when both were followed by radiotherapy: 100% of those having a biopsy being dead at 6 months from operation compared with 86% of those treated by excision being dead at 6 months and 96% being dead by 1 year.

The major proponents of radical excisional surgery have been Jelsma & Bucy (1967) who reported the outcome of 162 cases treated between 1945 and 1964 and later expanded this to 186 consecutive cases up to 1966 (Jelsma & Bucy, 1969). In their earlier report, the surgical mortality (death within 30 days of operation) was 21.7% overall, being least at 10.3% for patients undergoing extensive resection. The major factor in reducing surgical mortality, which was only 3% in 35 cases treated by extensive resection in the final 2 years of the study (Jelsma & Bucy, 1967), was the preoperative use of dexamethasone. Median survival from operation was 2 months for those patients having an external decompression (25 patients), 2.8 months for partial resection (19 patients) and 7.5 months for extensive resection (92 patients); partial resection was probably little more than an open biopsy. Only patients undergoing extensive resection survived more than 1 year from operation (27%), although whether they were symptom-free at that time was not recorded. This benefit of extensive resection was still apparent when only the patients in poor condition preoperatively were considered.

Jelsma & Bucy (1967, 1969) are the only authors reporting a major benefit from extensive resection possibly lasting longer than might be accounted for by the mere production of a large internal decompression. It is noteworthy that all their patients surviving longer than 2 years from operation were aged under 50 years, a powerful and favourable prognostic factor as shown repeatedly in the randomised trials of the Brain Tumour Group of the EORTC (1981) and the Brain Tumour Study Group (Walker et al, 1978). It is particularly unfortunate that Jelsma & Bucy (1967, 1969) did not give the age distribution of their treatment groups and this emphasises yet again the value of well-randomised trials over retrospective studies. Indeed, in two separate randomised trials designed to evaluate the effect of various chemotherapeutic agents on symptom free interval, the extent of surgery was not a prognostic factor (EORTC Brain Tumour Group, 1978, 1981). In another randomised trial of chemotherapy and radiotherapy (Walker et al, 1978) biopsy-only carried a worse prognosis than more extensive resection, but the former group was very small and 50% of the patients received ineffective chemotherapy as their only treatment.

If excisional surgery is at best of limited absolute value in malignant brain glioma what is its relative value in the therapeutic armamentarium? This question was addressed by Weir (1973) who performed a retrospective analysis of 248 cases operated upon by nine surgeons over the decade 1960 to 1970. Survival time from operation showed an apparent advantage from extensive resection in that 1 year survival was 28% of those undergoing 'total' excision compared to 18% for partial excision and 12% for biopsy, and there was a significant association between survival and extent of tumour removal. However, further analysis using a multiple regression equation showed radiotherapy to have a relative importance of 23.1% compared with age (5.9%) and all other factors including surgery (1.2%). Surgery would therefore seem *relatively* unimportant in prolongation of life in malignant brain glioma. This point was pursued by Saloman (1980) who extracted data on 2532 patients from 17 of the most frequently cited reports on malignant brain glioma appearing in the English literature and constructed survival curves from the fate of 1561 selected cases submitted to a major resection. The median survival was an unimpressive 6 months, only 7.4% surviving 2 years. Furthermore, for the 349 patients treated by extensive resection alone, the median survival was 4 months compared to 9.25 months in those receiving radiotherapy in addition to resection. The main determinant of survival in the first 18 months from operation is therefore not extirpation, but radiotherapy. This agrees with the experience of the population treated in Southampton; of 163 patients treated between 1965 and 1969 the average survival was 2.2 months for the whole group, and only 3.3 months for the 76 patients undergoing internal decompression (Garfield & Dayan, 1973).

If, therefore, excision is of limited benefit is 'second look' surgery of any value? The report of Roth & Elvidge (1960) included 13 patients having multiple operations, the interval between interventions ranging from 6 to 79 months. The survival from first operation extended from 8–83 months with a median of 31 months and a 2 year survival of 50%, compared with an overall median survival for their patients of 6 months and a 2 year survival of 8.8%. This apparently impressive result was hardly confirmed by the more modest achievements found in a detailed study of 24 patients by Young et al (1981); they reported a median survival of 62 weeks from first operation and 14 weeks from second operation and concluded that re-operation was only likely to produce a 'reasonable result' if the Karnofsky rating was 60 or over and the inter-operative period was greater than 6 months. Re-operation at the time of symptomatic recurrence would, therefore, seem to have little to offer in terms of delaying progression of the disease.

Does excision improve quality of survival?
Few would deny that rapid and gratifying improvement in a patient's condition may follow a timely internal decompression as advocated by McKenzie (1936) and reiterated by Taveras et al (1962). Jelsma & Bucy (1967) found that only amongst their group of patients undergoing extensive resection was there an absolute increase in the number able to enjoy life; preoperatively, only 8 out of 92 patients were able to work, but 3 months after extensive resection 40 were able to work and out of 25 still alive at 1 year from operation, 14 were still enjoying life. In a further analysis, Jelsma & Bucy (1969) found that even aphasic patients benefited from extensive resection, 67% showing postoperative improvement. They did not, therefore, share the views of Pennybacker et al (1950) and Hitchcock & Sato (1964) that biopsy was the only appropriate intervention in aphasic patients. I have only found patients under 60 years of age to show any great improvement in focal deficit following major excisional surgery and usually the greater proportion of this improvement has been achieved preoperatively by dexamethasone. The occasional relief of focal deficit by simple cyst drainage through a burrhole has already been mentioned. Re-operation for relief of symptoms is rarely justified except occasionally in younger patients with severe headache or incipient visual loss not controlled by acceptable doses of steroids. Young et al (1981) found that of patients who had achieved a symptomatic remission of 6 months from their first operation and who still had a Karnofsky rating of 60 or greater, only one third of those subjected to a second operation

would survive a further 6 months with Karnofsky rating greater than 60. At this level of function, patients are independent with assistance, but unable to work or go far from home unaided. Although Young et al (1981) did not condemn second operations, their observations lend little justification to the procedure.

Does excision affect the behaviour of malignant brain glioma?
The major achievement of extirpation is the reduction of tumour bulk to the point that radiotherapy and chemotherapy have a greater chance of success (Wilson & Hoshino, 1969). Unfortunately, these adjuvant therapies have failed to make much impact upon the disease, as discussed by Goldsmith & Carter (1974) and Saloman (1980), whose extensive analysis showed that excision plus radiotherapy achieved a median survival of 9.25 months extended to 10 months by addition of chemotherapy, compared to 4 months for excision alone. Clearly, the true potential of excision will only be realised when therapies are developed that take advantage of not just the bulk reduction achieved, but also the concomitant changes in growth fraction that accompany surgery (Hoshino et al, 1975; Norton & Simon, 1977). In the interim surely a more critical examination of the use of available treatments is called for?

As the main determinant of survival in the first 18 months from diagnosis is radiotherapy (Roth & Elvidge, 1960; Taveras et al, 1962; Weir, 1973; Saloman, 1980) should we abandon excision in our everyday, essentially palliative, management of malignant brain glioma? I am acutely aware that many physicians and surgeons feel that operative intervention should be limited to burrhole biopsy alone, further management whether aggressive or purely palliative proceeding according to the clinical state of the patient. In the light of the data reviewed, much of it drawn from retrospective and uncontrolled experiences spread over many years with little accounting for the known prognostic factors, there is ample justification for a randomised trial of biopsy plus radiotherapy versus maximal resection plus radiotherapy. As both groups would receive the most influential treatment available, namely radiotherapy, and as patients 'failing' on the biopsy arm could still procede to excisional surgery, there could be no objection that useful therapy was being witheld. Steroids would be used to provide early relief of distressing symptoms and given in a strictly scheduled way to both groups for a defined period. Both time from first symptom and time from surgery to either progression or death would be measured. Quality of survival would be closely followed using the Karnofsky scale (Karnofsky et al, 1948). Such a trial would examine critically both the 'curative' and the 'palliative' influences of excisional surgery.

CONCLUSION

Extensive resection of malignant brain gliomas, although widely practised, is probably only of palliative benefit. Whether the same palliation could be achieved by radiotherapy, based upon tissue diagnosis at burrhole biopsy, is not known because of the failure of surgeons to conduct randomised trials of surgical treatment. The full potential value of extirpation awaits the development of therapeutic modalities that are more effective in manipulating the changes that surgical intervention can induce in the complex and various cell pools of the tumour.

REFERENCES

Bender M B, Elizan T 1962 The non-surgical management of brain tumor. Transactions of the American Neurological Association 87: 20–24
Bennett A H, Godlee R J 1885 Case of cerebral tumour. The surgical treatment. British Medical Journal 1: 988–989
Cairns H 1935 The ultimate results of operations for intracranial tumours. Yale Journal of Biology and Medicine 8: 421–492
Cushing H 1932 Intracranial tumours. Notes upon a series of two thousand verified cases with surgical mortality percentages pertaining thereto. Thomas, Springfield
Davis L, Martin J, Goldstein S L, Ashkenazy M 1949 A study of 211 patients with verified glioblastoma multiforme. Journal of Neurosurgery 6: 33–34
EORTC Brain Tumour Group 1978 Effect of CCNU on survival rate, of objective remission and duration of free interval in patients with malignant brain glioma — final evaluation. European Journal of Cancer 14: 851–856
EORTC Brain Tumour Group 1981 Evaluation of CCNU, VM–26 plus CCNU and Procarbazine in supratentorial brain gliomas. Final evaluation of a randomised study. Journal of Neurosurgery 55: 27–31
Ferrier D, Macewen W, Horsley V, Jackson J H 1885 Discussion of paper by Bennett A H, Godlee R J Case of cerebral tumour. The surgical treatment. British Medical Journal 1: 988–989
Frankel S A, German U J 1958 Glioblastoma multiforme: review of 219 cases with regard to natural history, pathology, diagnostic methods, and treatment. Journal of Neurosurgery 15: 489–503
Garfield J S, Dayan A D 1973 Post-operative intracavitary chemotherapy of malignant gliomas. A preliminary study using methotrexate. Journal of Neurosurgery 39: 315–322
Goldsmith M A, Carter S K 1974 Glioblastoma multiforme: a review of therapy. Cancer Treatment Reviews 1: 153–165
Hitchcock E, Sato F 1964 Treatment of malignant gliomata. Journal of Neurosurgery 21: 497–505
Hoshino T, Wilson C B, Rosenblum M L, Barker M 1975 Chemotherapeutic implications of growth function and cell cycle time in glioblastomas. Journal of Neurosurgery 43: 127–135
Jelsma R, Bucy P C 1967 The treatment of glioblastoma multiforme of the brain. Journal of Neurosurgery 27: 388–400
Jelsma R, Bucy P C 1969 Glioblastoma Multiforme: its treatment and some factors affecting survival. Archives of Neurology 20: 161–171
Karnofsky D A. Abelmann W H, Craven L F 1948 The use of the nitrogen mustards in the palliative treatment of carcinoma with particular reference of bronchogenic carcinoma. Cancer 1: 634–656
Lorenz R 1940 Differential diagnose der arteriographisch darstellbaren, intrakraniellen Geschwulste: Glioblastom, Meningeom, Sarkom Zentralblatt fur Neurochirurgie 5: 30–61
McKenzie K G 1936 Glioblastoma. A point of view concerning treatment. Archives of Neurology and Psychiatry 36: 542–546
Marshall L F, Jennett B, Langfitt T W 1974 Needle biopsy for the diagnosis of malignant glioma. Journal of the American Medical Association 288: 1417–1418
Maxwell H P 1946 The incidence of interhemispheric extension of glioblastoma multiforme through the corpus callosum. Journal of Neurosurgery 3: 54–57
Moniz E 1931 Diagnostic des tumeurs cérébrales et épreuve de l'encéphalographie arterielle' Masson et Cie, Paris
Netsky M G, August B, Fowler W 1950 The longevity of patients with glioblastoma multiforme. Journal of Neurosurgery 7: 261–269
Northfield D W C 1973 The surgery of the central nervous system. Blackwell, London
Norton L, Simon R 1977 Tumour size, sensitivity to therapy, and design of treatment schedules. Cancer Treatment Reports 61: 1307–1317
Pennybacker J, Northfield D W C, Parsons-Smith G, Tutton G K 1950 Discussion on current treads in the management of the gliomata. Proceedings of the Royal Society of Medicine 43: 329–334
Roth J G, Elvidge A R 1960 Glioblastoma multiforme: a clinical survey. Journal of Neurosurgery 17: 736–750

Saloman M 1980 Survival in glioblastoma: historical perspective. Neurosurgery 7: 435–439

Scherer H J 1940 The forms of growth in gliomas and their practical significance. Brain 63: 1–35

Shackney S E, McCormack G W, Cuchural G J Jr 1978 Growth rate patterns of solid tumours and their relation to responsiveness to therapy: an analytical review. Annals of Internal Medicine 89: 107–121

Shetter A G, Bertuccini T V, Pittman H W 1977 Closed needle biopsy in the diagnosis of intracranial mass lesions. Surgical Neurology 8: 341–345

Taveras J M, Thompson H G Jr, Pool J L 1962 Should we treat glioblastoma multiforme? A study of survival in 425 cases. American Journal of Roentgenology 87: 473–479

Walker M D, Alexander E Jr, Hunt W E, MacCarty C S, Mahaley M S Jr, Mealey J Jr et al 1978 Evaluation of BCNU and/or radiotherapy in the treatment of anaplastic gliomas: a co-operative clinical trial. Journal of Neurosurgery 49: 333–343

Weir B 1973 The relative significance of factors affecting post-operative survival in astrocytomas grades 3 and 4. Journal of Neurosurgery 38: 448–452

White W H 1886 One hundred cases of cerebral tumour with reference to course, operative treatment, mode of death and general symptoms. Guy's Hospital Reports 43; 117–142

Wilson C B, Hoshino T 1969 Current trends in the chemotherapy of brain tumours with special reference to glioblastomas. Journal of Neurosurgery 31: 589–603

Young B, Oldfield E, H, Markesbery W R, Haach D, Tibbs P A, McComb P et al 1981 Reoperation for glioblastoma. Journal of Neurosurgery 55: 917–921

16. What has surgery to offer in cervical spondylosis?

Pauline Monro

Degenerative changes in the joints of the cervical spine are an almost inevitable accompaniment of ageing. On radiological evidence they occur in 75% of the population over 50 (Pallis et al, 1954) and are nearly universal by the age of 70 (Halt, 1954). Most of the time these changes are asymptomatic since joint pain (either local or referred) usually subsides with conservative measures, and immobility is not disabling with so many joints in the neck and the possibility of compensatory trunk movements.

Surgical treatment for cervical spondylosis is considered in those relatively few patients whose disability arises from secondary involvement of the soft tissues adjacent to the disordered joints; commonly the nerve roots, less frequently the spinal cord, and rarely the vertebral arteries. Is there any evidence that any of the surgical techniques are beneficial, and if so, when should they be used? Published results are conflicting. One reason is that the term 'cervical spondylosis' covers a wide range of radiologically demonstrated changes which (probably as a result of various combinations of distortion, compression and ischaemia, exacerbated by movement) produce the neurological disability that surgery is intended to alleviate.

PATHOGENESIS OF SPONDYLOTIC MYELOPATHY AND RADICULOPATHY

Distortion

Some degree of distortion of cord or root is always present and is due to tissue, either hard or soft, impingeing from any direction and at one or more vertebral levels. The cord is most frequently distorted anteriorly at an intervertebral level by thickening of the annulus fibrosus, extruded disc material, bony osteophytes or by anterior or posterior vertebral subluxation. These changes occur most frequently at the fifth, sixth or seventh cervical vertebral level where lordotic curvature and movement are greatest, but may occur throughout the cervical spine (Wilkinson, 1960; Friedenberg et al, 1959) and are often seen adjacent to congenitally, surgically or pathologically fused vertebrae. Posteriorly, thickening of the laminae and of the ligamentum flavum may produce cord distortion most

168

marked on neck extension when laminal overlap and ligamentous buckling can occur (Stoltmann & Blackwood, 1964; Adams & Logue, 1971c). Hypertrophy accompanying degeneration of the apophyseal joints is found less often and may occur independently of disc disease. It is most frequent in the upper cervical region where it may distort the cord postero-laterally (Epstein et al, 1978), whereas caudally these joints lie more antero-laterally.

Degeneration in the postero-lateral part of the intervertebral joint (the uncinate region) may distort the emerging nerve roots, most commonly the sensory roots, while the more inferiorly situated motor roots may be protected or differentially affected by protruding vertebral osteophytic ridges (Holt & Yates, 1966). Disordered apophyseal joints may involve the dorsal root ganglia at all levels.

Compression

In most people there is room in the cervical canal for adaptation to distorting tissues, and neuronal damage occurs only when there is severe disease, or congenital narrowing of the spinal canal. There is a close association between the acquired canal width and the development of myelopathy (Wolf et al, 1956; Payne & Spillane, 1957; Nurick, 1972a). Compression is most likely in the lower cervical region where the spondylotic changes are greatest and the cord and emergent nerve roots (which normally occupy about one-quarter of the exit foramina) are largest. However, there is a wide range of canal width in spondylotic myelopathy (Adams & Logue, 1971b) and although complete block of flow on myelography is common, it is frequently not seen and at surgery the cord may not appear compressed. Moreover, even in the presence of complete obstruction, surgery does not result in the same benefit which would be expected from the relief of a similar obstruction from some other cause. While this may in part reflect the chronicity of the lesion, it seems likely that other factors are of importance, as is also suggested by the often poor correlation between the site and extent of the compressing lesions and the clinical picture and the frequently diffuse pathological findings.

Movement

The cord may be traumatised by both anterior and posterior tissues as it moves a few millimetres rostrally and posteriorly on neck flexion and adapts to the change in shape and length of the cervical canal (Reid, 1960; Breig et al, 1966; Adams et al, 1971b). This effect may be exacerbated by 'tethering' of the cord anteriorly either by fibrosed and fixed nerve roots, which may be under tension especially if the kyphosis is exaggerated (Adams & Logue, 1971a), or by the dentate ligaments (Kahn, 1947), although the effect of the latter has been disputed (Stoltmann & Blackwood, 1966). Either fusion or disruption of intervertebral joints resulting in loss of normal alignment, angulation, or increased range of movement may exaggerate these effects on cord and roots.

Ischaemia

The pathological changes in the cord resemble those of ischaemia (Mair & Druckman, 1953) but there has been dispute as to whether the major contributing factor is anterior spinal artery compression, impairment of flow in the one or two radicular vessels which feed this artery below the third cervical segment (Taylor, 1964; Turnbull, 1973), or degenerative changes in the walls of those medullary and pial vessels shown by Breig et al (1966) to be distorted and attenuated on movement (Nurick, 1972a). Since the position of the anterior spinal artery makes it difficult to compress before distorting the smaller intrinsic vessels (Shimomura et al, 1968), since anterior spinal artery thrombosis is rare in association with cervical spondylosis (Hughes & Brownell, 1964; Scoville et al, 1976), and since the ischaemic changes may be in the boundary zone between anterior and posterior spinal arteries and not in the distribution of these vessels (Hawkins et al, 1975), it seems likely that local compression and ischaemia play an additive role in the production of cord pathology; experimental evidence supports this conclusion (Hukuda & Wilson, 1972; Gooding et al, 1975). The role of congestion, which is sometimes seen at surgery, has been disputed since it may be an artefact and venous drainage is very extensive.

Systemic factors
Theoretically, systemic disturbances which might impair cord perfusion could contribute to the pathology, particularly atherosclerosis. However, Nurick (1972a) showed that there was no association between spondylotic myelopathy and atherosclerosis elsewhere. The fact that the pathology in the spinal cord is confined to the cervical region and is closely associated with the degree of canal narrowing, distortion, and abnormal movement, and the rarity of major vessel occlusion makes it most likely that the major causes of spondylotic myelopathy are local and mechanical; hence the rationale for attempted surgical correction.

Trauma
It is likely that ageing of joint tissues together with a lifetime of minor traumas associated with neck movement, and the occasional more severe blow to the head or neck, contribute to the spondylotic changes. The role of surgery in acute cervical trauma will not be discussed. In the majority of patients over the age of 50 such trauma is likely to exacerbate any pre-existing spondylotic changes as well as possibly cause fractures, dislocation, disc prolapse or, more rarely, haematoma. Acute exacerbation of pre-existing myelopathy could, therefore, be due to any of these factors (Clarke & Robinson, 1956). Recovery to the pre-trauma level of disability may occur with conservative measures (usually steroids and immobilisation in a collar, or perhaps more effectively, traction). Deterioration presumably results from contusion in a chronically distorted, probably ischaemic, narrowly confined cord.

Prolapsed intervertebral disc
The diagnosis of prolapsed intervertebral disc is usually made only in the absence of spondylotic changes, and therefore usually under the age of 40, with acute onset of symptoms often after trauma. However, most reports of surgery for 'spondylotic' radiculopathy or myelopathy include patients with protruded disc material (e.g. Galera & Tovi, 1968, in 31 of 51 cases) and trauma is noted months or years before the onset of symptoms in 10–60% of cases. It is likely that local

170

osteophytic reaction to a prolapsed disc causes spondylosis at this level, and altered stresses in the vertebral column then predispose to similar changes at other levels.

SURGICAL TECHNIQUES

A number of different techniques have been used to treat the factors thought to be responsible for radiculopathy and myelopathy.

Radiculopathy
Soft or bony tissue distorting the nerve roots has been removed either posteriorly by laminectomy and foramenotomy at one or two levels, by partial removal of adjacent laminae, or by an anterior approach through the disc space. No difference in outcome has been shown whether the latter procedure has been followed by grafting with autologous bone dowell (Cloward, 1958), with a wedge (Smith & Robinson, 1955; Riley et al, 1969), using Kiel bone (Ramani et al, 1975), or by complete removal of the disc with no graft (Murphy & Gado, 1972; Harkinson & Wilson, 1975). Martins (1976), in a randomised study of 51 patients, found equally good fusion and results with or without grafting. Lunsford et al (1980a) found no difference between the results of any of the anterior techniques and favoured discectomy alone because of the lower morbidity.

Myelopathy

Posterior approach
Decompression. Laminectomy at the site of the major distortion gives poor results (Guidetti & Fortuna, 1969). It has been extended to levels above and below, to the level at which the dura no longer bulges posteriorly (Stoops & King, 1962), or to include the whole cervical spine (Aboulker, 1965). It has been combined with removal of the ligamentum flavum and sometimes of anteriorly situated hard or soft distorting tissue approached either transdurally or extradurally (Epstein et al, 1969). In attempts 'to give the cord more room' the dura has been opened and left open postoperatively, patched, and even attempts made to distend the space by nursing the patient head downwards postoperatively (Rodgers, 1961).
'Freeing the cord'. To give the cord more mobility the dentate ligament has been sectioned (Fager, 1973), a procedure subsequently stated to be of limited benefit and to carry increased risk of deterioration. Gorter (1976) collected the results of a number of series and quoted them as confirming this view, but since many reports of dentate section were published between 1952 and 1964, whereas other results were for subsequent years, no valid comparison is possible. Piepgras (1976) compared the results of laminectomy with and without dentate section carried out by a number of surgeons over 6 years at the same hospital and found neither additional benefit nor increased risk of deterioration (see Table 16.3b).
Improving the blood supply. Lateral extension of the laminectomy to include

the articular facets at one or more levels has been recommended on the grounds that freeing the fibrosed and tethered nerve roots would not only allow the cord to move posteriorly and obviate the necessity to remove anterior distorting tissue, but might also increase the radicular blood supply (Scoville, 1961; Stoops & King, 1962). The very variable position of the radicular feeding vessels must render the effectiveness of such a procedure unpredictable.

Immobilisation. Laminectomy has been combined with posterior fusion either locally or throughout the cervical spine (Gonzáles-Feria, 1975). Whether achieved by an anterior or posterior approach, immobilisation has been shown to promote resorption of osteophytes, as well as to diminish the movement of the cord.

Anterior approach
Intervertebral fusion, with or without removal of soft or hard distorting tissue using the anterior approach and the techniques previously described for radiculopathy, is also used in the treatment of myelopathy, the operation being carried out at up to four levels.

Multiple operations
Most series both for radiculopathy and myelopathy describe some patients who, having failed to benefit from one approach, show some improvement after a second or even third operation, either at different levels or using an alternative approach at the same level (e.g. Connolly et al, 1965).

THE ROLE OF SURGERY

Most clinicians treat spondylotic myelopathy or radiculopathy by immobilisation for varying periods, depending on severity and progression before considering surgery. The majority of surgical series do not question its role in radiculopathy and imply that it is mandatory in the presence of advancing myelopathy in order to 'prevent deterioration' and 'to give the best chance of improvement'. Do the results justify this approach?

Since there have been no randomised controlled trials of surgery versus non-intervention, any assessment of results, or the appropriate indications for its use, and indeed as to whether it would be justifiable to carry out such a trial, must be made by comparison of the non-random surgical series, which are often poorly documented, with the natural history about which information is sparse.

It is clear, from reports both of natural history and surgical series, that pure radiculopathy is seen more frequently than myelopathy (Mayfield, 1965) and that, while it is common for myelopathy and radiculopathy to occur together (Brain et al, 1952; Bradshaw, 1957; Wilkinson, 1960; Crandall & Batzdorf, 1966), the root disorder does not usually precede the myelopathy (Clarke & Robinson, 1956), and it is uncommon for patients presenting with pure radiculopathy to develop disabling myelopathy subsequently. None of Lees & Turner's (1963) 51 patients who presented with pure radicular features noticed any disabling cord disorder over a 2–19 year follow-up period, and only 1 of Nurick's 23 patients did so, and this patient had a narrow canal. It therefore seems likely that the absence of any later development of myelopathy in the many series of patients having surgery for radiculopathy is due mainly to the natural history of the disease, rather than a beneficial prophylactic effect of surgery, particularly if the canal is capacious.

The evidence suggests that pure radicular symptoms should be assessed and treated on their own merit, and not with a view to preventing the later development of myelopathy which, if not noted at presentation or shortly after, is unlikely to develop later. Pure radiculopathy will, therefore, be considered separately.

PURE RADICULOPATHY

Natural history
If there is no sensory or motor deficit it is not always clear whether pain radiating down the arm is referred from the joints of the cervical spine or is due to nerve root involvement. Whatever the aetiology the majority of such patients recover within a few weeks or months when treated conservatively. In a prospective study, the British Association of Physical Medicine (1966) showed that 75% of patients with such pain (with or without paraesthesiae) treated conservatively, improved markedly by 4 weeks, and there was no difference in those treated with traction or by a collar.

Lees & Turner (1963) showed that 22 of their 51 patients with pure radiculopathy were not only symptom-free within a few months, but remained so for the subsequent 2–19 years during which, although a further 15 had mild recurrent symptoms and 14 slightly more troublesome episodes, only 10 were described as 'moderately disabled' and only 1 had a more severe recurrence.

Surgery, therefore, has a limited role to play in the management of radiculopathy even if it can be shown to help the small number of patients with disabling symptoms persisting for more than a few months. There is obviously considerable variation in surgical practice as shown by the varying length of history in different series from only 1 week (Murphey et al, 1973) to years, and by Hunt's (1980) estimation that surgery is required for 0.3–2% of patients compared to Chirls' (1978) of 12%.

Results of surgery
Whichever approach is used, the results of surgery for pure radiculopathy are almost invariably good with 75–100% cure or improvement. The best results are those for soft disc protrusion and with the shortest history (Murphey et al, 1973) and follow-up period (Cloward, 1958). However, it is more than likely that many of these patients would have improved even if they had been managed conservatively. The length of history in the series in Table 16.1 suggests that surgery has been used mostly for patients with persistent disability, although in no paper is it clear whether the symptoms were unremitting or episodic. Symon (1971) suggested that 'soft' prolapsed intervertebral discs might have a better prognosis than 'hard' spondylotic changes, a suggestion supported by Connolly et al (1965) who showed 70% improvement with 'soft' discs compared to 30%

Table 16.1 Results of surgery for radioculopathy.

	n	Type	Length of history	Follow-up period	Outcome Excellent	Returned to work
Haft & Shenkin (1963)	29	Spondylotic	av 23 m	3–13 y	21	27
Laminectomy	21	Soft disc	av 8 m	3–13 y	16	20

					Improved %	Unchanged or worse %
Symon (1971) Laminectomy	129	From 4 reports			89	11
Gregorius et al (1976) Anterior approach	41	Mixed	1–12 y	2–10 y	76	24
Lunsford et al (1980a) Anterior approach	253	Soft Hard	av 15 m av 33 m	1–7 y	84	16

with 'hard'. However, neither Haft & Shenkin (1963) nor Lunsford et al (1980a) confirmed this. Lunsford et al (1980a), using an anterior approach for 253 patients showed that the overall results were not affected by the nature of the tissue removed, nor the number of levels operated on, although the morbidity was slightly higher in 'hard discs'. The recurrence rate in the follow-up period was the same at 38% and, although more patients with 'hard discs' sought medical attention for their symptoms, none required further surgery. The only clinical difference between the two groups was that the 'hard' discs had a longer preoperative history. Scoville et al (1976) used a posterior approach in 170 patients with radiculopathy of whom 28% had soft discs and reported 95% long-term improvement. Riley et al (1969) showed worse results if more than two levels were operated on.

Neither Gregorius et al (1976) nor Lunsford et al (1980a) found any significant correlation between the outcome and any preoperative factor including the length of history, trauma, severity of symptoms or the presence of neurological signs including muscle weakness or wasting. It should, however, be noted that only 36% of Lunsford's et al patients had any muscle weakness and only 6% atrophy, and return of muscle power occurred in more patients with soft (60%) than 'hard' (40%) discs. Moreover, 4 of the 24 patients described by Gregorius et al with impaired hand movements, due to sensory or motor deficit, were worse postoperatively. Brandt et al (1976), in a very poorly documented series, claimed that if muscle atrophy was present only 65% of patients with cervical spondylosis improved after surgery compared with 84% of patients with no atrophy, but their series included patients with combined radiculopathy and myelopathy, and they did not state whether the correlation was with respect to improvement in myelopathic or radiculopathic features.

Conclusion
The results of surgery for pure radiculopathy, both short- and long-term, indicate that it offers a good chance of improvement or cure whatever the nature of the distorting tissue and whichever surgical approach is used, with insignificant morbidity and negligible mortality. However, the natural history data and clinical

experience indicate that most patients treated conservatively recover after a few weeks or months. In some series the development of any neurological deficit has been taken as an indication for immediate surgery, but there is no good evidence that this or any other preoperative factor influences the outcome. The evidence, therefore, supports the practice of conservative treatment of patients with pain for a few months before considering surgery. It seems sensible to be guided as to the timing of surgical intervention in patients with functional disability by general principles, that is, by the severity of the disability, whether it be motor or sensory, in relation to the patients' everyday life, and by their ability to withstand surgery, and to operate on patients with disabling weakness before atrophy occurs. There is no evidence that early surgery to provide immediate relief of symptoms, which in the majority of patients improve with time, carries any long-term benefit.

Practice
When a patient presents with radicular symptoms, having taken X-rays to ensure that there is no foraminal enlargement or destruction, I follow these principles, taking particular care that the patient has a collar which efficiently immobilises the neck in a neutral position, that he can put it on himself, that it is sufficiently comfortable to wear continuously, and also that he has a soft collar for night-wear and analgesics for pain. While there is no statistical evidence to prove that a collar helps most patients appear to find relief. Very rarely indeed have persistent radicular symptoms led to myelography with a view to surgery which has been undertaken only when there is clear evidence, both clinically (or occasionally on electromyography) and radiologically, of the level(s) of the lesion(s).

MYELOPATHY

Natural history
Spondylotic myelopathy usually presents with spastic weakness of the legs. The arms may be similarly affected and, less commonly, there may be proprioceptive or spinothalamic loss, the latter occasionally either 'suspended', indicating a central cord lesion, or with a sensory level. These features may be unilateral but any associated radiculopathy, reported in 40–90% of cases, is commonly bilateral and at more than one level (Clarke & Robinson, 1956; Bradshaw, 1957; Crandall & Batzdorf, 1966).

The very few series analysing the natural history of myelopathy are of limited value since the numbers are small, all are retrospective, and most have been carried out during a period in which some other patients have been selected, on arbitrary criteria, for surgery. However, both Clarke & Robinson's (1956) and Lees & Turner's (1963) series confirmed the clinical impression that the natural history is variable, and that it is commonly episodic with periods of a few weeks to a few months or even years of deterioration interspersed with very long periods of stability, or sometimes of improvement. Such an episodic pattern was seen in 80% of Clarke and Robinson's 120 patients followed for 2–5 years, and in 41 of Lees and Turner's 44 patients seen for up to 40 years after the onset of symptoms.

Periods of slow continuous deterioration lasting 2–14 years were seen in 36% of Lees and Turner's and 20% of Clarke and Robinson's patients, of whom 1 in 5 showed late improvement after this period.

Effects of immobilisation
There have been no randomised controlled trials to show whether cervical immobilisation has any effect on the course of spondylotic myelopathy. Table 16.2 shows the few series that there are; the immobilisation was by a variety of methods, some of which are likely to be more efficient than others, for varying

Table 16.2 Outcome with conservative treatment.

	n	Follow-up (years)	Better	Unchanged	Worse
Clarke & Robinson (1956)	22	up to 5	14	8	0
Bradshaw (1957)	26	2	12	6	8
Lees & Turner (1963)	28	3–40	17	7	4
Roberts (1966)	24	up to 7	7	9	8
Nurick (1972b)	36	6–10	8	16	12
Total	136		58	46	32
%			43%	34%	23%

periods of time. The criteria for improvement or deterioration in these series were clearly stated and, except for Clarke and Robinson's patients, were based on the patients' mobility. All 8 patients in Lees and Turner's series who wore collars continuously for 1–10 years improved; the other patients wore collars for months only. Although these figures are of little value in assessing the effects of immobilisation, they indicate that patients who are not subjected to surgery may improve or remain unchanged, and that only a minority are likely to deteriorate.

The very long periods without any progression and the possibility of improvement led Lees & Turner (1963) to describe the myelopathy associated with spondylosis as 'relatively benign', a statement often quoted. However, at the end of their follow-up period, 39 patients (89%) were 'moderately' or 'severely' disabled; that is 21 had considerable difficulty in using their arms or walking, and 18 required assistance or were confined to a chair. In Roberts' series (1966) only those who showed a complete block on myelography were subjected to surgery, and of the remaining 24 patients treated conservatively 19 (79%) had markedly impaired mobility at the onset and at the end of 2–5 years the number had decreased to 15 (67%) of whom 7 required assistance in walking and 1 was chair-bound.

Prognostic indicators to the course of the disease
The very small numbers in these series, and in some the lack of information about accompanying myelographic findings, act against the identification of any

prognostic variables which might influence the outcome, and in most series none were found. Clarke & Robinson (1956) showed that whereas at *presentation* 76% of their patients had a spastic weakness in their legs, those who subsequently developed the most severe disability were the 20% whose *first symptoms* were sensory in the arms, while those whose *initial symptoms* were either of weakness in the legs (50%) or pain in the arms (20%) had a rather better prognosis. No other series reported this correlation.

Neither Nurick (1972b) nor Roberts (1966) found any correlation between the severity at presentation, the duration of history, the length of the follow-up and the outcome, thus reflecting the variable and episodic natural history previously described. Although trauma antedated, by varying periods, the onset of symptoms in some patients, in only very few was it associated with periods of deterioration (Lees & Turner, 1963). Bradshaw (1957) showed a significantly better outcome in those patients with radiological changes localised to one level, but Clarke & Robinson (1956) and Nurick (1972b) showed no association with the severity or extent of the radiological findings and the clinical picture. Nurick (1972b), who had shown a close association between the degree of narrowing of the spinal canal and the severity at presentation, found that neither the degree of narrowing nor the severity of obstruction to flow of contrast medium influenced the subsequent course; deterioration was linked only with age, occurring significantly more often in those over the age of 60.

Conclusion
From these limited data it seems that the disability at presentation may, in approximately equal numbers, remain unchanged, lessen or progress. In a few cases the progression is steady, but in most it is episodic with varying and often long periods of stability interspersed with shorter periods of deterioration, the cause of which is not known. It is against this unpromisingly sketchy background that the results of surgery must be evaluated. There is no firm evidence that any clinical or radiological features predict the prognosis except, possibly, the elderly, those with initial sensory symptoms in the hands, and those with multiple level disease are more likely to deteriorate. There are, therefore, no firm criteria on which to base either selection for surgery or assessment of the outcome.

Evaluation of the reports of surgery
Evaluation of the many small and retrospective series is extremely difficult because documentation has often been poor and there is no uniformity either between or within series in the preoperative clinical and radiological features of the patients, in the operative techniques used, and — of particular importance — in the criteria for assessment of outcome.

Preoperative variables
   Clinical features. The length of history varied from months to years, and it was usually assumed that steady deterioration had occurred before surgery and stability followed until the time of assessment. In only a few instances was the pattern of deterioration noted, information of particular importance in assessing the impact of surgery on a disease with such a variable course (Symon &

Lavender, 1967; Galera & Tovi, 1968; Gregorius et al, 1976; Adams & Logue, 1971c).

Patients with all gradations of disability have been operated on. Some had minimal defects while others were chronically bed-ridden. In some series no distinction was made between patients with pure radiculopathy and those with myelopathy, and others even included patients who, while they had radiological evidence of spondylosis, were eventually shown to have other diseases responsible for their neurological deficit, most commonly motor neurone disease or multiple sclerosis. Many authors stressed the possibility of mistakenly attributing myelopathy developing in patients over 50 to the spondylotic changes almost invariably found, and such false diagnoses vary in medical series between 10–17% (Clarke & Robinson, 1956; Bradshaw, 1957; Campbell & Phillips, 1960).

Some series excluded patients with a history of trauma but, in most, trauma at unspecified times preceding the symptoms was noted (10–60%).

Radiological features. In many series no details at all were given of the radiological findings. Although some stated the number of patients with block on myelography, no indication was given as to whether this was bony or soft, opposite a disc space, or situated anteriorly or posteriorly. If the canal was narrowed it was not stated whether this was due to diffuse congenital narrowing with superimposed focal distortion, multifocal degenerative disease, or subluxation. The range of movement was noted only by Adams & Logue (1971c).

Operative techniques
The multiplicity of techniques bears witness to the poor results. In some series, although patients had been subjected to the same operative approach at one or more levels, any combination of the additional procedures already mentioned may have been used, e.g. after laminectomy the dura may be opened, the dentate ligament sectioned, soft or hard tissue removed, or postoperative fusion carried out, and there is variation both between and within series. Similarly, with the anterior approach fusion alone may or may not be accompanied by removal of distorting soft or hard tissue. Selection criteria for subjecting patients to either an anterior or a posterior approach were not uniform; although the anterior approach was most often used for disease localised to two or three levels, this was not always so and patients with complete block may have been subjected to either approach.

Postoperative assessment
Follow-up varied from months to years and often information was based merely on patient self-assessment by post. Results were sometimes tabulated as 'good' or 'satisfactory' indicating lack of progression despite the fact that the natural history shows that this can occur spontaneously, even following prolonged periods of deterioration. The majority of patients were classified as 'improved', 'unchanged' or 'worse', but frequently no indication was given as to whether this applied to motor or sensory deficit or, most important of all, to the effect on radiculopathy or myelopathy. Some of these factors have exaggerated the benefits of surgery on myelopathy. In the carefully documented series in which attempts have been made to correlate the outcome with preoperative findings, the

small number of patients and the large number of variables has precluded any significant findings.

Conclusion
There must be considerable reservations about the interpretation of the results of many series and particularly of cumulative figures from the literature.

Hazards of surgery
The possibility not only of failure to improve, but of severe postoperative deterioration in myelopathy immediately or within 24 hours, particularly if attempts are made to remove anteriorly situated bony tissue whether this is done from a posterior or anterior approach, is well recognised, frequently mentioned, but poorly documented. Kraus et al (1975) described five cases and quoted five reports of such deterioration after Cloward's operation and suggested that this might result from interference with a radicular artery, as was also suggested by Sugar (1981). Mayfield (1966) suggested that the hazards were greater and the postoperative morbidity longer after the posterior approach, but gave no figures to support this. In many series for myelopathy one or two deaths attributed to surgery are reported (Stoops & King, 1962; Symon & Lavender, 1967; Epstein et al, 1969; Lunsford et al, 1980b).

Results of surgery for myelopathy
Although Nurick's cumulative figures (Table 16.3 a) are of limited value including, as they presumably do, a range from 25% improvement (O'Connell, 1956) to 83% improvement (Stoops & King, 1965), they do indicate that, despite the bias tending to exaggerate the benefits of surgery, the results after laminectomy in comparison to conservative management are not good. Nurick's own figures, which he collected from surgery performed at one hospital and categorised strictly according to mobility, were worse. Symon & Lavender (1967) carefully analysed their results after laminectomy followed by various other procedures (Table 16.3a) and concluded that surgery should be used for patients steadily deteriorating, despite the occasional postoperative deterioration, since some striking improvements were seen. Thirty of the 32 patients who had been steadily deteriorating were stabilised, and 14 of 16 patients stopped having episodes of deterioration. The significance of these findings is unclear since neither the length of history nor the postoperative period were stated. Phillips' (1973) poorer figures are not strictly comparable since patients were selected with diffuse disease on whom anterior surgery was considered impractical. The variable results claimed for laminectomy in the past decade shown in Table 16.3b are not well substantiated. There were no stated criteria for improvement except for Gonzáles-Feria's (1975) results after posterior fusion.

Since Galera & Tovi's (1968) report of improvement in only one and deterioration in 20 of 29 patients after anterior surgery, results in other reports have been very variable. Table 16.3c shows the results of three well-documented and carefully analysed series with strict criteria for improvement. Phillips (1973) compared his results with the natural history as recorded by Nurick and concluded that the anterior approach should be undertaken for patients with

Table 16.3 Myelopathy. Outcome after surgery.

	n	Length of history	Follow-up period	Better %	Unchanged %	Worse %
a. Laminectomy						
Nurick 1972b						
Cumulative figures	474			56	25	19
Own figures	36	?	?	37	44	18
Symon & Lavender (1967)	40	?	?	68	25	5
Bishari (1971)	59	weeks – 2 y	More than 5 y	61	25	13
Phillips (1973)	24	12<1 year 8>2 y	2–19 y	50	25	25
b. Laminectomy						
Fager (1973)						
Laminectomy & dentate section	37	?	1–7 y	68	26	6
Gonzáles-Feria (1975)						
Extensive laminectomy + immobilisation	20	months – 16 y	1–7 y	85	5	10
Piepgras (1976)						
Laminectomy	36	?	?	44	53	3
Laminectomy + dentate section	44	?	?	43	52	3
c. Anterior surgery						
Nurick (1972b) (Cum'tive)	123	43<1 y		55	41	4
Phillips (1973)	65	15>2 y	2–10 y	74	12	14
Gregorius et al (1976)						
Anterior + posterior	53	months – 25 y mean 4 y	10 y	33	44	22
Lunsford et al (1980b)						
Anterior	32	months – 2 years	1–7 y	50		50

disease localised to two or three levels. Lunsford et al's (1980b) figures were for eight surgeons removing bone and soft tissue from a varying number of levels, using different anterior techniques, without the aid of a microscope. Only half the patients improved and, since more than 70% showed deterioration of gait during follow-up, they were unconvinced of the benefits of surgery, either by their own results or by previous reports, and concluded that a randomised prospective trial should be undertaken. Gregorius et al's (1976) figures, which were very similar to those for cervical immobilisation, were combined results obtained by subjecting approximately half of their patients to laminectomy if they had disease at more than three levels, if the canal was less than 13 mm in diameter, or if there was laminal shingling (overlap), while patients with disease at one or two levels or with fixed kyphosis were subjected to anterior surgery.

Conclusion
The results of surgery for myelopathy using either the anterior or posterior approach are inconsistent and there is no uniformity of opinion. Some reports do

show a higher percentage of improvement and less deterioration than might be expected from the scanty natural history data. Is there any evidence of any factors before, at or after surgery which might explain these discrepancies, help to select patients who are likely to benefit, and indicate the appropriate operations?

Prognostic factors for outcome after surgery

Clinical. Most authors have shown no correlation between outcome and any preoperative feature, including age and length of history, but the most severely disabled tend to fare badly (Nurick, 1972b; Jefferson, 1970; Gregorius et al, 1976; Lunsford et al, 1980b). Nonetheless, many reports have included the occasional old, severely disabled patient who made a good recovery (e.g. Fager, 1973). Guidetti & Fortuna (1969) and Bishari (1971) thought the length of history was important in that, as might be expected, of the most severely disabled, those with the shortest history had the better prognosis, and in Phillips' (1973) series 86% of patients with symptoms for less than 1 year improved.

It has been suggested that a sensory level, either bilateral or more frequently as part of a Brown-Séquard syndrome, found in approximately 16% of patients with cervical spondylotic myelopathy, indicates soft disc protrusion, which might carry a better prognosis. However, this was found in only 3 of Scoville et al's (1976) 7 patients with soft discs, and it has been reported in 6 cases with 'hard' spondylosis (Jabbari et al, 1957), although the substantiation for such a diagnosis is poor in the only 2 cases they reported in detail. Only 3 of Jabbari et al's patients improved postoperatively. Although all Scoville et al's and Jabbari et al's patients with a sensory level showed a partial or complete block on myelography, such a block is frequently reported in its absence.

Galera & Tovi (1968) in their small series showed that postoperative deterioration was most likely to occur in patients with both root and cord dysfunction.

Radiological. No significant correlation has been shown between radiological features (e.g. the degree of block on myelography, the number of levels involved, and the degree of canal stenosis) and the outcome after surgery (Nurick, 1972b; Gregorius et al, 1976; Lunsford et al, 1980b), although Phillips' (1973) patients selected for anterior surgery on the basis of focal disease had a better outcome.

Type of operation. Although Gregorius et al (1976) showed no significant difference in outcome between those patients subjected to laminectomy for more generalised disease in comparison to those who had anterior surgery for focal disease, there was a tendency for the latter to do better, a trend also shown by Crandall & Batzdorf (1966) in a small number of patients, and by Phillips' markedly better results with an anterior approach. Comparison between series has little meaning for the reasons already given, but Piepgras' (1976) claims for laminectomy with or without dentate section were not as good as those of Gonzáles-Feria's (1975) very small series with posterior immobilisation after laminectomy (Table 16.3 b).

Tissue removed. The hazards of removing bone are frequently mentioned but there are only a few reports that the removal of soft disc material is followed by any better results (e.g. Scoville et al, 1976; Tedeschi et al, 1980).

Postoperative. In those series in which it has been described it is clear that the postoperative course is as variable as the preoperative one. Gregorius et al (1976) showed that the majority of patients who improved postoperatively had done so by 8 months, but that either improvement or deterioration could also occur after many months or years. Late deterioration has been observed after both the anterior and posterior approach (Galera & Tovi, 1968, Gregorius et al, 1976; Lunsford et al, 1980b). A possible explanation was put forward by Adams & Logue (1971c) who carried out laminectomy on 27 patients, followed them for 5 years postoperatively, and showed a significant increase in the range of movement in the sagittal plane in 6 of the 7 patients who deteriorated, compared to the 7 who improved.

Conclusion. The numbers of patients in the series are too small, the data too limited and the results too disparate to allow any soundly based conclusions. The results suggest only that age should not be a bar to surgery (particularly since the elderly are more likely to deteriorate if managed conservatively), patients with severe disability are more likely to improve if they have early surgery, and that those selected for anterior surgery on the basis of focal disease limited to a few levels may do better than those who have posterior surgery, particularly if soft tissue only is removed and if immobilisation of the spine is achieved and maintained.

What has surgery to offer patients with 'spondylotic' myelopathy?
The literature does not provide a clear answer. Although it is full of reports of patients who, having been deteriorating preoperatively, following surgery remain stable or improve, sometimes dramatically, this can occur with conservative management. These optimistic reports are balanced by others of deterioration, sometimes severe, and of occasional death. Uncertainty about the role of surgery will persist unless further attempts are made to assess carefully the effects of surgery on patients at different stages of disease, with different radiological findings, who may have different pathogenetic mechanisms requiring different, or possibly multiple, operative techniques for correction. Correlation is required of the effects of the various surgical approaches on the long-term radiological as well as clinical outcome since some surgery, while correcting one defect, may predispose to the development of others, e.g. hypermobility or degenerative changes adjacent to fusion. The minimum features to document are:

(1) *clinically* the pattern of deterioration, length of history, severity of involvement of motor and sensory, cord and root function; (2) *radiologically* the number of levels at which there is distortion, whether it is anterior or posterior, hard or soft, both the congenital and the acquired width of the canal at these levels, and the range of movement in the sagittal plane, and (3) *surgically* whether an anterior or posterior approach is used, the number of levels operated on, whether hard or soft tissue is removed and whether immobilisation is carried out.

Are the published results so equivocal in relation to the scanty knowledge of natural history that it would be justifiable to carry out a prospective randomised trial bearing in mind that recent advances in neurosurgery and anaesthesia might be expected to improve results (provided that the relevant pathogenetic mechanisms in the spine responsible for neurological dysfunction are being corrected or arrested)? Many surgical series have described patients who were deteriorating pre-operatively and most, but not all, series indicated a less than 25% chance of deterioration after surgery. Despite the known variability in the natural history it would, therefore, be difficult to justify withholding surgery from any patient who was continuing to deteriorate despite conservative management, particularly if independent mobility were threatened, and any trial would probably have to exclude such patients and offer them surgery.

The contradictory results and unpredictable outcome of surgery for multifocal disease with involvement of root and cord are such that it might be justifiable to randomise these patients for surgery, immobilisation in a collar, or no treatment. Although there is some evidence that patients with focal disease at one or two levels, and those with soft tissue distortion may have a good chance of improving after surgery, particularly if they have a short history, it is not known whether such patients have a similar outcome if managed conservatively. However, the ready amenability to surgery of the radiologically demonstrated abnormality and the possibly better results of surgery would make a randomised trial in such patients difficult to sustain.

The difficulties involved in any trial of the treatment of cervical spondylosis would be formidable in view of the large number of variables, the relatively few patients likely to be seen at any one centre, and the necessity for long-term follow-up with assessment of both clinical and radiological features. It is doubtful whether there would be sufficient participation from patients and clinicians to make such a trial feasible. However, even if no randomised trials were carried out, current medical and surgical practice is probably so variable that if sufficient physicians and surgeons at a number of centres were to document accurately the data previously indicated for patients treated medically and surgically, analysis of this might help to clarify the present confused picture. The analysis would not answer the question whether surgery benefited patients with myelopathy, but should indicate the probable outcome after particular operations carried out on patients with a particular radiological appearance at a particular stage of their disease. Such information would provide a firmer foundation of knowledge from which to predict the outcome and advise patients. It might also indicate those patients in whom a controlled trial would be justifiable and helpful.

Current practice

Faced with a patient with symptomatic spondylotic myelopathy, with or without radiculopathy, I advise myelography at presentation only if I think that surgical intervention will follow. The patient should be fit enough for surgery, and there must be the possibility that he would benefit from it, either by prevention of progression or by improvement of disability. Patients for whom I consider the hazards and discomforts of myelography outweigh any possibility of surgical benefit include those with a long history of cord disorder, with no recent deterioration, in whom independent mobility is not threatened, and who have *clinical* evidence of multi-level disease and, in addition *radiological* evidence of multi-level disease with sufficient bony narrowing of the canal to account for their neurological deficit. Clinical indications for myelography include a short progressive history, recent deterioration, significant difficulty in walking, and signs which can be accounted for by disease at one level only. Radiological indications for myelography in symptomatic cervical cord disorder include (1) disease at one or two levels only, (2) focal instability, (3) insufficient evidence of degenerative disease to account for the cord dysfunction with no narrowing of the canal, or (4) evidence of other pathology, e.g. widening of the canal or erosion of bone.

Those patients managed conservatively are fitted with collars with the same precautions previously described for those with radicular symptoms, and with particular care to ensure that the head is immobilised with the chin slightly down, a position which is often the most comfortable, and in which the antero-posterior diameter of the canal is widest. Although there is no proof that a collar helps, there is at least some theoretical justification. Any patient who does not have a myelogram at presentation is followed carefully, initially every 2 or 3 months but then at increasing intervals over a 2 or 3 year period, and investigation is undertaken if there is deterioration or no improvement.

The results of myelography are discussed with neurosurgical colleagues. In general, younger patients with focal anterior disease, those with a congenital narrow canal and with evidence of disc protrusion, or with localised subluxation and instability, and those with significant or progressive disability are more likely to have surgery. Patients with multi-focal diffuse disease are usually given a further 2 or 3 month trial period with a collar and surgery undertaken only if they continue to deteriorate.

REFERENCES

Aboulker J, Metzger J, David M, Engel P, Ballivet J 1965 Les myelopathies cervicales d'origine rachidienne. Neurochirurgie 11: 89–198
Adams C B T, Logue V 1971a Studies in cervical myelopathy. I Movement of the cervical roots, dura and cord and their relation to the course of the extrathecal roots. Brain 94: 557–560
Adams C B T, Logue V 1971b Studies in cervical myelopathy. II Movement and contour of the cervical spine in relation to the neural complications of cervical spondylosis. Brain 94: 569–586
Adams C B T, Logue V 1971c Studies in cervical myelopathy. III Some functional effects of operations for cervical spondylotic myelopathy. Brain 94: 587–595
Bishari S N 1971 The posterior operation — treatment of cervical spondylosis with myelopathy: long term follow up study. Journal of Neurology, Neurosurgery and Psychiatry 34: 393–395
Bradshaw P 1957 Some aspects of cervical spondylosis. Quarterly Journal of Medicine New Series XXVI 102: 177–208
Brain W R, Northfield D, Wilkinson M 1952 The neurological manifestations of cervical spondylosis. Brain 75: 187–225
Brandt R A, Fager C A 1976 Cervical spondylosis. Prognostic value of preoperative signs and symptoms. Arquives Neuro-Psiquiat (Sao Paulo) 34: 32–39
Breig A, Turnbull I, Hassler O 1966 Effects of mechanical stresses on the spinal cord in cervical spondylosis. A study in fresh cadaver material. Journal of Neurosurgery 25: 45–56
British Association of Physical Medicine 1966 Pain in the neck and arm: a multicentre trial of the effects of physiotherapy. British Medical Journal 1: 253–258
Campbell A M G, Phillips D G 1960 Cervical disc lesions with neurological disorder. British Medical Journal 2: 5197–5201
Chirls M 1978 Retrospective study of cervical spondylosis treated by anterior interbody fusion (in 505 patients performed by the Cloward technique). Bulletin of Hospital for Joint Disease 39: 74–82

Clarke E, Robinson P K 1956 Cervical myelopathy, a complication of cervical spondylosis. Brain 79: 483-510

Cloward R B 1958 The anterior approach for removal of ruptured cervical discs. Journal of Neurosurgery 15: 602-614

Connolly E S, Seymour R J, Adams J E 1965 Clinical evaluation of anterior cervical fusion for degenerative cervical disc disease. Journal of Neurosurgery 23: 431-437

Crandall P H, Batzdorf U 1966 Cervical spondylotic myelopathy. Journal of Neurosugery 25: 57-66

Epstein J A, Carras R, Lavine L S, Epstein B S 1969 The importance of removing osteophytes as part of the surgical treatment of myeloradiculopathy in cervical spondylosis. Journal of Neurosurgery 30: 219-265

Epstein J A, Epstein B S, Lavine L S, Carras R, Rosenthal A D 1978 Cervical myeloradiculopathy caused by arthrotic hypertrophy of the posterior facets and laminae. Journal of Neurosurgery 49: 387-392

Fager C A 1973 Results of adequate posterior decompression in the relief of spondylotic cervical myelopathy. Journal of Neurosurgery 38: 684-692

Friedenberg Z B, Edeiken J, Newton-Spencer H, Tolentino S C 1959 Degenerative changes in the cervical spine. Journal of Bone and Joint Surgery 41A: 61-70

Galera R, Tovi D 1968 Anterior disc excision with interbody fusion in cervical spondylotic myelopathy and rhizopathy. Journal of Neurosurgery 28: 305-310

González-Feria I 1975 The effect of surgical immobilisation after laminectomy in the treatment of advanced cases of cervical spondylotic myelopathy. Acta Neurochirurgica 31: 185-193

Gooding M R, Wilson C B, Hoff J T 1975 Experimental cervical myelopathy. Effects of ischaemia and compression of the canine cervical spinal cord. Journal of Neurosurgery 43: 9-17

Gorter K 1976 Influence of laminectomy on the course of cervical myelopathy. Acta Neurochirurgica 33: 265-281

Gregorius F K, Estrin T, Crandall P H 1976 Cervical spondylotic radiculopathy and myelopathy. A long term follow-up study. Archives of Neurology 33: 618-625

Guidetti B, Fortuna D 1969 Long term results of surgical treatment of myelopathy due to cervical spondylosis. Journal of Neurosurgery 30: 714-721

Hadley L A 1957 The covertebral articulations and cervical foramen encroachment. Journal df Bone and Joint Surgery 39: 910-920

Haft H, Shenkin H A 1963 Surgical end results of cervical ridge and disc problems. Journal of the American Medical Association 13: 312-315

Halt L 1954 Cervical dorsal and lumbar spinal syndromes. Acta Orthopaedica Scandinavica, Suppl. 17: 1-102

Hankinson H L, Wilson C B 1975 Use of the operating microscope in anterior cervical discectomy without fusion. Journal of Neurosurgery 48: 452-456

Hawkins J C, Yaghmal F, Gindin R A 1975 Cervical myelopathy due to spondylosis. Case report. Journal of Neurosurgery 48: 297-301

Holt S, Yates P O 1966 Cervical spondylosis and nerve root lesions. Incidence at routine necropsy. Journal of Bone and Joint Surgery 48B: 407-423

Hughes J T, Brownell B 1964 Cervical spondylosis complicated by anterior spinal artery thrombosis. Neurology 14: 1073-1077

Hukuda S, Wilson C B 1972 Experimental cervical myelopathy: effects of compression and ischaemia on the canine cervical cord. Journal of Neurosurgery 37: 631-652

Hunt W E 1980 Cervical spondylosis: natural history and rare indications for surgical decompression. Clinical Neurosurgery 27: 466-480

Jabbari B, Pierce J F, Boston S, Echol D E 1977 Brown Sequard syndrome and cervical spondylosis. Journal of Neurosurgery 47: 556-560

Jefferson A 1970 Myelopathy in cervical spondylosis: surgical treatment using a posterolateral approach. Journal of Neurology, Neurosurgery and Psychiatry 33: 716

Kahn C A 1947 The role of the dentate ligaments in spinal cord compression and in the syndrome of lateral sclerosis. Journal of Neurosurgery 4: 191-199

Kraus D R, Stauffer E S, 1975 Spinal cord injury as a complication of elective anterior cervical fusion. Clinical Orthopaedics and Related Research 112: 130-141

Lees F, Turner J W A 1963 Natural history and prognosis of cervical spondylosis. British Medical Journal 2: 1607-1610

Lunsford L D, Bissonette D J, Janetta P J, Sheptak P E, Zorub D S 1980a Anterior surgery for cervical disc disease. Part I Treatment of lateral cervical disc herniation in 253 cases. Journal of Neurosurgery 53: 1-11

185

Lunsford L D, Bissonette D J, Zorub D S 1980b Anterior surgery for cervical disc disease. Part 2 Treatment of spondylotic myelopathy in 32 cases. Journal of Neurosurgery 53: 12-19

Mair W G P, Druckman R 1953 The pathology of spinal cord lesions and their relation to the clinical features in protrusion of cervical intervertebral discs. Brain 76: 70-91

Martins A N 1976 Anterior cervical discectomy with and without interbody bone graft. Journal of Neurosurgery 44: 290-295

Mayfield E H 1965 Cervical spondylosis, observations based on surgical treatment of 400 patients. Post Graduate Medicine 38: 345-357

Mayfield E H 1966 Cervical spondylosis. A comparison of the anterior and posterior approaches. Clinical Neurosurgery 13: 181-188

Murphey F, Simmons J C H, Brunson B 1973 Surgical treatment of laterally ruptured cervical discs. Review of 648 cases 1939-1972. Journal of Neurosurgery 38: 679-683

Murphy M G, Gado M 1972 Anterior cervical discectomy without interbody graft. Journal of Neurosurgery 37: 71-74

Nurick S 1972a The pathogenesis of the spinal cord disorder associated with cervical spondylosis. Brain 95: 87-100

Nurick S 1972b The natural history and the results of surgical treatment of the spinal cord disorder associated with cervical spondylosis. Brain 95: 101-108

O'Connell J E A 1956 Cervical spondylosis. Proceedings of the Royal Society of Medicine 49: 202-208

Pallis C, Jones A M, Spillane J D 1954 Cervical spondylosis. Brain 77: 274-289

Payne E E, Spillane J D 1957 The cervical spine. An anatomico pathological study of 70 specimens using a special technique with particular reference to the problem of cervical spondylosis. Brain 80: 571-596

Phillips D G 1973 Surgical treatment of cervical spondylosis. Journal of Neurology, Neurosurgery and Psychiatry 36: 879-884

Piepgras D G 1976 Posterior decompression fdr myelopathy due to cervical spondylosis: laminectomy alone versus laminectomy with dentate ligament section. Clinical Neurosurgery 24: 508-515

Ramani P S, Kalbag R M, Sengupta R P 1975 Cervical spinal interbody fusion with Kiel bone. British Journal of Surgery 62: 147-150

Reid J D 1960 Effects of flexion-extension movements of the head and spine upon spinal cord and nerve roots. Journal of Neurology, Neurosurgery and Psychiatry 23: 214-221

Riley L H et al 1969 The results of anterior interbody fusion of the cervical spine. Review of 93 consecutive cases. Correlation with post operative movement. Journal of Neurosurgery 30: 127-133

Roberts A H 1966 Myelopathy due to cervical spondylosis treated by collar immobilisation. Neurology 16: 961-954

Rogers L 1961 The treatment of cervical spondylotic myelopathy by mobilisation of the cervical cord into an enlarged spinal canal. Journal of Neurosurgery 18: 490-492

Scoville W B 1961 Cervical spondylosis treated by bilateral facetectomy and laminectomy. Journal of Neurosurgery 48: 423-428

Scoville W B, Dohrmann G J, Corkill G 1976 Late results of cervical disc surgery. Journal of Neurosurgery 45: 203-210

Shimomura Y, Hukuda S, Mizuno S 1968 Experimental study of ischaemic damage to the cervical spinal cord. Journal of Neurosurgery 28: 565-581

Smith G W, Robinson R A 1955 Anterior cervical disc removal and interbody fusion for cervical disc syndrome. Bulletin of John Hopkins Hospital 96: 223-224

Stoltmann H F, Blackwood W 1964 The role of the ligamenta flava in the pathogenesis of myelopathy in cervical spondylosis. Brain 87: 45-50

Stoltmann H F, Blackwood W 1966 The role of the dentate ligament in the pathogenesis of myelopathy in cervical spondylosis. Journal of Neurosurgery 24: 43-46

Stoops W L, King R B 1962 Neural complications of cervical spondylosis, their response to laminectomy and foramenotomy. Journal of Neurosurgery 19: 986-999

Stoops W L, King R B 1965 Chronic myelopathy associated with cervical spondylosis: its response to laminectomy and foramenotomy. Journal of the American Medical Association 192: 281-284

Sugar O 1981 Spinal cord malfunction after anterior cervical discectomy. Surgical Neurology 151: 4-8

Symon L 1971 Surgical treatment. In: Marcia Wilkinson (ed) Cervical spondylosis, its early diagnosis and treatment, 2nd edn. Heinemann, London, ch 8, p 154

Symon L, Lavender P 1967 The surgical treatment of spondylotic myelopathy. Neurology 17: 117-127

186

Taylor A R 1964 Vascular factors in the myelopathy associated with cervical spondylosis. Neurology 14: 62–68

Tedeschi G, Cerillo A, Falivene R, Mottolese C, Vizioli L 1980 Cervical myelopathy by spondylosis, limits and results of decompressive laminectomy. Acta Neurologica (Italia) 35: 191–195

Turnbull I M 1973 Blood supply of the spinal cord, normal and pathological considerations. Clinical Neurosurgery, ch 5, 56–84

Wilkinson M 1960 The morbid anatomy of cervical spondylosis and myelopathy. Brain 83: 589–616

Wolf B, Khilnani M, Malis L 1956 Sagittal diameter of bony cervical canal and its significance in cervical spondylosis. Journal of Mount Sinai Hospital 23: 283–296

187

17. Uncertainties in degenerative lumbar spondylosis

John Garfield

INTRODUCTION

Degenerative lumbar spondylosis (DLS) is a term which conveniently emcompasses a number of pathological components and singly or in combination these components may contribute to a complex symptomatology. That is a naive and facile statement which has led to a correlation between pathology, radiology and symptomatology which is often without foundation, an observation which is supported by the frequent but incidental finding of the radiological features of severe DLS on plain radiographs or myelography in patients who have no symptoms of that disease. Furthermore, the natural process of ageing leads to the 'pathological' changes of DLS, which have been clearly documented in autopsy studies on subjects taken at random from a general population (Roberts, 1978). Those studies have been used (rightly) to illustrate the radiological features of the 'disease', and to draw a tacit conclusion about their relationship to symptoms. It is those aspects which make clinical assessment and its correlation with radiological findings, and decisions before and during surgery so difficult. With that background it is hardly surprising that the long-term results of surgery may be disappointing. It is these inconsistencies which may lead to confusion in physicians' and surgeons' minds about the nomenclature of degenerative disease of the lumbar spine, about their description of radiological features, and the indications for and against the type of surgery. Indeed some retrospective studies, and especially those of patients with 'prolapsed lumbar disc' are not even aware of this confusion. By the same token, what one surgeon may describe operatively as a disc protrusion, another will describe simply as one of the less significant features of DLS.

In an effort to clarify, or at least display these difficulties, the following aspects will be considered briefly in this chapter: the pathological components of DLS; the symptomatology and its mechanism; correlation between radiological abnormalities and symptoms; the indications for surgery; errors at surgery and results.

PATHOLOGY

The degree to which true *disc prolapse* contributes to DLS is often difficult to establish, even at operation. DLS is a disease of the middle-aged or elderly but the natural history and ageing of the intervertebral disc (Jonck, 1961) (with the dessication of the nucleus pulposus, and progressive fibrosis of the annulus) are not conducive to disc bulging, protrusion and extrusion. However, in the distant past there may have been an episode of acute low back pain with or without radiation to a lower limb; that episode may have been solitary or recurrent in bouts over the years. Although the initial episode may have been consistent with an acute disc protrusion, it is rare to find a true disc protrusion at surgery many years later. Instead the longitudinal ligament over the disc space (or what little remains of that space) may be displaced backwards smoothly, but not acutely, by a combination of thickened fibrotic annulus, fragments of dessicated fibrotic nucleus 'pulposus', and hard bony ridges extending across the full width of the contiguous posterior margins of the vertebral bodies. The word 'osteophyte' used to describe those changes is somewhat misleading; that is better reserved for more specific and circumscribed osteophytes related to the intervertebral foramina. Reactive bony lipping of the vertebral bodies is a more appropriate description, at least surgically, and may help to avoid an unwarranted and usually futile surgical attack upon the 'disc'.

The *posterior or interlaminar joints* have become in recent years the centre of much interest in the pathology and symptomatology of DLS (Epstein et al, 1972; Epstein et al, 1973). These synovial joints seem particularly prone to degenerative changes which may be described as osteoarthritis (Badgley, 1941), but that description is not entirely accurate, and does not emphasise the changes which are the most significant in contributing to the symptomatology of DLS. Thus the joint surfaces of the superior and inferior facets usually remain smooth and the joint space is preserved even when the disease is advanced; but there is gross and quite disproportionate enlargement of the facets and articular processes which bear them. These form solid masses of bone, often dense or 'ivory' rather than cancellous, which compress severely the structures at the intervertebral foramina (nerve roots and radicular arteries), and the main theca (Ciric et al, 1980). Whether these changes are secondary to degeneration and dessication of the intervertebral discs and subsequent weight-bearing by the interlaminar joints (Jonck, 1961), or whether the changes are primary, is a matter for speculation, but if the changes are not recognised preoperatively and are mistaken for disc protrusion, the results of surgery will be disappointing.

The *ligamenta flava* may also contribute to pathology. In anatomical diagrams the ligamentum is often represented as extending mid-way or perhaps three-quarters of the distance from the apex to the lateral angle of the cross-section of the canal. In fact the ligamenta flava may extend out to the lateral angles. Furthermore, they become thickened and buckled in DLS, and thus act as one of the elements compressing the theca and the nerve root sheaths. Indeed the final manoeuvre in achieving a thorough decompression of a root is the excision of the portion of ligamentum squeezed between the root and the overlying enlarged facet and articular process of the interlaminar joint.

The *pre-exising sagittal diameter* of the lumbar spinal canal has been the subject of careful studies in recent years (Roberts, 1978). When compression or constriction of the theca is the main pathology, the pre-existing diameter will increase that compression; when it is compression of the root sheaths by the interlaminar joints it is less likely to be a significant factor. It is therefore difficult to establish exactly what part the pre-existing sagittal diameter plays in the production of symptoms in an individual.

A degree of *spondylolisthesis* may occur in DLS, or at least on the lateral radiographs there may be an apparent forward movement of one vertebral body relative to the adjacent body. This is not associated with a defect in the pars interarticularis as occurs in 'congenital' spondylolisthesis (Fitzgerald & Newman, 1976). Whatever the precise causation, the effect of the malalignment is to aggravate the compression or constriction due to the factors already described.

SYMPTOMATOLOGY AND ITS MECHANISM

The symptoms of DLS may be considered under four headings: back pain; lower limb pain; neurological deficit and disturbance of bladder function.

Back pain
It is often difficult to establish accurately the pathology which is mainly responsible for back pain and, therefore, the results of surgery in that respect are disappointing. The interlaminar joints have a sensory nerve supply, as do any synovial joints, and therefore joints if disorganised may be largely responsible for the back pain. However, the evidence for this mechanism is not secure, although operations have been devised on that basis. It is realistic to accept that the precise mechanism of back pain in DLS cannot be established, so that the surgery for that particular symptom is assigned to a realistic and reserved position.

Lower limb pain
Pain of a root distribution is less common than in true disc protrusion. It is usually more diffuse and occurs particularly over the buttocks. It is often difficult to determine the roots which are selectively compressed because the compression may be a combination of central pressure upon the theca and root entrapment laterally (Epstein et al, 1972). There is good evidence that posture plays a part in the production of lower limb pain, in that a slight forward tilt of the trunk may lessen the pain, whereas full extension and thereby accentuation of the lumbar lordrosis may increase pain (Magnaes, 1982).

The symptoms variously called 'neurogenic claudication', 'intermittent claudication of the cauda equina', or 'neurogenic intermittent claudication' are of neurological interest and still of disputed physiology (Blau & Logue 1961, 1978; Wilson, 1969). Considering how common are the changes of DLS already described it is curious how rare these clinical symdromes are. It is the intermittency which has caused greatest dispute and it would seem reasonable to seek factors in addition to those of DLS. If a vascular basis, including 'steal' to the lower limbs on exercise is accepted, then the pathology must include compression of the ascending radicular arteries at the intervertebral foramina, and the presence of atheroma in the aorta, lumbar and radicular arteries. The factor of movement of an individual nerve root on exercise leading to irritation of the root at its intervertebral foramen, and reactive 'oedema' which increases the pressure upon the root, are less convincing. The presence of upper motor neurone signs in DLS is often difficult to assign to a specific pathology, particularly because cervical spondylotic myelopathy of a mild degree is not rare in this age group. However, that in conjuction with a mild sensory level higher than would be expected from the level of the skeletal changes shown on plain radiographs and myelography, supports a vascular disturbance through compression or atheroma of the ascending radicular arteries, which supply the cauda equina and the conus medullaris. These factors have implications for the extent and results of surgery.

Overt *neurological deficit* in the lower limbs is unusual in DLS, whether it be at rest or on exercise as in neurogenic intermittent claudication. Beyond impairment of pin prick in the L5 and S1 segments, or a more patchy and indefinite impairment below the groins, objective sensory loss is rare, even in those patients who present with disturbance of micturition (see below). Motor deficit is rarely more than a mild degree of foot-drop and although wasting of the buttocks may be observed, there is usually little disability due to weakness of these muscles. If motor or sensory deficit is marked, spinal tumour is a more likely diagnosis than DLS.

The relationship of *disturbance of micturition* to DLS remains something of a mystery, despite reports of urological presentation in DLS. Chronicity is striking, as is the uncomplaining attitude of the female who is prepared to accept urinary incontinence or retention, with or without backache for many years (Sharr, Garfield & Jenkins 1976). The usual pattern of disturbance is the atonic or lower motor neurone bladder. However, the uninhibited (hypertonic, upper motor neurone) bladder may occur, that implying a disturbance of the conus which is presumably secondary and ischaemic. In some patients the bladder symptoms occur in association with those of neurogenic intermittent claudication. Although a careful analysis of the urinary symptoms may indicate which type of neurological bladder disturbance is present, it is notable that the cystometrogram is unequivocally abnormal in less than a third of patients.

There are difficulties in correlating the severity of the spinal pathology in DLS with the presence or severity of the bladder symptoms. Some patients with severe skeletal changes are spared all urinary symptoms whereas others with very mild posterior compression of the theca have striking bladder symptoms of an atonic or hypertonic type. Since the majority of patients who present with bladder symptoms are female, in whom stress incontinence may be a feature, gynaecological disease such as pelvic prolapse may add further confusion to an already difficult problem. It is therefore not surprising that the indications for surgery are debatable, and the longer term follow-up after surgery does not always substantiate the earlier favourable results.

CORRELATION BETWEEN RADIOLOGICAL FINDINGS AND CLINICAL FEATURES

Pathological changes are responsible for characteristic radiological findings. Plain radiographs of the lumbar spine may show general degenerative abnormalities and especially enlargement and sclerosis of the posterior joints, loss of disc spaces, lipping of the posterior margins of the vertebral bodies, reduction of the sagittal diameter of the spinal canal, and mild degrees of spondylolisthesis; calcification in the wall of the abdominal aorta may also be relevant. Myelographic abnormalities include constriction of the contrast column opposite the disc spaces at several levels, often severe enough to produce fragmentation of the column. This 'wasting' or pinching is characteristic and may, quite erroneously, be called 'disc protrusion', thereby leading to errors of diagnosis and management. The myelographic abnormalities are, above all, due to the severe postero-lateral compression of the theca by the enlarged posterior (interlaminar) joints, and the associated thickening of the ligamenta flava.

In assessing the relevance of these radiological features great difficulties arise because such changes may be demonstrated in patients who have no symptoms of DLS. This is well seen in patients undergoing myelography for other reasons such as spinal tumour or cervical spondylosis and in whom the lumbar theca is examined. Certainly the abnormalities are more common in the elderly, and that is consistent with the pathological features being those of ageing, which may be more or less premature. This also poses the question: what, at the age of say 65, is an abnormal lumbar myelogram?

Conversely, as was found in patients presenting with bladder symptoms, the degree of deformity of the theca may be mild, and simply restricted to slight irregularities of its posterior aspect. Nevertheless some patients with such radiological features obtained relief of their urinary symptoms after decompressive lumbar surgery. Therefore in the light of our present knowledge it is not always possible to correlate the radiological findings with the presence or severity of symptoms. If symptoms warrant surgery, however, the severity of the radiological abnormalities gives some guide to the likelihood of surgery being effective; and the extent of the abnormalities are an essential guide to the extent of the surgery that is required.

SURGICAL ERRORS

The *decision to proceed to surgery* depends first and foremost upon the severity of symptoms and secondly upon the severity of the radiological abnormalities. Because of the difficulty in correlating the severity of clinical and radiological features, surgery for relatively mild symptoms with severe radiological abnormalities is usually unsuccessful. Unfortunately the converse is not always the case. A further difficulty arises with 'neurogenic claudication' in which it is often impossible to differentiate between the DLS and atheroma affecting the lumbar and radicular arteries. Often in the elderly the two coexist. Further confusion may arise when true 'intermittent claudication', that is ischaemic pain arising in the lower limb muscles on exercise, may also be present. The absence of distal lower limb pulses (e.g. post. tibials), while indicating the presence of atheroma, may not help to differentiate between the vascular and spinal components in neurogenic claudication, but will help to assess the factor of lower limb muscle ischaemia. Another difficulty is that the compression of the radicular arteries may be mainly at the intervertebral foramina, without much compression or 'waisting' of the theca seen myelographically.

The *technical errors in surgery* are mainly concerned with failures to deal adequately with all the compressive factors, and failure to cover the relevant levels. 'Laminectomy' is not sufficient to achieve a satisfactory decompression of the theca and nerve roots. That requires a painstaking and lengthy exposure of the main theca and the nerve roots, the major battle being with the 'granite-like' masses of bone which have developed from the pedicles and articular facets (Shenkin & Hash, 1976; Ciric et al, 1980). The initial step of removal of the central part of the laminae is not without its problems; the dura may be adherent to the thickened and buckled ligamenta flava and great care is needed in their separation. If the dura is torn and c.s.f. escapes, the dura collapses and bleeding from extradural veins may obscure the field and make thorough exposure of the nerve roots very difficult. Furthermore, once the dura becomes slack the risk of catching it in bone-nibbling instruments increases.

If the surgeon has been misled clinically and radiologically into a diagnosis of disc protrusion, he may spend fruitless hours trying to remove bony ridges and scanty fibrotic disc material from in front of the main theca. That may be not only irrelevant and technically impossible, but also dangerous because of retraction of the theca and pressure upon an already compromised cauda equina especially if a wide posterior and posterolateral decompression has not been done.

RESULTS OF SURGERY

Because of the diagnostic, radiological and surgical difficulties, it is not surprising that the results of decompressive surgery may be unpredictable and sometimes disappointing. That is not to deny that surgery may be very effective in relieving certain symptoms, but much depends upon the careful selection of patients for surgery and the thoroughness of that surgery (Verbiest, 1977). As with other degenerative diseases, the longer the postoperative follow-up, the more disappointing are the results, an aspect that is not always referred to in papers dealing with and often extolling the virtues of operation, and very few papers attempt to assess the quality and thoroughness of surgery and their influence upon results.

Backache is the symptom which is least helped by decompressive surgery. That is not surprising because the genesis and pathology of backache in DLS is not clear. If the pain arises in the diseased posterior joints, then excision of one or both facets might relieve pain; that is certainly an opinion which, so far, cannot be substantiated. However, there is no evidence that removal of facets in DLS contributes to any spinal instability (Shenkin & Hash, 1976) and if it is necessary to remove facets to expose roots, the surgeon should not hesitate to do so. Overall, if backache is the predominant symptom in DLS, decompressive surgery is not advisable, but moderation of activity, and the wearing of a well-fitting lumbar support may bring some relief.

Persistent root symptoms in the lower limbs, in the presence of severe radiological changes, are those most likely to be helped by decompressive surgery, provided that surgery is extensive and thorough. Buttock pain (which must be carefully differentiated from sacro-iliac joint pain), thigh pain, and lateral leg (peroneal) pain may be relieved dramatically, and thereby mobility much improved. Unfortunately improvement in mobility may bring backache to the fore later, but provided the decompression has been thorough, and atheroma is not a major feature 'neurogenic claudication' is not usually a later problem.

'Neurogenic claudication' may, in itself, merit surgery, but the difficulties of genesis and pathology have been discussed. The early postoperative results are reasonable but personal experience is that after the first 6 months the improvement is often not maintained. Whether that reflects arterial rather than skeletal disease as the main pathology is a matter of speculation.

Bladder symptoms may be relieved dramatically, for reasons which are still obscure, and with little correlation between the clinical and radiological findings (Sharr, Garfield & Jenkins 1976). Since bladder symptoms, and incontinence in particular, may be especially disabling and distressing, surgery is more than justified, provided there has been thorough urological assessment to exclude primary urological disease. Unfortunately the initial enthusiasm for surgery for these curious symptoms has been tempered by longer follow-up, because urological symptoms have recurred in some patients in whom the initial improvement was very difficult to understand.

CONCLUSIONS

As in so much of medicine and surgery correlation between pathology, radiology and symptomatology in DLS is often difficult. It is all too easy to invoke features which are no more than the effects of normal ageing in order to explain symptoms and, conversely, to dismiss those same findings as irrelevant in the absence of symptoms. Pain in the lower limbs is perhaps the least difficult to explain on the basis of compression or constriction of the cauda equina, but as soon as the factor of ischaemia is added, correlation becomes more difficult. The explanation of bladder symptoms is often pure speculation.

It is not surprising, therefore, that the results of surgery in the long-term are variable and unpredictable. The surgery itself is not for the 'amateur' because decompression must be done with great care and thoroughness, and is not concerned with 'disc protrusion', a term which is still erroneously applied to these cases. In the elderly this surgery is a major undertaking.

Nevertheless, provided that all features of the pathology are considered before and during operation, surgery may bring considerable relief of lower limb pain and bladder symptoms. Above all the decision to proceed to surgery should depend more upon the degree of disability than upon the severity of the radiological abnormalities.

REFERENCES

Badgley C E 1941 The articular facets in relation to low back pain and sciatic radiation. Journal of Bone and Joint Surgery 23: 481–496
Blau J N, Logue V 1961 Intermittent claudication of the cauda equina. An unusual syndrome resulting from central protrusion of a lumbar intervertebral disc. Lancet 1: 1081–1086

Blau J N, Logue V 1978 The natural history of intermittent claudication of the cauda equina. Brain 101 (part II): 211–222

Ciric I, Mikhael M A, Tarkington J A, Vick N A 1980 The lateral recess syndrome. A variant of spinal stenosis. Journal of Neurosurgery 53: 433–443

Epstein J A, Epstein B S, Rosenthal A D, Carras R, Lavine L S 1972 Sciatica caused by nerve root entrapment in the lateral recess: the superior facet syndrome. Journal of Neurosurgery 36: 584–589

Epstein J A, Epstein B S, Lavine L S, Carras R. Rosenthal A D, Sumner P 1973 Lumbar root compression at the intervertebral foramina caused by arthritis of the posterior facets. Journal of Neurosurgery 39: 362–369

Fitzgerald J A W, Newman P H 1976 Degenerative spondylolisthesis. Journal of Bone and Joint Surgery 58B: 184–192

Jonck L M 1061 The mechanical disturbances resulting from lumbar disc narrowing. Journal of Bone and Joint Surgery 43B: 362–375

Magnaes B 1982 Clinical recording of pressure on the spinal coad and cauda equina. Part 2 Position changes in pressure on the cauda equina in central lumbar spinal stenosis. Journal of Neurosurgery 57: 57–63

Roberts G M 1978 Lumbar stenosis. The significance of the narrow lumbar spinal canal and its diagnosis in spondylotic cauda equina syndrome. M. D. Thesis University of London

Sharr M M, Garfield J S, Jenkins J D 1976 Lumbar spondylosis and neuropathic bladder: investigation of 73 patients with chronic urinary symptoms. British Medical Journal 1: 695–697

Shenkin H A, Hash C J 1976 A new approach to the surgical treatment of lumbar spondylosis. Journal of Neurosurgery 44: 148–155

Verbiest H 1977 Results of surgical treatment of idiopathic developmental stenosis of the lumbar canal: a review of twent-seven years experience. Journal of Bone and Jount Surgery (British) 59B: 181–188

Wilson C B 1969 Significance of the small lumbar spinal canal: cauda equina compression syndrome due to spondylosis. Part 3 Intermittent claudication. Journal of Neurosurgery 31: 499–506

18. Antiviral and corticosteroid therapy in herpes simplex encephalitis

Maurice Longson

INTRODUCTION

Few titles for a book to include a chapter about herpes (simplex) encephalitis (HSE) can be more apt than one which carries the word 'dilemmas'. The virus of herpes simplex (HVS) was discovered by Gruter (1920) in 1913, and within 5 years its neurotropic role became the centre of fierce disputation, as distinguished physicians on both sides of the Atlantic argued about its possible involvement in encephalitis (Kling et al, 1922). Since then, impassioned debates about many aspects of HSE (primary or reactivation disease?, pathogenesis?, site and nature of any HVS latency in c.n.s. ? etc.) have never abated and it is probably true to say that HSE is as mysterious a disease today as ever it was — not many satisfactory answers to the controversies of the past 50 years have yet been tabled! We still do not understand how HVS spreads to the brain of man, whether it does so in everybody and why (with a virus which infects virtually 100% of mankind) HSE only occurs in 0.0001% of those at risk each year. Virus can be identified in affected parts of the brain but when pathogenesis is considered, it is probably the only thing we really know; beyond this relatively crude fact very little is understood, and many aspects of the clinical syndrome recognised as HSE defy explanation.

With such a back-drop, it is hardly surprising that of all controversies which surround HSE, amongst the most profound and intractable relate to treatment. From the stand point of design, for therapy to be successful we ought to know what we are treating. So, what is the real object of therapy? What pathological process are we trying to moderate? Why does HSE kill 70% of its victims and cripple the majority of survivors? The truth is that we have no answers to these questions. Undoubtedly, HSV *is* present in the brain of our patients, but is it in fact *responsible* for the cataclysmic brain destruction? In other words, are antivirals ever likely to cure our patients, or ought we to look at other pathological processes and attempt to control these. Perhaps our patients are more the victims of an aberrant immune response and of cerebral oedema; hence the main thrust of therapy might be better directed towards the restoration of normal physiology, in the knowledge that with a 'healthy' immunological response, HSV is rarely — if ever — a 'killer' and is soon brought to heel in a normal host.

196

Another debate revolves around methods for the diagnosis of HSE. All are agreed that therapeutic success can hardly be expected in cases of advanced brain destruction. Ergo, physicians and virologists must recognise the illness with precocity, before encephalitic damage is established and irreversible. Brain biopsy is the obvious tool but the practicalities and ethics of such an invasive technique in (as yet) mildly ill patients are dilemmas of magnitude.

Herpes encephalitis is a virological emergency. In this chapter, we will discuss some of the difficulties which have to be faced when, late on a Friday evening (why does the disease always present at the most inconvenient time?), a possible case is admitted to hospital.

CLINICAL DIAGNOSIS

It is not within the scope of this dissertation to describe the clinical presentation of HSE; suffice it to record that there are many excellent accounts elsewhere (Illis & Gostling, 1972; Whitley et al, 1982). The prodromal illness is protean, yet sufficiently characteristic for it to be useful as a pivot in differential diagnosis. Experienced neurologists will use clinical history, clinical examination, c.s.f. analysis, e.e.g., neuroradiology and acumen and achieve a specific diagnosis with noteworthy accuracy. The less experienced will be confused by many other brain diseases, which mimic HSE and confound the unwary. As the disease progresses and brain destruction gathers pace; the *clinical* diagnostic 'hit-rate' increases from 40% in mildly ill patients, to about 100% in the deeply comatosed. In all instances, confirmation of diagnosis is exclusively the province of laboratory tests.

BRAIN BIOPSY OR WHEN TO TREAT?

One way to manage and diagnose an illness is to treat it with a highly specific drug and use therapeutic success (or failure) as a diagnostic marker. Such 'therapeutic trials' send a shudder down the spine of the rigorist, but the humane doctor at the bedside of a mortally ill patient has responsibilities which go beyond the letter of the scientific code. It will be argued — and the argument is potently valid — that the 'therapeutic trial' is a licence to destroy the whole basis of rational therapeutics. Yet, human patients and their medical attendants are often faced with tragedies which cannot be codified or subjected to virtuous protocols. When the 'test' drug is toxic, dangerous or capricious, few doctors feel the urge to deviate from the 'straight and narrow' but with safer and more dependable agents, transgressions of the rule book become more and more difficult to police, and indict.

When idoxuridine was the only anti-HVS drug (Tomlinson & MacCallum, 1970), horrendous toxicity immediately limited its systemic use to laboratory confirmed cases of life-threatening HVS and varicella-zoster virus infections. No diagnostic acrobatics were too difficult or too demanding and, for possible HSE, a virological opinion on a specimen of brain was mandatory before the initiation of chemotherapy. In this way, HSE became a virological emergency and rapid diagnostic tests were devised, so as to allow the administration of the first dose to a proven case, at the very earliest opportunity, day-or-night, within 2 or 3 hours of craniotomy.

A few years later, two new antivirals appeared; cytarabine (Juel-Jensen & MacCallum, 1972) and vidarabine (Ch'ien et al, 1973). These retained substantial side-effects but in entirely manageable proportions and, particularly in the case of the former drug, they were easy to administer. Henceforth it was possible to envisage treatment of HSE without recourse to brain biopsy, and without previous laboratory confirmation of diagnosis. In centres where neurosurgical skills could readily be harnessed on an emergency basis, craniotomy remained a prerequisite to treatment; but even so, the administration of the first doses of drug was usually allowed to anticipate the virologist's report. It is hardly a surprise that when children were concerned, or when informed consent to operation was difficult to obtain, or in hospitals with no or deficient neurosurgical support, the 'give the drug and see what happens' philosophy began to develop. After all, even in 'Centres of Excellence', laboratory confirmation was being used only retrospectively, for 'scientific reasons' to measure drug efficacy, and no longer as a 'starter's signal'.

The discovery of the so-called second generation nucleoside analogues (see below) as remarkably safe, but potently effective and easy to administer anti-HVS drugs, is certain to make the life of the investigator even more difficult. In many European countries brain biopsy is simply no longer an acceptable procedure in most cases of HSE, and craniotomy is restricted to patients where there are other indications — for example, to deal with a possible brain abcess or tumour.

The problem actually goes deeper than has been described so far. During the mid-seventies, there were two double-blind drug trials in HSE. One in Europe studied cytarabine, the other in the USA used vidarabine. The protocols for both trials were broadly similar and in each instance, brain biopsy was mandatory. The results of these studies have been published, the American experience very fully (Whitley et al, 1977) and subsequently expanded (Whitley et al, 1981); the European experience in less detail (Longson et al, 1980). The trials have not solved anything, but may in fact have deepended controversies (Alford et al, 1982). However, one judgement is that brain biopsy may, in some circumstances, be harmful to the patient's cause. The operation itself is reasonably safe, but it can induce a nefarious delay in the sequence of events which could save the patient's brain. One thing is certain, the outcome of HSE is directly related to the depth of brain dysfunction at the beginning of treatment. Patients not in coma when admitted for treatment, but only lethargic — about 12 points on the 'Glasgow Coma Scale' (Teasdale et al, 1979) — fare *very* much better than patients treated in the same way, but already in coma (3–11 points, Glasgow Coma Scale) (Johnson, 1982). Although in some centres, in the USA and elsewhere, neurosurgeons are prepared to biopsy mildly ill patients and will do so as an emergency procedure without delay, the same attitude does not apply universally. In the European trial of cytarabine, and in the experience of members of the British Herpes Encephalitis Working Party, mandatory brain biopsy is more often than not a positive disincentive to the early institution of treatment. For various reasons (ethical misgivings, failure to obtain consent, shortage of operating time, wait-and-see mentality, etc.) the act of brain biopsy is postponed and postponed, and when at last it is performed, the damage to the brain of the patient is extensive and more or less irreversible. The different strategies are well illustrated by a comparison of the results of biopsy as described in American reports, and of British experience. In USA Centres where emergency brain biopsy of HSE is routine, 45% of biopsied patients do not in fact have the disease (Whitley et al, 1981), and are presumably sampled at an early stage of the illness when the differential diagnosis at the bedside is difficult. By contrast, in the UK, barely 5% of biopsies fail to confirm the preoperation diagnosis of HSE, which suggests that biopsies are undertaken at a later point in the illness when the clinical diagnosis is more certain.

The arguments for and against brain biopsy in HSE are fully debated elsewhere (Kaplan, 1980; Barza & Pauker, 1980; Whitley et al, 1981; Klapper & Longson, 1981) and the case for the procedure is strong. Lest there be any confusion in the reader's mind, it must be emphasised that the argument is *NOT* a plea to abandon brain biopsy. The technique remains the best method — and is the reference method — for the diagnosis of HSE, and it is often a vital step in the diagnosis of diseases which mimic HSE. The debate concerns the over-riding importance of early treatment. Brain biopsy must not be allowed to interfere with this goal. 'If thy hand scandalize thee, cut it off' (Mark 10:42). If craniotomy can be performed without prejudice to early initiation of treatment, then an ideal situation exists. Otherwise, this ideal must be sacrificed.

As the chapter develops, it will become clear that nothing is yet resolved in the matter of treatment of HSE. Similarly, there are huge gaps in our knowledge of the natural history of the disease. If students of neurovirology are to be deprived of data accumulated on soundly diagnosed cases simply because the best available test is 'out of fashion', how will progress be maintained and answers to fundamental questions obtained? This is a formidable challenge, and the glove lies at the virologists' feet.

LABORATORY DIAGNOSIS

The abandonment of brain biopsy in HSE poses serious problems; unless impregnable diagnoses can be achieved, in the future it will be impossible to make any assessment about the efficacy of any form of treatment. Already, a potentially dangerous situation has developed. Abuse of the licence described earlier has encouraged libertine physicians to treat vague encephalopathic illnesses with acyclovir. When the patient has recovered this has, in the mind of both doctor and patient, confirmed the diagnosis of HSE, although laboratory endorsement has never been obtained (or in some cases, even sought). Such behaviour is reprehensible; it is not only unscientific, but it can only bring disrepute upon a potentially very useful compound.

The techniques used to diagnose HSE are described in the specialist literature.

199

The disease *cannot* be recognised by assay of serum antibody alone, but measurement of intrathecal synthesis of autochnal specific anti-HVS immunoglobulin is a reliable and precise tool (Levine et al, 1978), particularly if it incorporates an assessment of brain: c.s.f. barrier function. The *Antibody Index* (AI) proposed by Klapper, Laing & Longson (1981) forms the basis of a useful diagnostic test. Although in terms of specificity and sensitivity it may not quite match the best results from biopsy (Alford et al, 1982; Nahmias et al, 1982), the differences are small and for practical purposes are of minor importance. (It must be remembered that even brain biopsy can yield false negative information.) The main shortcoming of the c.s.f. antibody methods lies in their inability to provide an answer during the acute phase of the illness. In most instances, the AI does not yield a diagnosis until about the tenth day of neurological illness. Clearly this is totally useless for treatment decisions, but is perfectly adequate for the (retrospective) assessment of efficacy. Doubtless, the future will generate better and more rapid tests (by, for example, the detection of trace amounts of virus proteins in lumbar fluid), but in the meanwhile there can be no excuse for not submitting each and every case of encephalopathy treated with a HSE regimen to virological scrutiny.

ANTIVIRALS

The classical theory holds that HSE — otherwise known as acute necrotising encephalitis (Van Bogaert et al, 1955) — is caused by a destruction of neurones and glial cells by a cytolytic infection with HVS. In other words, the pathology is a typical form of polioclastic encephalitis (Greenfield, 1947). If this is correct, HSE must be treated with the best possible anti-HVS compound. Table 18.1 lists

Table 18.1 Relative in vitro potencies of antivirals against HSV (arbitrary units).

Idoxuridine = 100 (H. simplex)	
Phosphonoacetic acid	5
Sodium phosphonoformate	5
Vidarabine	10
Trifluorothymidine	70
Idoxuridine	100
Cytarabine	500
Acyclovir	1000

the available drugs in order of efficacy. Of these, four agents merit attention. Idoxuridine is very toxic and is now only of historical interest (Longson, 1977). Cytarabine was shown to be ineffective in HSE under the conditions of a European double-blind study (Longson, 1979). Vidarabine is currently licensed in the USA for the treatment of HSE, but is *not* so licensed in Britain. The difference between the two countries perhaps highlights the disaccord which exists about the interpretation of data collected by the NIAID Group in the USA (Campbell et al, 1982). The controversy is profound but it can be summarised very briefly. The American authors believe vidarabine to be effective, but such is not the experience in the UK. According to the NIAID Group, vidarabine reduces the mortality of HSE from 70% (figure not in dispute), to 28% (Whitley et al, 1977). The original American double-blind study was terminated rather prematurely, largely because of politico-ethical pressure (McCartney, 1979) and the results were considered by some to be precarious for statistical reasons (Peto, 1977; Tager, 1977). In the circumstances, further data was accumulated, but on open trial basis. The results with this expanded group of patients (132) largely confirmed the earlier data, but the difference between the treated cases and the original (10) placebo cases, was somewhat less impressive (Whitley, 1981). Because of the ethical lobby in the USA, it has been impossible for our American colleagues to submit HSE to further double-blind scrutiny.

When USA claims for vidarabine reached Europe these, together with our own bad results using cytarabine, stimulated many physicians in the UK to prescribe vidarabine for HSE patients ('Named Patient' provision of the 'Medicines Act'). Results anecdotaly reported to the Herpes Encephalitis Working Party have failed to validate the efficacy of the drug (Campbell et al, 1982). In many UK and European hands, vidarabine appears to behave rather like idoxuridine or cytarabine and has very little impact on the natural history of HSE; the mortality of vidarabine treated cases remains about 70%.

Whatever the role of antivirals, it is undeniable that in some American hospitals, patients with HSE who are treated with vidarabine fare better than their counterparts in Europe, who might receive idoxuridine, cytarabine, vidarabine or no antiviral at all. Our American colleagues hold vidarabine to be the cause of their success, but there might be other factors responsible for the better survival rates. In this context, it will be noted that when patients treated with vidarabine have died, virus has been recovered from necropsy brain, thus revealing a certain ineffectiveness for the drug (Longson, 1981; Johnson, 1982).

Before these differences are further explored, it is necessary to look at the British cytarabine and American vidarabine studies, in more detail. In the NIAID studies, although about 60% of patients survived, only about half of these returned to a fairly normal life, with good neurological function or only moderate disability. As has already been emphasised, pretreatment brain biopsy was mandatory in both study protocols. In the USA, it was possible to biopsy (and treat) a significant number of patients when they were only mildly ill (lethargic); it is precisely from this group that the best results (survival with minimal sequalae) were obtained. When patients were recruited, biopsied (and treated) in an advanced stage of disease (coma), they fared very badly (high mortality, or tragic crippling in survivors). The situation in Britain was that over 60% of patients recruited to the cytarabine study were already, at the time of craniotomy and admission to the study, in coma.

Returning now to possible differences between the UK and USA studies; perhaps (1) the American strategy of early biopsy unintentionally selected a group of patients with an inherently good prognosis, the so called 'mild HSE' cases (Campbell et al, 1982) or, (2) the American treatment regimen (vidarabine excepted) involving intra-cranial pressure control, respiratory and circulatory support, etc., was in some US Centres more sophisticated and more effective than the similar, but possibly different, treatment protocol on mortally ill patients in

Britain. Interestingly, even in the USA, there was a very marked difference in the vidarabine study results when these were stratified according to the participating centres.

One of the main problems associated with vidarabine has been its insolubility and the large amount of fluid required to carry an intravenous dose. There have been fears that this might exacerbate cerebral oedema. Vidarabine monophosphate (ara-AMP) is a soluble derivative which has been shown to have antiviral activity similar to the parent compound. An unverified report from the USA suggests that ara-AMP is not effective in HSE.

In summary therefore, it does not look as though we yet have at hand any antiviral drug of proven efficacy in HSE. It is impossible to escape the conclusion that nothing will be resolved without further controlled double-blind studies. The advent of acyclovir may be providing the opportunity for this, and indeed, a multi-centre study of the new drug is currently underway in the UK. Not surprisingly, the propriety of further double-blind studies with placebo in HSE have been brought into question (Lancet, 1981), and the views expressed about this controversy command respect (Campbell et al, 1982). However, an ethical problem arises only if there is scientifically sound evidence that an effective antiviral drug already exists. If such evidence is lacking, then further well monitored, controlled studies are not only ethical, but are compelling and inescapable.

Acyclovir, a novel and very exciting compound, belongs to a range of so-called 'second generation' nucleoside analogues. These anti-HVS drugs are themselves biologically inactive and as a direct consequence of this property, are remarkably non-toxic. In this way they differ from the 'first generation' nucleoside analogues (idoxuridine, cytarabine and vidarabine) described (Lancet, 1981; Timbury, 1982). The compounds are not substrates for mammalian enzymes, but *are* phosphorylated by HVS encoded thymidine kinases. The triphosphate derivatives inhibit (competitively, or by premature chain termination) the synthesis of viral DNA, thus making the parent compounds very safe, but highly selective antivirals.

Acyclovir is the first of these compounds to be licensed for human use (not, it must be stressed, for HSE). Reference to Table 18.1 will show how effective an anti-HSV drug, it is. Bromovynil deoxyuridine and fluoro-iodo-arabinosylcytosine may soon be available for clinical trial. The world literature now contains an impressive array of studies which all add up to a striking endorsement of acyclovir for the treatment of some forms of human infections caused by HVS and varicella-zoster virus (Timbury, 1982). Not surprisingly, acyclovir has been proposed as the ideal antiviral for the treatment of HSE. Two small clouds on the horizon, crystaluria in patients with renal impairment and the emergence of (thymidine kinase deficient) resistant strains of HVS, are not likely to interfere with any role acyclovir might have in the management of encephalitis.

Although the enthusiasm for acyclovir in HSE is entirely understandable and predictable, it must be emphasised over and over again that, at the time of writing, there is not one scrap of published evidence to show that the drug is actually of any value in this disease. Anecdotes abound, but many neurologists and virologists are sufficiently long in the tooth to remember exactly analogous excitement 20 and 10 years ago with respect to idoxuridine and cytarabine. Only results of carefully planned studies will yield the answer so earnestly desired. Meanwhile, enthusiasm for acyclovir in HSE should be tempered with wisdom and scientific integrity, together with meticulous documentation of every facet of each treated case (Lauter, 1980).

At this stage of the discussion, it might appear cynical to question the very place of antivirals in the therapy of HSE. But this student of the disease, after many years in the game, is beginning to wonder whether the lure of antivirals is not making us lose sight of the right path. The problem was clearly brought to light 3 years ago by Dr Roman-Campos and his colleagues (1980).

STEROIDS, AND OTHER THERAPEUTIC MEASURES

What is the pathogenesis of HSE? Is it in fact a simple acute polioclastic virus encephalitis, or could it be a much more complex affair? When the imagination is given free rein, many models merit discussion. These range from a relatively banal reactivation of latent HVS in the c.n.s. followed by a rare but catastrophic 'allergic' type of immune reaction to virus protein, which henceforth becomes the practical cause of the disease which maims or kills, to the concept of a neurological disease of unknown — probably non-viral — aetiology during which an incidentally present latent HVS genome in brain cells, is fortuitously induced and expresses itself. This last situation would be somewhat analogous to the peripheral reactivation of herpes labialis during an unrelated illness, say after a severe burn or following trigeminal rhizotomy.

Were mechanisms such as these to be the actual cause of HSE, then it is a pity that our search for a cure is being misdirected with work on antiviral agents. Our efforts might be better expended in other directions, for example in the area of immunosuppressive therapy. It is salutory to note that acyclovir appears to be very much more clinically useful in the treatment of primary (initial) HVS disease, than it is in the case of reactivation problems. The involvement of the virus in HSE is, in the majority of instances, a reactivation and prospects for antivirals are perhaps forlorn. The comments by Chin & Edis (1982) are very much apropos.

General supportive care

Few would doubt the importance attached to life support techniques in the management of HSE (Longson, 1977). The disease has a profound effect on the respiratory, cardiovascular and endocrine systems and these are perhaps as vulnerable as the brain itself. It is salutory to study the variation in survival rates from hospital to hospital, whether or not patients receive specific chemotherapy. The treatment schedules for a disease as protean and complex as HSE are of course themselves very capricious and the paucity of cases makes any analysis of the variables well nigh impossible. For example, might therapeutic success or failure be directly related to the quality of nursing care, or to the impact of cerebral oedema control, or to management of the patient's immune response?

Cerebral oedema control

Most patients with HSE are given dexamethasone, usually in high initial doses. The naive assumption is that this will control the oedema, which is often believed to be the main cause of brain damage (Reulen et al, 1973; Longson, 1977). Remarkably little is known about the effect of corticosteroids on inflammatory oedema. They promote diuresis by increasing glomerular filtration rate, and suppress inflammation. Both these effects endow dexamethasone with a very potent role in the control of the vasogenic oedema associated with cerebral tumours and brain abcesses, and a much less significant place in the reduction of the oedema caused by head injuries and stroke (Fishman, 1975; Reulen, 1976; Mulley et al, 1978). There is no suggestion that this steroid has any place in the management of either cytotoxic or interstitial cerebral oedema, and the precise mechanisms of inflammatory oedema in general, and HSE oedema in particular, are very moot points. In all probability, dexamethasone has little if any effect on the oedema of HSE. Certainly, the necropsy appearances of many HSE brains, even after full dexamethasone schedules, appear to give the lie to this form of decompressive therapy. The arguments in favour of dexamethasone are largely emotional, but of course the steroid may have other parts to play, for example in the treatment of shock (very doubtful) or in the manipulation of the immune or inflammatory response (see below).

Osmotherapy (urea, mannitol or glycerol) can be used to 'shrink' the brain, but this is unlikely to be particularly useful in HSE. Hypertonic solutions may well remove water from normal parts of the brain, but will probably not influence oedematous foci. In any event, the decompressive effect is bound to be only temporary and may be followed by rebound oedema. At best, osmotherapy may buy time before surgical decompression, or will temporarily reduce intra-cranial pressure during lumbar puncture. Lauter (1980) has once again raised the possibility that brain biopsy by craniotomy may have a beneficial therapeutic role by its decompression mechanism, a point already discussed by Illis & Gostling (1972). Hyperventilation and elevation of the bed head have also been found to be useful adjuncts in management. Clearly, little is known about the impact of intracranial pressure in patients with HSE and this warrants careful study. Would it be ethical and useful to use intraventicular pressure monitors in all cases of HSE?

Immunosuppressive treatment

Cytarabine is immunosuppressive and yet does not appear to have a useful role in HSE (Farris & Blaw, 1972; Longson et al, 1980). Corticosteroids have a potent effect on membranes, they prevent the rupture of lysosomes and inhibit both fibroblasts and macrophages. These marked immunosuppressive properties have led to many anecdotal and uncontrolled claims for the value of dexamethasone in HSE (see Illis & Gostling, 1972; Longson, 1977), but there have been no properly conducted studies. In the UK trial of cytarabine (Longson et al, 1980), dexamethasone was given to *all* patients in fairly high doses. The mortality was 70% and the steroid was certainly not beneficial, and could in fact have been harmful. When the original 28 patients in the US vidarabine study were stratified according to dexamethasone status, no useful information could be construed.

Whitley (1981) concluded that dexamethasone was not substantiated as effective. Obviously, further studies are now necessary. How these might be constructed is difficult to imagine — yet, we cannot until such studies answer the simple question, do we or do we not give dexamethasone to our patients? For theoretical reasons, steroids may in fact be harmful (Longson & Beswick, 1971).

One of the great difficulties in the area of immunological control of HSE, is that we do not really know whether.we ought to suppress or stimulate the patient's T (or B) lymphocytes. Otherwise we might be tempted to use drugs such as azathioprine or cyclophosphamide as suppressants, and levamisole, BCG or interferon as stimulators. These would be new avenues in the treatment of the disease, but they could be rewarding. However, the first thing is to learn more about pathogenesis.

SUMMARY

Herpes encephalitis was first described in 1941. It was soon known to be a catastrophic illness associated with a mortality of about 70%. Modern methods of care and antivirals may be moderating the mortality, but at a high price in terms of neurological crippling (Wolman & Longson, 1977; Johnson, 1982; Chinn & Edis, 1982) and only if treatment is started on mildly-ill, non-comatose patients (Lauter, 1980). Brain biopsy is still the best route to diagnosis, but the procedure must not delay the initiation of treatment. Further improvements in prognosis will probably not be achieved through the medium of newer antivirals, but only by a better knowledge of the pathogenesis of the disease and a different therapeutic approach. For example, fundamental questions, such as those raised by Dr Whitley and his colleagues (Whitley et al, 1982), need to be fully explored and we need to know whether HSE is caused by the same virus which might provoke a patient's recurrent labial herpes, or whether it can be the result of an independent super infection with an unrelated strain of HVS.

ACKNOWLEDGMENTS

This work is supported by the Carl Barnett Encephalitis Research Fund and by the Clinical Research Committee of the North Western Regional Health Authority. Acknowledgments are due to Mr P. Klapper for advice and criticism and to Mrs C. Bradburn for secretarial assistance.

REFERENCES

Alford C A, Dolin R Hirsch M S, Karchmer A W, Whitley R J 1982 Herpes simplex encephalitis and clinical trial design. Lancet 1: 1013
Barza M, Pauker S G 1980 The decision to biopsy treat or wait in suspected herpes encephalitis. Annals of Internal Medicine 92: 641–649
Campbell M, Klapper P E, Longson M 1982 Acyclovir in herpes encephalitis. Lancet 1: 38
Ch'ien L T et al 1973 Effect of adenine arabinoside on severe herpesvirus homonis infections in man. Journal of Infectious Diseases 128: 658–663

Chinn D, Edis E 1982 Acyclovir for herpes simplex encephalitis: the price of survival? Lancet 2: 870

Farris W A, Blaw M E 1972 Cytarabine treatment of herpes simplex encephalitis. Archives of Neurology 27: 99–102

Fishman R A 1975 Brain oedema. Physiology in Medicine 203: 706–711

Greenfield J G 1947 The clinical and postmortem pathology of encephalitis. Recent Advances in Clinical Pathology: 426

Gruter W 1920 Experimentelle und klinische Untersuchungen uter den sogenannten Herpes Cornea. Bericht Zusammenkumft Deutchen Ophtalmologischen Gesellochaft 42: 162–166

Illis L S, Gostling J V T 1972 Herpes simplex encephalitis. Scientechnica, Bristol

Johnson R T 1982 Viral infections of the nervous system. Raven Press, New York

Juel-Jensen B E, MacCallum F O 1972 Herpes simplex and varicella. Heinemann Medical, London

Kaplan L R 1980 Brain biopsy in herpes simplex encephalitis. New England Journal of Medicine 303: 700

Klapper P E, Laing I, Longson M 1981 Rapid non-invasive diagnosis of herpes encephalitis. Lancet 2: 607–609

Klapper P E, Longson M 1981 Acute viral encephalitis. British Medical Journal 283: 1544

Kling C, Davide H, Liljenquist F 1922 Nouvelles investigation sur la pretendue relation entre le virus herpètique. Comptes Rendus Séances Societé de Biologie 87: 1179–1183

Lancet 1981 Acyclovir 2: 845–849

Lauter C B 1980 Herpes simplex encephalitis; a great clinical challenge. Annals of Internal Medicine 93: 696–698

Levine P, Lauter C B, Lerner A M 1978 Simultaneous serum and CSF antibodies in herpes simplex virus encephalitis. Journal of American Medical Association 240: 356–360

Longson M 1977 The treatment of herpes encephalitis. Journal of Antimicrobial Chemotherapy 3 (Sup. A): 115–123

Longson M 1979 Le defi des encephalites herpetiques. Annales de Microbiologie (Institut Pasteur) 130 A: 5–6

Longson M 1981 Personal observation

Longson M, Bailey A S, Klapper P 1980 Herpes encephalitis. In: Waterson A P (ed) Recent advances in clinical virology, vol 2. Churchill Livingstone, Edinburgh

Longson M, Beswick T S L 1971 Dexamethasone treatment in herpes simplex encephalitis. Lancet 1: 749

McCartney J J 1979 Encephalitis and adenine arabinoside. Hastings Centre Report, August 46–47

Mulley G, Wilcox R G, Mitchel J R A 1978 Dexamethasone in acute stroke. British Medical Journal 2: 994–997

Nahmias A J et al 1982 Herpes simplex virus encephalitis. Laboratory evaluations and their diagnostic significance. Journal of Infectious Diseases 145: 829–836

Peto J 1977 Personal communication

Reulen H J 1976 Vasogenic brain oedema. British Journal of Anaesthesia 48: 741–752

Reulen H J, Hadjidimos A, Hase U 1973 Steroids in the treatment of brain oedema. In: Schurmann M et al (eds) Advances in Neurosurgery, I. Springer, Berlin

Roman Campos G, Phillips C A, Poser C M 1980 Herpes simplex encephalitis. Lancet 1: 489

Tager I B 1977 Ara-A for herpes encephalitis. New England Journal of Medicine 297: 1289

Teasdale G, Skene A, Parker I, Jennett B 1979 Adding up the Glasgow coma score. Acta Neurosurgica Suppl. 28: 140–143

Timbury C 1982 Acyclovir. British Medical Journal 285: 1223–1224

Tomlinson A H, MacCallum F O 1970 The effect of iododeoxyuridine on herpes encephalitis in animals and man. Annals of the New York Academy of Science 173: 20–24

Van Bogaert L, Radermecker J, Devos J 1955 Sur une observation mortelle d'encéphalite aigue nécrosante. Sa situation vis à vis due groupe des encéphalites transmises par arthropodes et de l'encéphalite herpètique. Revue Neurologique 92: 329

Whitley R J 1981 Diagnosis and treatment of herpes simplex encephalitis. Annual Review of Medicine 32: 335–340

Whitley R J et al 1977 Adenine arabinoside therapy of biopsy-proven herpes simplex encephalitis. New England Journal of Medicine 297: 289–294

Whitley R J et al 1981 Herpes simplex encephalitis. Vidarabine therapy and diagnostic problems. New England Journal of Medicine 304: 313–318

Whitley R J et al 1982 Herpes simplex encephalitis clinical assessment. Journal of American Medical Association 247: 317–337

Wolman B, Longson M 1977 Herpes encephalitis. Acta Paediatrica Scandinavia 66: 243–246

19. Normal pressure hydrocephalus — to shunt or not to shunt?

J.D. Pickard

'The advisability of surgical intervention with some by-pass procedures must be considered carefully in these patients because of the tendency of the hydrocephalus to recompensate at a point where disability is minimal . . . a shunt can bring great relief . . . not foolproof procedure . . . not recommended unless disability is severe or progression of the condition is rapid and undoubted.'   (McHugh, 1964)

When McHugh wrote this he accurately summarised much of the present conventional attitude to patients with occult forms of hydrocephalus. Each clinician concerned with these patients sees a different facet of the problem. The physician, neurologist, geriatrician or psychiatrist would like clearly defined clinical criteria with which to select those patients presenting with dementia and/or a gait disorder who have a disturbance of the circulation of the c.s.f. The neuroradiologist would like reassurance that there is a reasonable possibility that a CT scan will reveal remediable pathology in patients presenting with dementia and would like in return to be able to distinguish accurately between hydrocephalus and cerebral atrophy on the scan. The neurosurgeon would like to know the natural history of these patients and at what point he can usefully intervene with a shunt. He would like to know which type of shunt would give optimal relief with minimal risk of complications both in the short and the long-term. Given the fragile state of many of these patients, and the need in some of them for repeated investigation over some years, the neurosurgeon would also like some guidance as to how best to deploy his limited bed resources. For a more detailed review of adult communicating hydrocephalus including its pathophysiology the reader is referred to a recent review (Pickard, 1982).

PRESENTING SYMPTOMS

Adult hydrocephalus may be entirely asymptomatic and a chance finding on investigation of unrelated problems. McHugh (1964) presented a series of case histories to illustrate the various more chronic presentations of hydrocephalus and some of his patients fell into the group later to be known as normal pressure hydrocephalus as described by Hakim (Hakim & Adams, 1965). Typically such patients presented with dementia, gait disturbance and urinary incontinence without any clinical evidence of raised intracranial pressure and with normal c.s.f. pressure on isolated observation at lumbar puncture. In fact the c.s.f. pressure is now known to be neither low nor normal and prolonged intracranial pressure monitoring techniques have revealed periods of intermittently raised pressure. The term normal pressure hydrocephalus will be used although the term intermittently raised pressure hydrocephalus would be preferable. Many of these patients responded to c.s.f. drainage with a shunt but subsequent experience has been less happy, perhaps because the clinical and diagnostic criteria were not well-defined. In an attempt to be precise about the nature of the presenting symptoms, various authors have analysed the clinical features of patients who have improved with shunting.

Although there are many exceptions, the pattern of the early dementia is of impairment of memory associated with inertia. Patients are slow in thought, vague and indecisive. They lose their intellectual grasp, become superficial and incapable of abstraction. They are dull, apathetic and careless with depressed vigilance and arousal. Such features are not always constant. Whilst agitation is unusual it by no means excludes the diagnosis. Initially there is no cognitive defect, aphasia or specific cortical defect. Finally severe dementia supervenes and the patient becomes unable to care for himself and enters an akinetic mute state leading to coma (McHugh, 1964; Hakim & Adams, 1965; Crowell et al 1973; Fisher, 1977; Katzmann, 1977).

'The mechanism that allows a 6 foot tall human to walk on his two hind legs is imperfect, but the nature of the imperfection has yet to be identified' (Fisher 1977). The characteristic of the very variable gait disturbance is that the disability is in excess of the fragmented neurological signs. There is usually hardly any weakness of voluntary movement, spasticity, sensory loss or cerebellar ataxia and the plantar responses may be flexor or extensor. Initially the disturbance may be little more than a slowing of gait but eventually the patient may be completely bed-bound, unable to either walk or stand or even turn over in bed. The gait is typically but not invariably wide-based with a shortened step and tandem walking along a straight line is impossible. There is a slowness in correcting a potential instability and unsteadiness with a tendency to fall. In some patients the feet appear to be glued to the floor and in others the resemblance to the flexed posture and shuffling gait of Parkinsonism is very striking (Messert & Baker, 1966; Chawla & Woodward, 1972; Sypert et al, 1973; Botez et al, 1975; Fisher 1977; Estanol, 1981)

The urinary incontinence is very much of the frontal lobe type with lack of appropriate concern and it may be profuse. Faecal incontinence particularly in the early stages is much less common.

These clinical features may have been slowly progressive over some years by the time the patient presents. Of course they are not pathognomic of one condition and a CT scan is required to confirm the presence of ventriculomegaly once the basic investigations have been completed. However, it is as well to remember (Vide infra) that only patients in whom dementia is preceded or accompanied by a disturbance of gait have a reasonable chance of responding to a shunt. Occasional patients may present in particularly bizarre fashions with status epilepticus, spontaneous hypothermia, recurrent dehydration from depressed thirst sensation and visual field defects due to an enlarged third ventricle for example.

CT SCANNING

A cause for the ventriculomegaly may be shown such as aqueduct stenosis, a tumour, ectatic basilar arteries or aneurysm, or basal cistern calcification suggestive of previous tuberculous meningitis. The presence of either a large fourth ventricle or particularly of periventricular low density are good prognostic signs for successful response to shunting. Low attenuation areas may be seen in the white matter in patients with subcortical arteriosclerotic encephalopathy or Binswanger's disease, but such areas are different in form and extent from true periventricular oedema (Moseley & Radii, 1979; Zeumer et al, 1980). There is no difference neuropathologically between the brains of these patients with Binswanger's disease and those with multi-infarct dementia (Dr Reuck et al, 1980). Unfortunately, despite early promise that the demonstration of widened sulci on the CT scan confirms the presence of cerebral atrophy rather than hydrocephalus this has not been born out in practice (Jacobs & Kinkel, 1976; Laws & Mokri, 1976; Crockard et al, 1977; Greenbert et al, 1977; Gunasekera & Richardson, 1977; Black, 1980; Borgesen & Gjerris, 1982). Unlike the measurement of total ventricular size from CT scans which is now a well-defined problem (Wyper et al, 1979) the quantification of cerebral atrophy remains controversial (Roberts et al, 1976). Thus it is uncertain which tomographic slices should be interrogated and whether the Sylvian fissures should be included in estimates of the width and length of more superficial sulci. It is common experience that occasional patients with widened superficial sulci respond well to a shunt.

INTRACRANIAL PRESSURE MONITORING

There is now a consensus that when B waves of intracranial pressure are found to occupy at least 5% of the day then there is a good chance of such patients responding to a shunt (Symon et al, 1972; Chawla et al, 1974; Belloni et al, 1976; Brock, 1977; Crockard et al, 1977; Hartmann & Alberti, 1977; Jeffreys, 1978; Jensen & Jensen, 1979; Lamas & Lobato, 1979; Gucer et al, 1980; Pickard et al, 1980; Borgesen & Gjerris, 1982). Such spontaneous periodic waves occur with a frequency of 0.5 — 2.0 per minute and they can be of very variable height. The mean intracranial pressure in patients who respond to a shunt is in the upper range of normal (for example 12.5 ± 6 mm Hg in responders and 7.5 ± 2mm Hg in non-responders). However, the overlap of these two values is too great for it to be useful in practice. c.s.f. pulse pressure is statistically greater in responders than in non-responders but again the overlap is too great to be useful. One practical point is that to see low amplitude B waves reliably I need to use an intraventricular catheter for pressure monitoring but other authors claim that subdural and extradural techniques give good results in their hands.

Fisher (1978) and Wikkelso et al (1982) have shown that with removal of some 50 ml of c.s.f. by lumbar puncture some patients will make an immediate but transient clinical improvement and that this is a good indication that the patient will improve after a shunt. It remains to be shown in a properly controlled study how many patients, in whom improvement is delayed after a shunt, would be missed with this simple test.

Lumbar air encephalography and isotope cisternography will confirm that in communicating hydrocephalus there is little passage of the air or marker over the convexities (convexity block) with accumulation within the ventricles which may persist for over 48 hours (ventricular stasis). Although these tests will show an abnormality they do not differentiate well between shunt responders and non-responders (Stein & Langfitt, 1974; Katzmann, 1977; Pickard et al, 1980). CT metrizamide cisternography will give similar information (Ostertag & Mundinger, 1978).

There has been a resurgence of interest in the use of c.s.f. infusion tests. The ability of c.s.f. absorption to increase with rising c.s.f. pressure is impaired in communicating hydrocephalus (Lorenzo et al, 1974). The Katzmann-Hussey test in which artificial c.s.f is infused into the lumbar subarachnoid space at twice the normal rate of c.s.f formation has not been found to be a useful discriminant test in chronic hydrocephalus (Katzmann, 1977). However, a recent modification by Borgesen & Gjerris (1982) involves a lumbo-ventricular perfusion system in which Ringers lactate is infused at a constant rate into a lumbar cannula and the pressure level is controlled by the height of the out-flow tip of the catheter from the ventricle. The unabsorbed fluid is measured and the conductance to out-flow of c.s.f. determined. Patients with a value below 0.12 ml/minute/mm Hg were all shunted and improvement only occurred in patients with a value below 0.08. They confirmed that no patients with B waves for less than 5% of the time improved after shunting and B wave activity could be significantly correlated with reduced c.s.f. outflow conductance. However, a low value for c.s.f. outflow conductance did not necessarily imply frequent B waves. Unfortunately, their test did not predict the extent of improvement with shunting. No test at present appears to give that information.

PROBLEMS OF MANAGEMENT

The incidence of complications following anaesthesia and insertion of a shunt into these relatively elderly and fragile patients is alarming. Most surgeons have horror stories and can remember vividly providing prolonged in-patient care for some patients. Most series report a mortality rate of 5–12% and a morbidity rate of 33–51% reflecting the complications of subdural haematomas (2.5–23%), shunt revisions (up to 27%), shunt infections (6–18%), pneumonia, pulmonary emboli, epilepsy (6.5% in one series), intracerebral haematoma caused by insertion of a ventricular catheter, non-haemorrhagic stroke and low pressure headaches (Illingworth et al, 1971; McCullough & Fox, 1974; Udvarhelyi et al, 1975; Greenberg et al, 1977; Hughes et al, 1978; Black, 1980; Pickard 1980; Borgesen & Gjerris, 1982).

It is not sufficient merely to insert a shunt. These patients have to be followed long-term with repeat CT scanning and clinical re-assessment. Where patients have not improved or continue to deteriorate, their shunt is often not working. This population of patients presents a considerable clinical load. It should be stressed that inserting a shunt into patients with cerebral atrophy is not a benign procedure and may make them worse. Occasional cases of Alzheimer's disease have been reported in the literature where transient improvement has occurred after a shunt but such benefit has rapidly been vitiated with the natural progressive deterioration of the basic disease (Salmon, 1972; Katzmann, 1977).

There are no controlled studies of the relative merits of various shunts in the treatment of normal pressure hydrocephalus. Selman et al (1980) have published an impressive account of the low morbidity associated with lumbo-peritoneal shunting in the short-term but the value of its long-term use remains to be established.

The least complicated shunt system is usually used to reduce the risk of colonisation, infection and blockage. Obsessional attention to surgical technique is required if a useful shunt is to be established in these fragile patients (Jeffreys & Wood, 1978). Some subdural haematomas may be provoked by rapid initial decompression of the ventricles and it is common practice to keep the patient flat in bed for the first 2 to 3 days. In order to avoid the syphon effect when the patient becomes erect the antisyphon device has been developed which shuts off with negative pressure gradients. Unfortunately such antisyphon devices do not always avert the formation of subdural haematomas (Portnoy et al, 1973; McCullough & Fox, 1974; Hughes et al, 1978). The optimal opening pressure and pressure flow characteristics for the valve have not been determined and it is salutary to find that even high pressure valves do not prevent subdural haematomas (Hughes et al, 1978). At present in Wessex we use either the simplest low pressure valve systems or no valve at all for the lumbo-peritoneal or ventricular-peritoneal shunt, and use ventriculo-atrial shunting mainly in obese patients.

THE RESULTS OF SURGICAL TREATMENT

Much of the literature is confused by incomplete reporting of the clinical details of patients. Only recently has the change in mental state been quantified with psychometry (Jeffreys & Wood, 1978; Crockard et al, 1980; Wikkelso et al, 1982; Borgesen & Gjerris, 1982; Caltagirone et al, 1982). In patients with the typical triad of dementia, gait disturbance and incontinence of urine and in whom the aetiology of normal pressure hydrocephalus is known, there is a broad consensus that useful improvement with shunting occurs in up to 65% with complete recovery in 30%. The results in the idiopathic group vary widely between series: in patients with a typical triad, a return to normal activity occurs in 10-39%; if incontinence is not present only 10% of patients appear to return to normal activity. In patients with dementia alone or in whom dementia precedes gait problems, the results are very poor. In subjects with the whole clinical picture, the prognosis for gait and incontinence is better than for intellectual function.

Surprisingly, age, duration of symptoms and degree of disability do not correlate well with the outcome (Stein & Langfitt, 1974; Fisher, 1977; Greenberg et al, 1977; Katzmann, 1977; Hughes et al, 1978; Black, 1980; Pickard et al, 1980; Crockard et al, 1980; Borgesen & Gjerris, 1982; Wikkelso et al 1982). A paradox revealed by follow-up of these patients is that some improve despite the ventricles remaining large after operation and the degree of reduction in ventricular size does not correlate well with outcome (Shenkin et al, 1975; Jacobs & Kinkel, 1976).

In summary, there is much scope for detailed long-term studies of the natural history of this condition and its various clinical manifestations. The finding of patients with an atypical clinical picture will require greater availability of CT scanning services (Crowell et al, 1973; Rice & Gendelman, 1973; Sypert et al, 1973). There is a place for a careful controlled study of the relative merits of various shunting systems with reference both to clinical outcome, incidence of complications and objective changes on the CT scan. In the absence of data from such controlled studies my present practice is to offer a shunt to patients with the typical triad, a predisposing cause for their hydrocephalus and the demonstration of periventricular lucency on their CT scans. Patients in whom there is no known aetiology for the ventricular enlargement, the cerebral sulci are widened, or the complete triad is not present have their intracranial pressure monitored for 24–48 hours. Increasingly brain biopsy is being performed at the time of pressure monitoring or at the time of insertion of the shunt. The patients are followed up long-term and a CT scan is routinely performed some 6 months later.

REFERENCES

Belloni G, di Rocco C, Focacci C, Galli G, Maira G, Rossi G F 1976 Surgical indications in normotensive hydrocephalus. A retrospective analysis of the relations of some diagnostic findings to the results of surgical treatment. Acta Neurochirurgica 33: 1–21
Black P McL 1980 Idiopathic normal pressure hydrocephalus. Results of shunting in 62 patients. Journal of Neurosurgery 52: 371–377
Borgesen S E, Gjerris F 1982 The predictive value of conductance to outflow of CSF in normal pressure hydrocephalus. Brain 105: 65–86
Botez M I, Leveille J, Berube L, Botez — Marquard T 1975 Occult disorders of the cerebrospinal fluid dynamics. Early diagnosis criteria. European Neurology 13: 203–223
Brock M 1977 Klinik und therapie des intermittierend normotensiven hydrocephalus. Radiologe 17: 460–465
Caltagirone C, Gainotti G, Masullo C, Villa G 1982 Neurophysiological study of normal pressure hydrocephalus. Acta Psychiatrica Scandinavica, 65: 93–100
Chawla J C, Woodward J 1972 Motor disorder in normal pressure hydrocephalus. British Medical Journal 1: 485–486
Chawla J C, Hulme A, Cooper R 1974 Intracranial pressure in patients with dementia and communicating hydrocephalus. Journal of Neurosurgery 40: 376–380
Crockard H A, Hanlon K, Duda E E, Mullan J F 1977 Hydrocephalus as a cause of dementia: evaluation by computerized tomography and intracranial pressure monitoring. Journal of Neurology, Neurosurgery and Psychiatry 40: 736–740
Crockard A, McKee H, Joshi K, Allen I 1980 ICP, CAT Scans and psychometric assessment in dementia: a prospective analysis. In: Shulman et al (eds) Intracranial pressure IV, Springer Verlag, Berlin, p 501–504
Crowell R M, Tew J M, Mark V H 1973 Aggressive dementia associated with normal pressure hydrocephalus: report of two unusual cases. Neurology 23: 461–464
De Reuck J, Crevits L, De Coster W, Sieben G, vander Ercken H 1980 Pathogenesis of Binswanger chronic progressive subcortical encephalopathy. Neurology, Mineapolis 30: 920–928

Estanol B V 1981 Gait apraxia in communicating hydrocephalus. Journal of Neurology, Neurosurgery and Psychiatry 44: 305-308

Fisher C M 1977 The clinical picture in occult hydrocephalus. Clinical Neurosurgery 24: 270-284

Fisher C M 1978 Communicating hydrocephalus. Lancet 1: 37

Greenberg J O, Shenkin H A, Adam 1977 Idiopathic normal pressure hydrocephalus — a report of 73 patients. Journal of Neurology, Neurosurgery and Psychiatry 40: 336-341

Gucer G, Viernstein L, Walker A E 1980 Continuous intracranial pressure recording in adult hydrocephalus. Surgical Neurology 13: 323-328

Gunasekera L, Richardson A E 1977 Computerized axial tomography in idiopathic hydrocephalus. Brain 100: 749-754

Hakim S, Adams R D 1965 The special clinical problem of symptomatic hydrocephalus with normal cerebrospinal fluid pressure. Journal of Neurological Sciences 2: 307-327

Hartmann A, Alberti E 1977 Differentiation of communicating hydrocephalus and presenile dementia by continuous recording of cerebrospinal fluid pressure. Journal of Neurology Neurosurgery and Psychiatry 40: 630-640

Hughes C P, Siegel B A, Coxe W S, Gado M H, Grubb R L Coleman R E, Berg L 1978 Adult idiopathic communicating hydrocephalus with and without shunting. Journal of Neurology Neurosurgery and Psychiatry 41: 961-971

Illingworth R D, Logue V, Symon L, Uemura K 1971 The ventriculocaval shunt in the treatment of adult hydrocephalus: results and complications in 101 patients. Journal of Neurosurgery 35: 681-685

Jacobs L, Kinkel W 1976 Computerized axial transverse tomography in normal pressure hydrocephalus. Neurology 26: 501-507

Jeffreys R V 1978 The complications of ventriculo-atrial shunting in hydrocephalus. In: Wüllenweber R (ed) Advances in Neurosurgery 6: 17-22

Jeffreys R V, Wood M M 1978 Adult non-tumourous dementia and hydrocephalus. Acta Neurochirurgica 45: 103-114

Jensen F, Jensen F T 1979 Acquired hydrocephalus II. Diagnostic and prognostic value of quantitative isotope ventriculography, lumbar isotope cisternography, pneumoencephalography and continuous intraventricular pressure recording. Acta Neurochirurgica 46: 243-257

Katzmann R 1977 Normal pressure hydrocephalus. Contemporary Neurology 15: 69-92

Lamas E, Lobato R D 1979 Intraventricular pressure and CSF dynamics in chronic adult hydrocephalus. Surgical Neurology 12: 287-295

Laws E R, Mokri B 1977 Occult hydrocephalus: results of shunting correlated with diagnostic tests. Clinical Neurosurgery 24: 316-333

Lorenzo A V, Bresnan M J, Barlow C F 1974 Cerebrospinal fluid absorption deficit in normal pressure hydrocephalus. Archives of Neurology 30: 387-393

McCullough D C, Fox J L 1974 Negative intracranial pressure hydrocephalus in adults with shunts and its relationship to the production of subdural haematoma. Journal of Neurosurgery 40: 372-375

McHugh P R 1964 Occult hydrocephalus. Quarterly Journal of Medicine 33: 297-308

Messert B, Baker N H 1966 Syndrome of progressive spastic ataxia and apraxia associated with occult hydrocephalus. Neurology 16: 440-452

Moseley I F, Radii E W 1979 Factors influencing the development of periventricular lucencies in patients with raised intracranial pressure. Neuroradiology 17: 65-69

Ostertag C B, Mundinger F 1978 Diagnosis of normal pressure hydrocephalus using CT with CSF enhancement. Neuroradiology 16: 216-219

Pickard J D 1982 Adult communicating hydrocephalus. British Journal of Hospital Medicine 27: 35-44

Pickard J D, Teasdale G, Matheson M, Lindsay K, Galbraith S, Wyper D, MacPherson P 1980 Intraventricular pressure waves — the best predictive test for shunting in normal pressure hydrocephalus. In: Shulman K et al (eds) Intracranial pressure IV Springer-Verlag, Berlin p 498-500

Portnoy H D, Schulte R R, Fox J L, Croissant P D, Tripp L 1973 Anti-siphon and reversible occlusion valves for shunting in hydrocephalus and preventing post-shunt subdural haematomas. Journal of Neurosurgery 38: 729-738

Rice E, Gendelman S 1973 Psychiatric aspects of normal pressure hydrocephalus. Journal of the American Medical Association 223: 409

Roberts M A, Caird F I, Grossart K W, Steven J L 1976 Computerized tomography in the diagnosis of cerebral atrophy. Journal of Neurology, Neurosurgery and Psychiatry 39: 909-915

Salmon J H 1972 Adult hydrocephalus. Evaluation of shunt therapy in 80 patients. Journal of Neurosurgery 37: 423-428

Selman W R, Spetzler R F, Wilson C B, Grollmus J W 1980 Percutaneous lumboperitoneal shunt: review of 130 cases. Neurosurgery 6: 255–257

Shenkin H A, Greenberg J O, Grossman C B 1975 Ventricular size after shunting for idiopathic normal pressure hydrocephalus. Journal of Neurology, Neurosurgery and Psychiatry 38: 833–837

Stein S C, Langfitt T W 1974 Normal pressure hydrocephalus. Predicting the results of cerebrospinal fluid shunting. Journal of Neurosurgery 41: 463–470

Symon L, Dorsch N W C, Stephens R J 1972 Pressure waves in so-called low pressure hydrocephalus. Lancet 2: 1291–1292

Sypert G W, Leffman H, Ojemann G A 1973 Occult normal pressure hydrocephalus manifested by parkinsonism — dementia complex. Neurology 23: 234–238

Wikkelso C, Andersson H, Blomstrand C, Lindquist G 1982 The clinical effect of lumbar puncture in normal pressure hydrocephalus. Journal of Neurology, Neurosurgery and Psychiatry 45: 64–69

Wyper D J, Pickard J D, Matheson M 1979 The accuracy of ventricular volume estimation. Journal of Neurology, Neurosurgery and Psychiatry 42: 345–350

Udvarhelyi G B, Wood J H, James A E 1975 Results and complications in 55 shunted patients with normal pressure hydrocephalus. Surgical Neurology 3: 271–275

Zeumer H, Schonsky B, Sturm K W 1980 Predominant white matter involvement in subcortical arteriosclerotic encephalopathy (Binswanger's disease). Journal of Computer Assisted Tomography 4: 14–19

20. Should chronic subdural haematomas always be evacuated?

John R. Bartlett

INTRODUCTION

It is well known that in symptomatic cases early evacuation of chronic subdural haematomas (CSDH) leads to a rapid recovery in the majority of patients so treated. Indeed, there is no other intracranial disorder which has such a favourable prognosis. However, it is not possible to establish with certainty the existence of a CSDH on clinical criteria alone. Until the advent of computerised axial tomography (CT scanning) the unpleasant nature and the risks of investigations to prove the diagnosis made it necessary to accept informed clinical opinion rather than to insist on accurate anatomical knowledge in those cases without a clear mandate for operation. CT scanning has changed everything. Previously the investigation of patients who had received head injuries involved invasive procedures; burrhole exploration, angiography and occasionally ventriculography. All these procedures carried a significant risk and were therefore not used lightly. CT scanning provides a non-invasive and risk-free method for diagnosing haematomas within the cranial cavity. Moreover, it has been possible to follow the removal of blood from the subdural space and it is now known that blood entering the subdural space at the time of injury is usually absorbed and the formation of a CSDH is a rare event.

Understanding something of the possible mechanisms of the formation and natural history of CSDH could affect attitudes to methods of management, including surgical treatment. Virchow (1857) suggested that CSDH's were the result of an inflammatory process in the dura and described the condition as pachymeningitis haemorrhagica. Trotter (1914) drew attention to the association of the disorder with mild, often forgotten, head injury. More recently it has become appreciated that 'injury' need not necessarily imply a blow to the head itself; CSDH's have followed whiplash injury (Ommaya & Yarnell, 1969), shaking of the head of an infant (Guthkelch, 1971), and even lumbar puncture (Edelman & Wingard, 1980). In these cases the mechanism seems to be tearing of the bridging veins between the cerebral hemispheres and the sagittal sinus. Occasionally a CSDH may form when blood has entered the subdural space following the rupture of an intracranial aneurysm or arteriovenous malformation and very rarely from a tumour.

What then are the mechanisms involved in the formation of chronic subdural haematomas, what are the criteria for suspecting the diagnosis, when should patients be investigated, what are the indications for treatment, and what form should this take?

PATHOLOGY

A chronic subdural haematoma is not a static entity but a dynamic process which is still not fully understood. There is an initiating factor, usually an injury, which leads to the entry of blood into the subdural space. Other factors play a part and the formation of a CSDH is unusual unless one is present. All have in common the property of allowing a large quantity of blood to enter the cranial cavity. The factors are conveniently divided into two groups — mechanical, and those affecting the coagulability of the blood. The mechanical factors increase the potential space into which bleeding may occur. Cerebral atrophy and the ageing process reduce the size of the brain; loss of c.s.f. from any cause, for example a c.s.f. fistula from a skull fracture or the treatment of hydrocephalus, may provide potential space into which blood can spill; and the soft malleable skull and unfused sutures of an infant can permit enlargement of the head to contain a haematoma. Disorders of blood coagulation, such as anticoagulant therapy and haemophilia, also favour the formation of large haematomas once bleeding has been initiated. The bleeding eventually ceases as a result of blood coagulation and counter pressure from the rise in intracranial pressure.

The natural history of haematomas in the subdural space is usually divided into three phases: acute, the first week; subacute, the second and third weeks, and chronic (CSDH) starting with the fourth week, but the distinction is far from absolute, each phase merging imperceptibly into the next. Broadly speaking these phases correspond to the hyper-, iso-, and hypodense CT scan appearances. Resolution of the haematoma or death from cerebral compression may occur during any phase.

As time passes the haematoma becomes 'encapsulated' — the characteristic feature of a CSDH. The dura reacts to blood in the subdural space with an intense response characterised by capillary growth, formation of sinusoids resembling veins (but without the normal investing layers) and fibroblastic activity. As the haematoma ages the number of capillaries is reduced and the fibroblasts mature. In those cases that resolve the haematoma is gradually absorbed and the inner endothelial layer adjacent to the pia-arachnoid approximates against the inner membrane which is ultimately indistinguishable from normal dura. Not all cases resolve this way. Some progress and the haematoma enlarges producing signs due to distortion of the brain or raised intracranial pressure. Two theories have been put forward to explain the increase in size of CSDHs. In one, the capsule acts as a semipermeable membrane and as the haematoma is broken down into smaller particles fluid is drawn in and increases the volume (Gardner, 1932). This theory, on which the rational use of osmotic dehydrating agents depends, cannot be the full explanation. Fresh erythrocytes are regularly found in the haematoma fluid. Ito et al (1976) studied this using chromium 51 labelled red cells and have shown that daily fresh haemorrhage may amount to 10% of the volume of the haematoma. Furthermore, Weir (1980) has shown that the osmotic pressure of the haematoma fluid is the same as the c.s.f. which effectively disposes of the theory and studies of the ultra structure of the 'membrane' make it clear that to think of a haematoma capsule as a simple semipermeable device is naive. The alternative theory postulates that from time to time bleeding takes place into the cavity from the outer vascular membrane (Putnam & Cushing, 1925). This theory explains why fresh red cells and albumen are found in the fluid aspirated from haematomas, and gives a convincing reason for the growth of a CSDH: the arguments are discussed in the excellent reviews by Markwalder (1981) and Guthkelch (1982).

The vascular neomembrane of the CSDH provides the means for removal of the haematoma. What determines why some CSDH enlarge and others resolve is not clear but there is no doubt that absolute size is an important factor. Apfelbaum, Guthkelch & Shulman (1974) have pointed out that the larger the volume the smaller proportionately is the surface area. If the rate of absorption is directly related to surface area then the larger haematomas will take relatively longer to absorb and it is possible that haematomas must reach a critical size to become chronic and progressive. Recurrent haemorrhages could interrupt the process of absorption at any time and lead to increase in size of the haematoma. Neurosurgeons know that evacuation of CSDH through burrholes is not a complete process; the brain often fails to expand immediately and indeed a CT scan carried out days after such a procedure often reveals very little change in the shape or disposition of the brain. Why removal of the bulk of this liquid haematoma does not precipitate further bleeding from the fragile capillaries into the cavity is also unclear but the removal of the fibrinolytic activity and the fibrin degredation products may be important. It is as if this minor procedure — a burr or twist drill hole and aspiration — tips the balance back in favour of the normal healing process.

RELATIONSHIP BETWEEN PATHOLOGY AND CLINICAL PRESENTATION

Intracranial space occupying lesions (CSDH being one of the largest encountered in clinical practice) produce symptoms and signs in three interrelated ways — distortion, destruction and raised intracranial pressure — each of which may exist singly or in various combinations. Chronic subdural haematomas are extracerebral and exert pressure over a large area of brain — sometimes the best part of the convexity of a cerebral hemisphere — and the local forces on the cerebral cortex are small. Intrinsic damage to the immediately underlying brain itself is, therefore, slight so focal signs relating to the site of the haematoma are usually minimal and may be absent altogether. When present the early signs generally suggest a diffuse malfunction of the brain — confusion, intellectual deterioration — combined with headache.

As has already been emphasised, conditions that favour the development of

CSDH are just those which also make it possible for large lesions to exist without an inordinate rise of intracranial pressure. For this reason the distortions and shifts of the intracranial structures are often very large and have their maximum effect on the brain stem as it passes through the tentorial hiatus where the forces are concentrated. Many of the clinical features of CSDH depend on this fact and a knowledge of the anatomy and function of the brain stem at this level will help the clinician to identify cases which are most likely to have a CSDH that requires treatment.

Within the tentorial hiatus the midbrain is surrounded by subarachnoid cisterns, the prepontine anteriorly traversed by the third nerves, the narrow ambiens on each side, and the cistern of the great cerebral veins posteriorly. A section of the midbrain at this level passes through the superior colliculi, tegmentum, third nerve nucleus, reticular formation, red nucleus, substantia nigra and the cerebral peduncles. Compression may affect the function of any of these structures and the pattern varies from case to case. However, there are some points that merit particular attention. The oculomotor nuclear complex is arranged with the elevators of the eye and eyelids above those which control other movements and compression affects these components first leading to defective upward gaze and ptosis. The nucleus which controls accommodation and the light reflexes is in close proximity so that pupillary abnormalities are common. The reticular formation is composed of neurones which lie outside the major nuclear groups. This system has a very widespread network of connections with the cerebral hemispheres, hypothalamus and the spinal cord and its integrity is necessary for maintaining normal levels of activity and arousal in the nervous system. Impairment of function leads to drowsiness and reduced responsiveness to all kinds of stimuli, and ultimately coma. The pyramidal tracts lie in the peduncles. When the brain stem is displaced transversely against the sharp edge of the tentorium the function of the pyramidal tract from the hemisphere on the opposite side to that of the haematoma is compromised producing a hemiparesis on the same side as the haematoma. (See Johnson, 1957 for a review of the tentorial pressure cone.)

WHAT ARE THE CLINICAL CRITERIA FOR SUSPECTING THE DIAGNOSIS?

If we always had to rely on clinical criteria alone the diagnosis of CSDH would be very difficult. The discussion on pathophysiology has emphasised the varied way in which CSDH may present. Diffuse symptoms of a cerebral disorder (personality change and intellectual failure) are common; focal signs may occur (such as mild hemiparesis) but hard signs, signs of focal tissue destruction, like hemiplegia, hemianopia and global aphasia are very rare; signs of brain stem compression (altered consciousness, defective ocular movements particularly loss of upward gaze which is difficult to assess in the elderly, and anisocoria) are relatively common. Certain conditions favour the development of CSDH: age (infancy and the sixth and seventh decades); mild head injury; hydrocephalus; c.s.f. fistula due to disease, injury or therapy; severe epilepsy which causes repeated injury as well as atrophy from hypoxic episodes; regular inebriation from excessive consumption of alcohol; factors which affect blood coagulability. Insidious neurological deterioration occurring in the presence of any of these should alert the clinician to the possibility of a CSDH. Most patients present with a history of about 6–8 weeks; symptoms of more than 3 months are very unusual.

Many patients who have a persistent headache without any physical signs following a head injury are sent for investigation, but CSDH is very rarely the explanation. Routine investigation of such patients is not justified. When a significant CSDH is present patients are clearly unwell and minor signs are always present. It is much harder to differentiate CSDH from diffuse cerebrovascular disease and tumours but there is one feature which, if present, is very characteristic of CSDH, namely a very marked fluctuation in the level of consciousness. When papilloedema is present there is a clear mandate for investigation.

ESTABLISHING THE DIAGNOSIS

The method used to establish the diagnosis and its accuracy depends to some extent on the training of the clinician and access to specialist methods of investigation. Some of the conditions which favour the formation of CSDH may also be responsible for similar symptoms and signs, for example, cerebral atrophy due to cerebrovascular disease. This is an important fact to take into account for it will have a profound effect on prognosis and therefore should affect the clinician's approach to investigation. Clearly it is unrealistic to investigate every elderly dementing patient with a CT scan and there are patients who, even if a CSDH were detected and evacuated, would not improve with treatment. This fact, and the fear that missing a CSDH in such circumstances could still lead to criticism, is a source of misunderstanding between doctors whose differing points of view merit a brief examination. The physician's view is based solely on the clinical data; the radiologist bases his diagnosis on demonstrating a circumscribed shadow lying between the brain and skull vault using one or other of the various imaging techniques at his disposal; the neurosurgeon bases his diagnosis on finding the characteristic fluid beneath the dura at operation; and finally the pathologist's view is based on finding an encapsulated haematoma partly solid and partly liquid lying between the dura and brain. Inevitably occasions arise when there are disagreements between those responsible for the care of patients and those who control access to and the means of definitive diagnosis on whether, how far and by what means the investigation of some patients should be pursued. This problem will increase as doctors are made increasingly aware that, under the present system of cash limits, spending money for one purpose means that it will not be available for something else. Quality of care and diagnostic certainty have a price.

The investigations available in the average general hospital are limited in scope. The plain skull radiograph may reveal displacement of a calcified pineal. When a fracture is present the injury is usually a significant feature of the history. Lumbar puncture is mentioned only to emphasise that if brain stem signs are present with impairment of consciousness then this procedure may be very dangerous. The value of isotope imaging techniques has proved disappointing for routine use and does not replace careful clinical appraisal and a CT scan if indicated. If CSDH is a probable diagnosis, transfer to a specialist unit for a CT scan is usually justified.

The CT scan has proved to be a very reliable method of making the diagnosis but it is still possible to miss bilateral haematomas and it may be necessary to resort to angiography or isotope studies in an exceptional case. In neurosurgical practice exploratory burrholes have less risk than angiography for the elderly and are often the preferred alternative although this may lead to a negative exploration and it is still possible to miss a haematoma if an insufficient number of holes are made.

TREATMENT — WHO, WHEN AND HOW — IS THERE AN ANSWER?

The literature on treatment presents a wide variety of approaches, but despite this it is almost universally accepted that symptomatic CSDH should be evacuated (Markwalder, 1981; Loew & Kivelitz, 1976). It has already been emphasised that the formation of a progressively enlarging intracranial space occupying lesion in the form of a chronic subdural haematoma is an unusual result of injury, the 'healing process' working in some ill understood way to the patient's disadvantage. In symptomatic and progressive cases the purpose of treatment is twofold — first to save life when this is threatened by midbrain compression, and second to tip the balance of the 'healing process' back in favour of resolution.

Bender & Christoff (1974) who reported 100 cases of subdural haematomas treated conservatively blurred the distinction between subacute and chronic haematomas but their study does demonstrate unequivocally that all do not need removal. Attempts to distinguish between a CSDH with progressive symptoms and signs, and a resolving haematoma in the subdural space which has been present for several weeks as if these are fundamentally separate pathological entities prevents clarity of thought. When a CSDH is detected the problem of management should be solved by identification of those haematomas which are enlarging and causing progressive disturbance of brain function, from those which are resolving. Fundamentally the pathological processes in the haematoma itself must be qualitatively the same though the effect on the cranial contents may differ. If this fact is accepted the management of the patient must depend on the natural history of the particular haematoma and the adverse effects, if any, it is producing. Bender and Christoff's paper shows that patients whose life is threatened by brain stem compression should still be treated by operation and that those where the haematoma is discovered early, simply because the means of diagnosis has become readily available, can safely be managed conservatively unless there is evidence of clinical deterioration.

Suzuki & Takaku (1970) treated 23 cases with daily infusions of 500–1000 ml 20% mannitol. The average duration of treatment was about 6 weeks and only one patient failed to improve and was cured by evacuation of the haematoma. When Gjerris & Schmidt (1974) attempted to confirm these results in a controlled trial, mannitol treatment failed and the study could not be completed. Suzuki (1974) criticised Gjerris and Schmidt on the grounds that it is often important to 'wait patiently for the true results and effects of a new method before drawing final conclusions, rather than terminate a trial prematurely'. Whether mannitol really reduces the size of a haematoma by osmosis, or whether it reduces the size of the brain and so removes the immediate threat of death by midbrain compression and buys time for resolution is, in the author's opinion, an open question. In any event a treatment which takes on average 6 weeks when, by alternative surgical means, many patients will be cured in a fraction of the time is unlikely to gain great favour especially now that escalating costs of health care are of increasing concern. At one time it was thought that unless the membrane of a CSDH was excised healing of the brain would not occur, or in the case of infants normal development would be prevented. This is not the case. Indeed it is now well known that the best results from surgery follow the simplest procedure — aspiration through a drill hole (Tabaddor & Shulman, 1977) or a burrhole. Some advocate continuous drainage through a closed system either external or in the case of infants internal with a tube between the subdural space and peritoneal or pleural cavity. Craniotomy is now reserved for those cases where the haematoma is almost completely solid or reaccumulates rapidly.

CONCLUSIONS ON MANAGEMENT

It is inevitable that any attempt to tackle the question raised by the title of this chapter must to some extent be a personal opinion. Those cases with clearly progressive disease and whose lives are threatened by the effects of brain stem compression must be treated by evacuation. A second episode of brain stem compression after initial relief may have a disastrous effect on the prognosis — particularly in the elderly — and this observation provides the reason for continuous drainage in the initial phase, either with a closed system or even suturing the burrholes open for the first 48 hours.

When a CSDH is detected during an uninterrupted recovery from a head injury there is no need to intervene though most clinicians will wish to follow the progress of resolution with a CT scan and see that this is complete before lifting restrictions on physical activities. It is my practice to observe patients with mild diminishing symptoms in the expectation of resolution.

It is much harder to know what to do when a patient has a large CSDH and yet there is fairly clear evidence that the primary fault and cause of neurological disability is the predisposing cause to the formation of the CSDH. Indeed, it is easy to find oneself on a treadmill of treatment; failure of the simple burrhole evacuation leads on to craniotomy and further disappointment and utimately, at best, a technical triumph but therapeutic failure. Despite this we fall for the trap, perhaps because excessive zeal is unlikely to lead to censure, but an autopsy 'revelation' will raise the question of professional ineptitude or even negligent stupidity, particularly in the minds of those with limited practical experience of the disorder. If there is a way to solve this dilemma, which hangs on the sound assessments of probabilities, it will be through mutual trust and frank discussion with the families of those patients concerned and an acknowledgement that they have understood the issues and been an informed party to the decision on management.

REFERENCES

Apfelbaum R I, Guthkelch A N, Shulman K 1974 Experimental production of subdural hematomas. Journal of Neurosurgery 40: 336–346
Bender M B, Christoff N 1974 Nonsurgical treatment of subdural hematomas. Archives of Neurology 31: 73–79
Edelman J D, Wingard D W 1980 Subdural hematomas after lumbar dural puncture. Anaesthesiology 52: 166–167
Gardner W J 1932 Traumatic subdural hematoma with particular reference to the latent interval. Archives of Neurology and Psychiatry 27: 847–858
Gjerris F, Schmidt K 1974 Chronic subdural hematoma — surgery or mannitol treatment. Journal of Neurosurgery 40: 639–642
Guthkelch A N 1971 Infantile subdural haematoma and its relationship to whiplash injuries. British Medical Journal 2: 430–431
Guthkelch A N 1982 The aetiology and evolution of chronic subdural haematoma. In: Rice Edwards J M (ed) Topical reviews in neurosurgery vol 1. Wright, Bristol, ch 6, p 122–133
Ito H, Yamamoto S, Komai T, Mizukoshi H 1976 Role of local hyperfibrinolysis in the etiology of chronic subdural hematoma. Journal of Neurosurgery 45: 26–31
Johnson R T 1957 Pattern of mid-brain deformity in expanding intracranial lesions. In: Williams D (ed) Modern Trends in Neurology (Second Series). Butterworth, London, ch 20, p 274–286
Loew F, Kivelitz R 1976 Chronic subdural haematomas. In: Vinken P J, Bruyn G W (eds) Handbook of clinical neurology, vol 24, Injuries of the brain and skull Part II. North-Holland Publishing Company, Amsterdam, ch 16, p 297–327
Markwalder T M 1981 Chronic subdural hematomas: a review. Journal of Neurosurgery 54: 637–645
Ommaya A K, Yarnell P 1969 Subdural haematoma after whiplash injury. Lancet 2: 237–239
Putnam T J, Cushing H 1925 Chronic subdural hematoma: its pathology, its relation to pachymeningitis hemorrhagica and its surgical treatment. Archives of Surgery 11: 329–393
Suzuki J 1974 Mannitol treatment of subdural haematomas. Journal of Neurosurgery 41: 785–786 (letter)
Suzuki J, Takaku A 1970 Nonsurgical treatment of chronic subdural hematoma. Journal of Neurosurgery 33: 548–553
Tabbaddor K, Shulman K 1977 Definitive treatment of chronic subdural hematoma by twist-drill craniostomy and closed-system drainage. Journal of Neurosurgery 46: 220–226
Trotter W 1914 Chronic subdural haemorrhage of traumatic origin, and its relation to pachymeningitis hemorrhagica interna. British Journal of Surgery 2: 271–291
Virchow R 1857 Das haematom der dura mater. Verhandlungen Physikalisch-Medizinisch Gesellschaft zur Wuerzburg 7: 134–142
Weir B 1980 Oncotic pressure of subdural fluids. Journal of Neurosurgery 53: 512–515

21. Aggressive medical care of severe head injury — is it justified, ethically and economically?

J. Douglas Miller

THE BASIC ISSUES

A notable development in medical practice in many countries during the past 10 years has been increasing involvement of anaesthetists, neurosurgeons and others working in intensive care in the management of severely head injured patients, and the adoption of a more aggressive, anticipatory approach as compared with the previous practice of admitting head injured patients for observation and acting only when there was a deterioration in neurological status. Have these changes had a significant influence on the outcome after severe head injury, and has the effort been worthwhile in humanitarian and economic terms? This chapter represents an endeavour to answer these difficult questions.

Aggressive medical care of the severely head injured is now extremely expensive, and involves high-technology diagnostic methods such as CT scanning and cerebral angiography as well as intensive monitoring and therapy. This is justified only if the mortality from severe head injury can be reduced without producing a corresponding increase in severe morbidity. If specific medical therapies are applied to head injured patients, it must be demonstrable that the treatment carries greater benefits than risks, and that definite conclusions about effectiveness of therapy can be drawn. Continued application of ineffective therapy may deny the patient another, perhaps more effective, form of treatment.

CURRENTLY AGREED PRINCIPLES OF CARE

Only since the widespread adoption by neurosurgeons throughout the world of the Glasgow Coma Scale (Teasdale & Jennett, 1974) and the Glasgow Outcome Scale (Jennett & Bond, 1975) has it been practicable to state the outcome of patients with head injuries of a given severity (Table 21.1). Jennett and his colleagues (1976, 1979) have defined a 'severe head injury' as one which results in the patient becoming unable to open his eyes, obey commands, or to speak intelligible words for a period of 6 hours or more. In such patients a mortality of 50% was recorded and 10% remained vegetative or severely disabled for at least 6

Table 21.1 Glasgow Coma Scale (Teasdale & Jennett, 1974) and Glasgow Outcome Scale (Jennett & Bond, 1975). Coma on the scale is defined as E1, M5, V2 or below.

Coma scale/score			Outcome scale
Eye opening:	Spontaneous	4	Good recovery
	To command	3	(to previous level of activity)
	To pain	2	
	Nil	1	Moderate disability
			(below previous level but
			independent for ADL)
Best motor response:	Obeys commands	6	
	Localises pain	5	
	Normal flexor	4	Severe disability
	Abnormal flexor	3	(dependent on others for
	Extensor	2	ADL
	Nil	1	
			Permanent vegetative state
Verbal response:	Oriented	5	(unresponsive to changes
	Confused	4	in environment)
	Words	3	
	Sounds	2	Death
	Nil	1	

months. Jennett's group compared their results with those of several other authors who had provided sufficient clinical details to ensure that their cases were of comparable severity (Overgaard et al, 1973; Pagni, 1973; Rossanda et al, 1973; Pazzaglia et al, 1975). The mortality in all of these series was close to 50%, being consistently higher in the sub-group of comatose patients who also required surgical decompression of intracranial haematomas.

In 1977, Becker and his colleagues at the Medical College of Virginia published a series of cases of severe head injury managed by a standardised regimen of immediate resuscitation and then ventriculography, angiography or CT scan to identify any intracranial mass lesion as soon as possible after admission. In this series, therefore, serial neurological observations were not used to detect deterioration and so identify patients with an intracranial haematoma. The criteria for immediate CT or other contrast studies were simply that after resuscitation the patient could not speak or obey commands. In the first series of 160 patients, 40% were found to be harbouring intracranial mass lesions producing at least 5 mm of brain shift. These patients were all submitted to immediate surgical decompression. The mortality in this series of cases was 30% overall, and the incidence of severe disability or permanent vegetative state in surviving patients was 10% of the entire series, a similar proportion to that recorded in the previously mentioned series of severely head injured patients (Table 21.2).

The publication of these results started a wide controversy concerning the claim that this change from an expectant management policy to a more anticipatory approach had resulted in a true fall in mortality in comparable patients. The opposing view was that the apparent fall in mortality merely indicated that the series included many less severely injured patients who had a better chance of survival in any case. Since then, however, other authors have published similar series aggressively managed in the same anticipatory way and mortality rates of

Table 21.2 Comparison of morbidity and mortality rates in reported series of cases of severe head injury.

	Number of cases	% with intra-cranial haematoma	Outcome % Severely disabled/ vegetative	Dead
Expectant management series				
Jennett et al (1979) a	593	54	12	48
b	239	28	9	50
c	168	56	19	50
Rossanda (1973)	223	39	—	52
Pagni (1973)	1091	61	—	52
Pazzaglia et al (1975)	282	41	11	49
Anticipatory management series				
Becker et al (1977)	148	40	11	32
Marshall et al (1979)	100	25	12	28
Clifton et al (1980)	124	32	—	29
Miller et al (1981)	225	41	10	34

between 30 and 40% have been confirmed (Bowers & Marshall, 1980; Clifton et al, 1980). In 1981, Miller and Becker and their colleagues published a further series of 225 comatose patients with a 34% mortality. Included in this series were 147 patients whose head injury was at least as severe as those reported by the Jennett group. These patients were unable to open their eyes even to pain, were unable to obey commands, and unable to utter recognisable words, both on admission and on re-examination between 6 and 24 hours later, but included patients who died in the interim period. The mortality in this sub-set of 147 cases was 40%. This is virtually the same as has been reported from Glasgow in cases managed in a similar way (early CT scan and urgent decompression) over the same period of time (Teasdale, personal communication). The application of predictive data from Glasgow to cases from the Medical College of Virginia resulted in the correct prediction of the actual outcome in all but 1 of 50 patients (Teasdale & Miller, unpublished data).

There now appears to be worldwide consensus on the expected mortality and morbidity after severe head injury and agreement on many of the general principles of care. These principles include the use of immediate CT scanning on all comatose patients (in whom there is a 40–50% risk of harbouring an intracranial haematoma producing significant brain shift; Miller et al, 1981), urgent evacuation of such space occupying lesions, and management of patients in an Intensive Care Unit. This 'aggressive' anticipatory approach does *not* result in a greater proportion of severely disabled and vegetative survivors. The proportion of vegetative patients remains about the same in all series — between 1 and 3%. Severely disabled patients account for 8–12% of all reported series. The anticipatory approach is, therefore, justified on ethical and economic grounds.

There is also considerable accord concerning the prognostic significance of the clinical variables recorded in severely head injured patients. The patient's age, presence of an intracranial haematoma, the level of consciousness on the Glasgow Coma Scale with special emphasis on the motor response, and the presence of clinical signs of impaired brain stem function (bilateral pupillary abnormalities and impaired or absent reflex eye movements) are the most important factors determining outcome, followed closely by the presence and severity of hypoxia, arterial hypotension or intracranial hypertension (Stablein et al, 1980; Narayan et al, 1981). In severely head injured patients, raised intracranial pressure (ICP) occurs in just over 50% of cases managed in an Intensive Care Unit and receiving artificial ventilation, including postoperative patients. The outcome is closely related to the highest level of ICP recorded, with no surviving patients when ICP exceeds 60 mm Hg for any time (Table 21.3).

Table 21.3 Relationship between the highest level of intracranial pressure and mortality. (Data from Miller et al, 1981.)

Highest intracranial pressure	n (%)	Mortality (%)
Less than 20 mm Hg	102 (47)	18
More than 20 mm Hg	113 (53)	45
More than 40 mm Hg	39 (18)	74
More than 60 mm Hg	18 (8)	100

Within diagnostic groups, a further important factor in survival is the time delay between injury or loss of consciousness and evacuation of an intracranial haematoma. This is true for both extradural and acute subdural haematoma where delay of more than 4 hours is associated with a steep rise in mortality and morbidity (Mendelow et al, 1979; Seelig et al, 1981).

Many other aspects of head injury remain highly controversial, however: which other patients should have CT scanning on a prospective basis? Which patients should be artificially ventilated? In which patients should ICP be monitored and, if it is increased, at what level of ICP should treatment begin, and which treatment should be given? Is raised ICP most safely and best controlled by osmotherapy, c.s.f. drainage, hyperventilation, barbiturate therapy, or by some other short acting anaesthetic agents such as althesin, gamma hydroxybutyrate or etomidate? These questions will be addressed in the remainder of this chapter.

CT SCANNING IN HEAD INJURY

Over the past few years it has been accepted that in a patient who is already comatose (at or below E1, M5, V2 on the Glasgow Coma Scale) it is no longer acceptable practice to await further deterioration in conscious level before applying the diagnostic measures required to find an intracranial haematoma. Coma signifies brain failure just as uraemia can signify renal failure. To await further deterioration in brain function is to invite irreversible brain damage. Patients who are admitted comatose following head injury to a hospital that contains a CT scanner should be scanned just as soon as it is considered safe to move the patient from the Accident and Emergency Department to the X-ray Scanning Suite. This means that the patient's airway, respiration, blood pressure and circulation must be adjudged stable and safe before making such a move.

Approximately 50% of comatose head injured patients also have major injuries requiring the services of other surgical departments, 30% are hypoxic on admission to hospital, and 15% have arterial hypotension (Miller et al, 1978, 1981). These insults are associated with doubling of the mortality rate and increased morbidity (Price & Murray, 1972).

What are the other indications and degrees of urgency for CT scanning in head injured patients? If a head injured patient has a skull fracture the overall risk of an intracranial haematoma is about 10% rising to 15 or 20% if the patient is also exhibiting persisting drowsiness and/or abnormal neurological signs. In my opinion, when the risk of an intracranial haematoma reaches 20%, the patient, if he is not already in a hospital with a CT scanner, should be transferred for this investigation to the nearest centre that has this facility. This recommendation may be considered controversial by some but it should be viewed in the light of the recent article by Jeffreys & Jones (1981) who found that 33% of head injury deaths occurring in hospitals in their region, but not in the regional neurosurgical unit, were due to undiagnosed, but potentially treatable, intracranial haematomas.

In which patients is the risk of intracranial haematomas so low as to make CT scanning, or even admission for observation, unnecessary? Patients over the age of 14 who are conscious and alert with no abnormal neurological signs, who are not complaining of headache or vomiting, and who have no visible signs or X-ray evidence of skull fracture, have such a small risk of developing an intracranial haematoma that they may be safely sent home from hospital with no CT scan (Mendelow et al, 1982). Because very young children may develop intracranial haematomas without an accompanying skull fracture, a greater proportion of these patients require to be admitted for at least overnight observation. This statement is not meant to imply, however, that intracranial haematomas do not develop in adult patients in the absence of a skull fracture. They do, but are virtually always accompanied by some degree of persisting drowsiness, abnormal neurological signs, headache and vomiting, or impairment in conscious level, any of which criteria should lead to the patient's admission for observation. The usual criterion for admission following head injury is a history of loss of consciousness, even if the patient when seen is alert and oriented with no abnormal neurological signs. The yield of intracranial haematomas detected early by admitting all such patients is extremely low, to the point where the policy should be modified on the lines suggested (Mendelow et al, 1982).

ARTIFICIAL VENTILATION IN HEAD INJURY

In view of the strong adverse influence of hypoxaemia and hypercarbia on the outcome from severe head injury, a strong argument has been made for early endotracheal intubation of all comatose head injured patients. The obvious extension of this is to apply artificial ventilation to all such patients as well. The risk: benefit ratio of this policy depends very much on the facilities and expertise available in individual treating centres. To date there has been no conclusive evidence that artificial ventilation per se results in a definite reduction in mortality or morbidity of severe head injury, despite strong claims that this is the case (Gordon, 1971; Rossanda et al, 1973).

Artificial ventilation usually entails administration of sedative or muscle relaxant drugs to prevent spontaneous respiratory efforts in opposition to the ventilator. Such efforts can produce severe increases in intracranial pressure. Furthermore, such agents, particularly muscle relaxants, prevent adequate serial neurological examination of the patient and allow for the worrying possibility of undetected neurological deterioration due to brain swelling or cerebral ischaemia in the aftermath of head injury. There are few occurrences more upsetting to the therapeutic team than instituting artificial ventilation in a head injured patient who is exhibiting bilateral pupillary light responses and bilateral flexor motor responses to pain, yet who on reversal of the muscle relaxants is found to have dilated fixed pupils with no motor response whatsoever and clinical evidence of brain death. The possibility of the undetected development of this catastrophic situation is one of the strongest arguments in favour of the institution of continuous monitoring of ICP in all comatose head injured patients who are subjected to artificial ventilation.

MONITORING OF INTRACRANIAL PRESSURE

The high frequency of raised ICP in comatose head injured patients — 53% overall and as high as 80% in patients with intraparenchymal haemorrhagic lesions associated with brain shift — the loss of neurological signs during artificial ventilation aided by muscle relaxants, and the strongly adverse prognostic significance of raised ICP have all proved powerful arguments in favour of applying continuous monitoring of ICP in cases of severe head injury (Miller & Sullivan, 1979). ICP monitoring permits early detection of raised pressure and allows a close watch to be kept on the efficacy of therapy directed at controlling raised ICP. If one therapeutic modality proves ineffective, it can quickly be changed for another (Miller er al, 1977; Miller, 1978). This is no longer regarded as very controversial, nor is there dispute as to the risks of ICP monitoring. These risks include haemorrhage along the track of an intraventricular cannula or under a subarachnoid screw, a rising incidence of intracranial infection with increasing duration of monitoring, becoming significant after 5 days, and the danger of misdirected therapy because of erroneous ICP measurements.

While ICP monitoring eases patient management, there is less evidence that the application of ICP monitoring does, in fact, result in a saving of lives or a better quality survival in severely head injured patients. While the question may to some extent be an unfair one (Miller et al, 1981) it has been at least partly answered by Bowers & Marshall (1980) and Clifton and his colleagues (1980) who noted a lower mortality in patients managed by an aggressive regime that included ICP monitoring than in comparable head injured patients managed similarly but without this modality.

The prognostic value of information from ICP monitoring has been carefully studied (Miller et al 1981; Narayan et al, 1981). The highest level of ICP observed during monitoring is closely related to head injury mortality, with no survivors in patients in whom ICP has ever exceeded 60 mm Hg (Table 21.3). In addition, patients with moderate intracranial hypertension (20–40 mm Hg) that has been successfully treated have a significantly higher incidence of severe disability (25% of survivors) than is observed in patients with normal ICP (11% of survivors).

'STANDARD METHODS' OF MANAGEMENT OF RAISED INTRACRANIAL PRESSURE

The threshold level of raised ICP at which it is recommended that treatment be started has fallen over the past few years. Most neurosurgeons today would agree that when ICP exceeds a mean of 25 mm Hg for more than 5 minutes, measures should be taken to reduce it. Many neurosurgeons feel that if therapy begins as soon as ICP exceeds 15 mm Hg better control of ICP is obtained. This proposition has never been proven. A suitable randomised trial would compare control of intracranial pressure in cases where therapy is begun only when ICP exceeds 25 mm Hg, versus those cases where treatment is begun as soon as ICP exceeds 15 mm Hg. Before specific therapy against intracranial hypertension is started, however, extracranial causes of raised ICP must be sought and corrected. These include airway obstruction, compression of neck veins, hypoxaemia, hypercarbia or hyperthermia (Miller, 1978).

The protocol for managing raised ICP that was advocated by Becker et al (1977) consisted first of hyperventilation to arterial PCO_2 levels of 3.0–3.5 kPa (20–25 mm Hg). If this was not successful, and ICP was being monitored by an intraventricular catheter, then continuous c.s.f. drainage was established always against a positive pressure of 20 cm water. This was necessary to prevent ventricular collapse. If ICP again became elevated or c.s.f. drainage could not be established, intravenous mannitol was given in an initial dose of 0.5–1.0 g/kg body weight. This was infused rapidly. Later doses were adjusted in quantity and timing according to the initial ICP response and its duration. The aim was to produce a satisfactory level of ICP, below 20 mm Hg, with the smallest dose of mannitol. Continuous administration of mannitol is not recommended because of difficulties with fluid balance and increasing serum osmolality. If baseline serum osmolality rises above 330 mmol/kg further mannitol is unlikely to produce significant reduction of ICP. At this point osmotherapy is declared to have failed. Further doses of mannitol not only fail to reduce ICP but lead to renal failure and metabolic acidosis. Osmotherapy demands meticulous replacement of fluids and electrolytes to avoid the twin hazards of hypovolaemia leading to arterial hypotension, and hyponatraemia leading to brain swelling.

In recent years there has been a growing reluctance to use large quantities of osmotic agents. The role of adjunctive diuretics such as frusemide has not been clearly established, although advocated by some (Cottrell et al, 1977). Superiority of other hypertonic agents, such as urea or glycerol, over mannitol has been claimed but not proven (Miller 1979a and b).

Nowadays, the most common approach to dealing with resistant intracranial hypertension in the short term is to turn to short-acting anaesthetic agents. While helping in some ways to control ICP, this form of therapy has introduced many other problems into head injury management and remains a highly controversial issue. Before dealing with this, however, another contentious issue must first be discussed, namely the role of steroid therapy in the management of head injured patients with respect to control of intracranial hypertension and overall outcome.

STEROID THERAPY IN HEAD INJURY

Ever since the introduction of powerful glucocorticoids into clinical neurosurgery in the early 1960s, there have been controversies concerning the indications for these agents, many of which have not yet been settled. As soon as clinicians observed the dramatic benefits afforded by steroids to patients with brain tumours with peritumoural oedema and some cases of brain abscess, many were anxious to apply the same agents to patients with acute stroke and head injuries. In head injury, the initial results were not encouraging and most neurosurgeons remained unconvinced of the benefits of dexamethasone in a dosage schedule of 4 mg 6-hourly in severely head injured patients. In 1976, however, two papers, by Gobiet, and by Faupel and their colleagues from two West German centres, made the claim that high doses of dexamethasone, 100 mg per day in the initial phase, reduced the incidence of resistant intracranial hypertension and significantly improved the outcome of head injured patients. These reports came at a time when clinicians involved with brain tumour patients were successfully using very large doses of dexamethasone to regain control of brain swelling in patients who had 'escaped' at a lower dosage schedule. These two favourable reports on the use of steroids in severe head injury led the majority of neurosurgeons in West Germany and the United States to adopt the administration of steroids as part of the routine management of all severely head injured patients. The practice of administering steroids to head injured patients was, in fact, so widespread in the United States as to make it virtually impossible in many parts of the country to embark on a randomised trial of steroid therapy that included a non-steroid arm.

Despite these difficulties, several trials have been carried out to study the effect of high-dose steroid therapy on intracranial pressure and outcome in severely head injured patients. In the last 2 years these results have become available and uniformly indicate that corticosteroid therapy, whether in the form of dexamethasone or methyl prednisolone, and whether given in standard dosage or high dosage, fails to produce any overall impression on intracranial hypertension or on outcome in severely head injured patients. These are patients defined as scoring between 3 and 8 on the Glasgow Coma Scale for a period of 6 hours or more after injury or deterioration. The reasons for this failure of observable effect have been widely debated but one thing seems clear, that in patients with severe diffuse brain injury who are in deep coma, scoring 3, 4 or 5 on the Coma Scale, steroid therapy has absolutely no effect (Jennett et al, 1980; Gudeman et al, 1979; Cooper et al, 1979; Pitts & Kaktis, 1980; Braakman et al, 1983).

Before the role of steroids in head injury is discounted completely, one important question remains to be answered. That is whether steroid therapy has a beneficial effect on focal brain contusion. This lesion, being focal, and often associated with perifocal oedema, is, in theory at least, the one most likely to benefit from steroids. There is no reliable information on the effect of steroid therapy in such cases. A randomised trial is badly needed.

230

THE USE OF ANAESTHETIC AGENTS IN SEVERE HEAD INJURY

The agents that have been most widely applied to control intracranial pressure and to protect the brain in severe head injury have been the barbiturate drugs thiopentone and pentobarbitone. By using pentobarbitone in a series of severely head injured patients with intracranial hypertension, and in whom other measures had failed Marshall et al (1979) and Rockoff et al (1979) claimed to have saved the lives of several patients who, had they been treated only by the ICP management protocol of Becker et al (1977), would surely have died. This claim has been examined in detail by Miller (1979a) who considered that at that time there was not sufficient proof for the effectiveness of barbiturates in severely head injured patients to warrant the widespread use of this drug regimen. Barbiturate therapy is not without dangers and drawbacks. The principal danger is in production of severe arterial hypotension by administration of barbiturates to hypovolaemic patients. Such patients should have central pressures carefully monitored, preferably by means of a Swan-Ganz catheter. Prolonged administration of barbiturate over a period of several days renders the patient inaccessible to neurological evaluation and most evoked potential activity is lost. Even when barbiturate therapy is stopped, several more days must ensue before the patient's central nervous system is free of barbiturate. Unfortunately, blood levels of barbiturate are not always an accurate guide to the tissue level.

Partly in response to these cautions, several trials of barbiturate therapy in severe head injury have been started and currently most remain in progress. Preliminary results suggest that the benefits of barbiturate therapy in terms of long-term control of intracranial hypertension and overall outcome from severe injury will not be very striking if demonstrable at all (Becker, personal communication; Schwartz, personal communication).

In a similar vein, there have been encouraging preliminary reports about the use of althesin, etomidate and gamma hydroxybutyrate in the management of ICP in severely head injured patients. Clearly randomised trials of these agents are also badly needed before a final verdict can be given.

CONCLUSIONS

In the management of patients with severe head injury a major stride forward was the adoption in the 1970s of a common terminology by many workers throughout the world to describe the clinical status and outcome of patients with head injury. Only then could realistic comparisons of treatment between centres even be contemplated. Several multi-centre and international studies have been completed and more are in progress. This is crucial for the future research in this area. Because of the disparate nature of head injury it becomes crucial to break cases down into specific sub-categories because, for example, the clinical presentation, management, complications and outcome of patients with diffuse white matter damage and acute subdural haematoma are so very different. Only by combining series from different centres is it possible to accumulate sufficient numbers. This very cooperation, however, is crucially and critically dependent upon rigid adherence to an agreed objective terminology.

The aggressive approach to head injury management is based on recognition of two key factors — that intracranial haematoma is the commonest cause of preventable death after head injury, and that intracranial hypertension is closely associated with increased morbidity and mortality after injury (Rose et al, 1977; Jeffreys & Jones, 1981; Miller et al, 1977, 1981). Early detection and urgent evacuation of haematoma by craniotomy, continuous monitoring and control of intracranial pressure have reduced the mortality from severe head injury without increasing the incidence of severe dependent disability, and are therefore justified in both ethical and economic terms.

REFERENCES

Becker D P, Miller J D, Ward J D, Greenberg R P, Young H F, Sakalas R 1971 The outcome form severe head injury with early diagnosis and intensive management. Journal of Neurosurgery 47: 491–502
Bowers S A, Marshall L F 1980 Outcome in 200 consecutive cases of severe head injury treated in San Diego County: a prospective analysis. Neurosurgery 6: 237–242
Braakman R, Schouten H J A, Van Dis Hoeck M W, Minderhoud J M 1983 Megadose steroids in severe head injury. Journal of Neurosurgery 58: 326–330
Clifton G L, Grossman R G, Makela M E, Minder M E, Handel S, Sadhu V 1980 Neurological course and correlated computerised tompgraphy findings after severe closed head injury. Journal of Neurosurgery 52: 611–624
Cooper P R, Moody S, Clark W K, Kirkpatrick J, Maravilla K, Gould A L, Drane W 1979 Dexamethasone and severe head injury. Journal of Neurosurgery 51: 307–316
Cottrell J E, Robustelli A, Post K 1977 Furosemide and mannitol induced changes in intracranial pressure and serum osmolality and electrolytes. Anaesthesiology 47: 28–30
Faupel G, Reulen H J, Müller D, Schurmann K 1976 Double blind study on the effects of steroids on severe closed head injury. In: Pappius H M, Feindel W (eda) Dynamics of Brain edema. Springer-Verlag, Berlin, p 337–343
Gobiet W, Bock W J, Liesgang J, Grote W 1976 Treatment of acute cerebral edema with high dose dexamethasone. In: Beks J W F, Bosch D A, Brock M (eds) Intracranial Pressure III. Springer-Verlag, Berlin, p 231–235
Gordon E 1971 Some correlations between the clinical outcome and the acid-base status of blood and cerebrospinal fluid in patients with traumatic brain injury. Acta Anaesthetic Scandinavica 15: 209–228
Gudeman S K, Miller J D, Becker D P 1979 Failure of high dose steroid therapy to influence intracranial pressure in patients with severe head injury. Journal of Neurosurgery 51: 301–306
Jeffreys R V, Jones J J 1981 Avoidable factors contributing to the death of head injury patients in general hospitals in Mersey Region. Lancet 2: 459–461
Jennett B, Bond M R 1975 Assessment of outcome after severe brain damage. Lancet 1: 480–484
Jennett B, Teasdale G M, Braakman R et al 1976 Predicting outcome in individual patients after head injury. Lancet 1: 1031–1034
Jennett B, Teasdale G M, Braakman R, Minderhoud J, Heiden J, Kurze T 1979 Prognosis of patients with severe head injury. Neurosurgery 4: 283–289
Jennett B, Teasdale G M, Fry J, Braakman R, Minderhoud J, Heiden J, Kurze T 1980 Treatment for severe head injury. Journal of Neurology, Neurosurgery and Psychiatry 43: 289–295
Marshall L F, Smith R W, Shapiro H M 1979 The outcome with aggressive treatment in severe head injuries. I. The significance of intracranial pressure monitoring. II. Acute and chronic barbiturate administration in the management of head injury. Journal of Neurosurgery 50: 20–25 and 26–30
Mendelow A D, Campbell D A, Jeffrey R R, Miller J D, Hessett C, Bryden J, Jennett B 1982 Admission after mild head injury: benefits and costs. British Medical Journal 285: 1530–1532
Mendelow A D, Karmi M Z, Paul K S, Fuller G A G, Gillingham F J 1979 Extradural haematoma: effect of delayed treatment. British Medical Journal 1: 1240–1242
Miller J D 1978 Intracranial pressure monitoring. British Journal of Hospital Medicine 19: 497–503
Miller J D 1979a Barbiturates and raised intracranial pressure. Annals of Neurology 6: 189–193
Miller J D 1979b Clinical management of cerebral oedema. British Journal of Hospital Medicine 20: 152–166

Miller J D, Becker D P, Ward J D, Sullivan H G, Adams W E, Rosner M J 1977 Significance of intracranial hypertension in severe head injury. Journal of Neurosurgery 47: 503-516

Miller J D, Butterworth J F, Gudeman S K, Faulkner J E, Choi S C, Selhorst J B, Harbison J W, Lutz H, Young H F, Becker D P 1981 Further experience in the management of severe head injury. Journal of Neurosurgery 54: 289-299

Miller J D, Sullivan H G 1979 Management of severe intracranial hypertension. International Anesthesiology Clinics 17: 19-75

Miller J D, Sweet R C, Narayan R, Becker D P 1978 Early insults to the injured brain. Journal of the American Medical Association 240: 439-442

Narayan R K, Greenberg R P, Miller J D, Enas G G, Choi S C, Kishore P R S, Selhorst J B, Lutz H L, Becker D P 1981 Improved confidence of outcome prediction in severe head injury. Journal of Neurosurgery 54: 751-762

Overgaard J, Christensen S, Jansen O, Haase J, Land A M, Pederson K K, Tweed W A 1973 Prognosis after head injury based on early clinical examination. Lancet 2: 631-635

Pagni C A 1973 The prognosis of head injured patients in a state of coma with decerebrated posture. Journal of Neurosurgical Sciences 17: 289-295

Pazzaglia P, Frank G, Frank F, Gaist G 1975 Clinical course and prognosis of acute post-traumatic coma. Journal of Neurology, Neurosurgery and Psychiatry 38: 149-154

Pitts L H, Kaktis J V 1980 Effect of megadose steroids on ICP in traumatic coma. In: Shulman K, Marmarou A, Miller J D, Becker D P, Hochwald G M, Brock M (eds) Intracranial Pressure IV. Springer-Verlag, Berlin, p 638-642

Price D J E, Murray A 1972 The influence of hypoxia and hypotension on recovery from head injury. Injury 3: 218-224

Rockoff M A, Marshall L F, Shapiro H M 1979 High-dose barbiturate therapy in man. A clinical review of sixty patients. Annals of Neurology 6: 194-199

Rose J, Valtonen S, Jennett B 1977 Avoidable factors contributing to death after head injury. British Medical Journal 2: 615-618

Rossanda M, Selenati A, Villa C, Beduschi A 1973 Role of automatic ventilation in treatment of severe head injuries. Journal of Neurosurgical Sciences 17: 265-270

Seelig J M, Becker D P, Miller J D Greenberg R P, Ward J D, Choi S C 1981 Traumatic acute subdural haematoma: major mortality reduction in comatose patients treated within four hours. New England Journal of Medicine 304: 1511-1518

Stablein D M, Miller J D, Choi S C, Becker D P 1980 Statistical methods for determining prognosis in severe head injury. Neurosurgery 6: 243-248

Teasdale G, Jennett B 1974 Assessment of coma and impaired consciousness. A practical scale. Lancet 2: 81-84

22. Which operation for trigeminal neuralgia?

Michael M. Sharr

INTRODUCTION

There can be little doubt that the pain known as trigeminal neuralgia, or tic douloureux, must be one of the worst that man can suffer. This was graphically illustrated by Pennybacker (1961) who quoted an elderly doctor who had had acute osteomyelitis of the tibia, biliary colic, renal colic, and trigeminal neuralgia, but he was in no doubt that the trigeminal neuralgia was immeasurably the worst.

The problem of deciding which operation is best for the condition begins immediately it is realised that there is still a basic lack of knowledge regarding its aetiology; hence the variety of operations that have been used to treat the unfortunate patients. Another important aspect is the way that a particular neurosurgeon has been trained, this being an important factor in whether an open root section may be preferred or a more conservative approach such as root or ganglion alcohol injection or radiofrequency lesion. Not only must it be acknowledged that an individual neurosurgeon will not have all the available operations in his repertoire, but of equal importance is that the obtaining of good results with one technique does not necessarily mean that similar or even better results could not be achieved with other techniques. Indeed, the type of operation performed by a particular neurosurgeon may influence the type of patients referred to him. It may therefore seem strange, bearing in mind the title of this chapter, to have to admit that there is no ideal operation for trigeminal neuralgia, for if there was then there would not be so many diverse opinions as to which is the best.

WHAT SHOULD THE IDEAL OPERATION OFFER?

The ideal operation should offer the following:

1. A very good chance of producing immediate pain relief.
2. Prolonged relief, although this may not always be as important as immediate relief. Those who doubt this should ask themselves what the patient wants during an acute attack, the answer being that relief from the pain is the

priority. This is not to negate the importance of preventing further attacks of pain but there will be instances where a patient will need a 'tiding over' procedure whereas other patients will need, or indeed demand, a once and for all cure.

3. Nil, or minimum mortality and morbidity.
4. The risk of undesirable side-effects should be as low as possible.
5. Reasonably flexible indications.

WHAT OPERATIONS ARE AVAILABLE?

For the purposes of this discussion any procedure that is used when conservative measures have failed will be regarded as an operation. Such conservative measures usually mean drug therapy with Carbamazepine, Phenytoin, or Clonazepam.

The operations that are available are:

1. Peripheral blocks of the branches of the trigeminal nerve, usually using alcohol.
2. Peripheral nerve branch section or avulsion.
3. Injection of the ganglion or root using alcohol, phenol, or boiling water.
4. Thermocoagulation, electrocoagulation, or radiofrequency lesions of the root or ganglion.
5. Open root section:
    a. Middle fossa or temporal approach, either extradural or intradural.
    b. Posterior fossa or suboccipital approach.
    c. Retrolabyrinthine approach (really a refined form of the posterior fossa approach).
    d. Retrogasserian transtentorial approach, this being a sophisticated extension of the middle fossa intradural operation.
6. Posterior fossa microvascular decompression of the nerve root.
7. Other manoeuvres on the ganglion such as 'decompression' or 'compression'.
8. Medullary tractotomy.

Most, but not all the above forms of treatment are fully discussed by Stookey & Ransohoff (1959), Penman (1968), and White & Sweet (1969).

Peripheral nerve blocks

Schlösser (1903) was probably the first to carry out blocks of the nerves at their exit foramina and Patrick (1912) was another early pioneer. Grant (1936) certainly believed in the place of injection and, in the discussion that followed his paper, he made it clear that he disagreed with the comments of Dandy who had claimed that radical operation was the primary treatment of choice.

There may be a number of circumstances under which peripheral injection is useful. Firstly, when immediate pain relief is required but more radical treatment is not available. Secondly, if the diagnosis is in doubt, the success of the procedure may differentiate true trigeminal neuralgia from other forms of facial pain. Thirdly, the ensuing sensory loss will enable a patient to experience the sensory loss on the face if there is apprehension about this in the long-term. A further indication may be when treating the second side in bilateral trigeminal neuralgia.

There has been some controversy regarding the place of a preliminary injection prior to more radical treatment to enable the patient to adjust to the sensory loss, although Cushing (1920) and many other workers (listed by White & Sweet, 1969) had no doubt that it did help, and moreover established the diagnosis. More recently Pennybacker (1961) reaffirmed the practice of giving a peripheral injection prior to a root section and, of all the published series of root section results, his remains one of the most impressive not only in terms of pain relief but the very low rate of postoperative facial sensory disturbances. However, equally eminent surgeons including Dandy (1932), Olivecrona (1939), and Stookey & Ransohoff (1959) have doubted the value of peripheral injections in this context.

The major objection to a peripheral injection is that it will not produce longstanding relief. However, accepting that, a 'tiding-over' procedure may be all that is required in some circumstances, it is worth noting the results of Horrax & Poppen (1935). They showed an average of 14 months relief for third division pain, the shortest being 9 months and the longest 8 years; apart from supraorbital injection the other nerve injections produced relief of an average of at least 1 year. Grant (1936) produced similar figures, again the duration of relief for third division pain being the best and first division the worst (16 months and 11 months respectively).

There is, therefore, no doubt that there is a place for peripheral nerve injection, both as temporising procedure and (although somewhat controversial) as a procedure to enable a patient to experience the numbness that will result from a more radical operation.

Peripheral neurectomy
In some ways the indications are the same as those for peripheral injections. However, Grantham & Segeberg (1952) were convinced of the value of this form of treatment as opposed to peripheral injections and they were able to show a greater duration of pain relief. The average duration following a peripheral injection was 15½ months with a range from 0–9 years; the average following neurectomy was 33 months with a range from 5 months – 8 years. Of course, the neurectomies were those of the supraorbital and infraorbital branches. Horrax & Poppen (1935) limited neurectomy to the supraorbital nerve and reported a period of relief varying from 2–4 years. Those who doubt the value of peripheral neurectomy would do well to remember that this period is longer than that of follow-up of some series of radiofrequency thermocoagulation that are discussed later.

It would, therefore, appear that if supraorbital injection gives the shortest duration of pain relief (see above), then neurectomy could be reserved for first division pain whilst injection may be favoured for third division and possibly second division pain. Certainly either technique was the initial favoured method used by Morgan, Cast & Wilson (1977). The advantage of neurectomy is that it is less painful than an injection, and the result is more predictable because the failure rate is lower. Moreover, avulsing the supraorbital nerve is a relatively simple operation that can be carried out by a non-neurological surgeon, whereas injection does require some expertise. Two other aspects of treatment should be mentioned: firstly whether injection or neurectomy is performed, it is the trigger area that should be treated and not the area to which the pain radiates (Patrick, 1912). Secondly, if a neurectomy is carried out, then the more the nerve can be twisted and pulled the better, in that the longer the removed segment the closer to the ganglion that removal will have been, and the smaller the risk of regeneration.

Neurectomy or injection may be a very acceptable compromise for both patient and doctor if pain returns after more radical treatment, and the patient declines further surgery. In summary, manoeuvres on the peripheral branches of the trigeminal nerve can certainly be worthwhile, and most neurologists and neurosurgeons seem to underestimate their value.

Ganglion or root injection

Whether the injected substance is alcohol (Taptas, 1911; Harris, 1912; Härtel, 1914), phenol (Putnam & Hampton, 1936), or boiling water (Jaeger, 1957), this treatment has been used for a long time. It is difficult to be sure whether the ganglion or root is being injected but Henderson (1965) explained much of the anomaly by showing that there was anatomical variation; some individuals have a long root and short nerves (pre-fixed) and others a short root and a long nerve (post-fixed). The obtaining of c.s.f. from the needle is not a necessary prerequisite to a successful injection (Garfield, 1977). Härtel first used the technique of ganglion or root injection in 1912 for obtaining facial anaesthesia and it was 2 years later that he used it to treat trigeminal neuralgia. Harris (1912) carried out more than 1000 injections, a figure that is unlikely ever to be surpassed.

Whilst the initial pain relief is usually good, the possible side-effects and complications have continued to be a significant factor in preventing the procedure being more widely used. However, their precise frequency has been somewhat controversial. For example, although early reports included mention of the problems of facial sensory disturbance and keratitis, the actual incidence seemed very variable and was not always quoted. In Hofer and Trauner's series of 116 patients (quoted by White & Sweet, 1969), nearly 10% actually lost the sight of an eye. Yet Kulenkampff (1942) reported 800 ganglion injections and claimed to have prevented keratitis by ensuring that the patients wore glasses. Ramb (1949) analysed his results using the Härtel technique and was pessimistic about the risk of keratitis. Some other frightening figures were also noted, namely, those of Von Brücke (1938) and Shimizu (1937). However, in a recent series (Sharr & Garfield, 1977) the ophthalmic complication rate was extremely low with only 2 out of 85 alcohol injections leading to tarsorrhaphy, 1 of which was permanent. It is worth noting that in only three series of root sections was the incidence of ophthalmic complications lower than this (Olivecrona, 1947; Stookey & Ransohoff, 1959; Pennybacker, 1961). It is evident that, provided the patient is given careful instructions about observing the eye for any reddening and not neglecting any evidence of early infection, the complication of keratitis should be very low.

The various sensory symptoms in the face that can follow any destructive surgery to the trigeminal nerve (including the root and ganglion) have been given various names such as dysaesthesiae, paraesthesiae, anaesthesia dolorosa (really a very severe form of dysaesthesia), but as far as the patient is concerned there is little point in dividing them up and claiming dogmatically that one is really worse than the other. The interpretation of these symptoms by the doctor will inevitably vary and there is much to be gained by simply accepting them as unreal and unpleasant sensations in the face and calling them 'trigeminal causalgia' (Harris, 1940). The reported incidence is variable but it is not insignificant (Ecker, 1974; Sharr & Garfield, 1977). However, it is very rare for the patient to claim that the original neuralgia was preferable to the causalgia. Intolerance to the numbness is another problem that may follow an injection but, again, the interpretation of this by both the doctor and the patient may be such that there is only a thin red line between this and causalgia. In Jefferson's series (1963) a small number of patients who had previously had a successful injection of alcohol needed further treatment; the numbness that resulted from a phenol injection seemed more tolerable than that which had resulted from the previous alcohol injection.

Although cranial nerve palsies may occur following alcohol injection, the incidence is low. Such palsies usually result from spillage of the alcohol into the c.s.f. pathways (hence Jaeger, 1957, resorted to using hot water), and can largely be prevented by keeping the needle vertical and the patient's head extended for a few minutes following the injection. Although there have been some frightening examples of multiple cranial nerve palsies (Dandy, 1929; Tonis & Kreissel, 1951; Stookey & Ransohoff, 1959), the few reported by Sharr & Garfield (1977) ultimately improved and disappeared in 24 hours to 2 years.

Having discussed the side-effects it is clearly essential to consider the question of pain relief. Even in the recent literature it is claimed that relief for more than a year is rare (Loeser, 1978). Such an inaccurate statement is not uncommon and similar comments are made about many of the other forms of treatment. Certainly the statement in relation to the treatment under discussion is untrue, Ecker (1976) reporting an 81% incidence of pain relief for at least 7 years or until death, and Sharr & Garfield (1977) an 84% incidence of pain relief for a follow-up period of 4–7 years. Indeed, the patients in the latter series have continued to be free of pain for up to 12 years (Garfield, 1982). Both Ecker (1976) and Sharr & Garfield (1977) produced some evidence that recurrence of pain was not related to any lack of complete sensory loss in either the divisions affected by pain, or in the whole side of the face. In the largest series ever reported 316 out of 457 (65%) patients were relieved of pain from 3–31 years, the few patients with partial sensory loss still having satisfactory pain relief (Harris, 1940). Jefferson (1963) also achieved very good pain relief without producing total sensory loss and the injection rate for recurrent pain was only 10%. Of Henderson's (1965) patients who developed a recurrence of their trigeminal neuralgia, 50% did so in the first year after the injection. This is a rather high recurrence rate and compares with Härtel's (1914) figures where the recurrent pain that occurred in 70% of the patients with partial sensory loss did so during a period ranging from 6 months to 4 years. However, in those with total sensory loss only 4% developed recurrent pain. Whether, therefore, it is worth struggling to achieve total sensory loss depends on whose evidence one chooses to be influenced by, but on the whole it it seems reasonable to adopt the philosophy that, unless easily attainable, it is probably unwise to pursue total sensory loss.

The final comment relates to the technique of the procedure which is essentially based on that of Penman (1971). Provided the procedure is carried out in an unhurried fashion with care and good, although not necessarily sophisticated, radiology and some attempt is made to titrate the aliquots of alcohol, the results can be rewarding; certainly the disasters reported by Dandy (1929) and Tonnis & Kreissel (1951) should be rare. Any suggestion that the procedure should be carried out in outpatients (Miles, 1980) is to be condemned, as is attempting to carry it out in the anaesthetic room between cases. I once witnessed such an attempt to pass the needle through the foramen ovale without any X-ray control and the screams from the patient remain firmly imprinted in my mind.

The main criticisms of the treatment are related to the uncertainty of the degree and extent of the sensory loss that is produced. It is because of this that some patients may not agree to have the procedure carried out although they may have very severe neuralgia. I think it may be wrong to 'call the patient's bluff' (Garfield, 1972) and assume that the pain cannot be that bad if the patient seems to prefer it to the anticipated sensory loss.

Thermocoagulation, electrocoagulation and radiofrequency lesions of the root or ganglion

First introduced by Kirschner in 1931 (Kirschner, 1942), the refinements of the technique, including stimulation, have made the procedure popular, not least because light touch is frequently preserved. Moreover, with prior stimulation, not only can dissociated sensory loss be achieved but the part of the face that has never been the site of pain can be spared. Some previous workers have been against the technique, especially Tonnis & Kreissel (1951) who saw some unpleasant complications; however, they were seeing patients who had been treated at other clinics and may, therefore, have reached distorted conclusions. Thiry (1962) achieved excellent pain relief although many others prior to 1970 were less successful, with a failure rate that varied from 10–30%.

Before assessing the results of more recent series it is well to remember that some of the technical problems are no more or less than directing a needle for ganglion or root injection. A protagonist of radiofrequency and gangliolysis (a refinement of electrocoagulation of the ganglion) has stated that in the hands of a highly skilled operator alcohol block may be safe yet pain relief rarely lasts more than a year and repeated blocks have even lower success rates (Loeser, 1978). Such a biased and inaccurate statement belies the fact that it still requires some skill to get the needle into the right position whether a current is to be passed or a substance injected. This point is laboured, together with the obvious error relating to the duration of the relief of pain following alcohol injection, because many accounts that praise radiofrequency treatment tend to combine the advantages with unjustified criticism of alcohol injection. Critical appraisal of the results of thermocoagulation and electrocoagulation does reveal that the problems occurring after alcohol injection may also occur after these newer techniques; any idea that they do not is quite erroneous.

The long-term follow-up results in the published series have not matched the success of the immediate pain relief even though the latter has been impressive. For example, Sengupta & Stunden (1977) had a follow-up of only 2–20 months and during that time there was an 8% recurrence rate. Nugent & Berry (1974) reported an average follow-up period of 13 months, the maximum being 41 months; recurrent pain occurred in 11% of the patients. Menzel, Piotrowski & Penholz (1975) had a higher recurrence rate and repeat of the procedure was frequently necessary. Onofrio (1975) reported excellent results but not the duration of follow-up. In a more recent series Burchiel et al (1981) reported that 78 patients required 92 procedures, meaning that technical failure or failure to achieve pain relief amounted to nearly 20%; in addition, 18 of the 78 patients (23%) had such severe pain recurrence that further procedures were necessary. Interestingly enough, although it is frequently stressed that the procedure can be easily repeated, more than half the patients had an alternative procedure carried out and not a repeat of the radiofrequency procedure. The authors pointed out that their follow-up was longer than most other series and their total recurrence rate of 64% might be related to the long follow-up period, which was up to 6 years. They also pointed out that 15% of their recurrences were beyond 2 years, this being longer than the follow-up period of some of the previously mentioned series. These results certainly seem worse than most others and cannot be entirely attributed to the long period of follow-up since Sweet & Wepsic (1974) had a follow-up of 6 years and their recurrence rate was 22% (still not small). Burchiel et al (1981) suggested that their poor results could be accounted for by the fact that the small lesions that were made could have been a mixture of ganglion and nerve rather than ganglion and root. The incidence of trigeminal causalgia was only 4% and this seemed to compare reasonably well with the figures of 0.7–12% in other series quoted by them. Perhaps the most impressive results are those of Tew (1979) who had 500 patients with only 5 failing to obtain initial pain relief; however, a further 12% needed another operation and 3% had to take drugs to control recurrent pain. If one adds these to the 2% with trigeminal causalgia then a total of 18% were not totally free of symptoms in the face. It is worth comparing these results with, for example, the Krayenbühl (1969) series of extradural middle fossa root sections where initial pain relief occurred in 95% of the patients but subsequently dropped to 82% at follow-up.

In summary, it appears that this technique is safe and has a relatively low risk of side-effects (although carotid artery injury leading to death has occurred, as stressed by Nugent & Berry, 1974), but is certainly not devoid of them. However, the most serious objection, if more than 'tiding over' is required, is that recurrence of the pain is not uncommon; this is likely to be related to the tendency towards a selective and dissociated lesion. Therefore, unlike some of the other methods of treatment, it has not yet withstood the test of time.

Open root section

The classical approach is the extradural temporal route and it is usually assumed that Spiller developed the idea and Frazier carried it out (Spiller & Frazier, 1901). In fact, Ferrier (1890) had already developed the concept and Hartley (1893) had actually carried out the operation. However, Horsley (1891) had performed an intradural approach before any description of the extradural approach. The latter approach is still probably the one most favoured by neurosurgeons, although the intradural approach has had its protagonists, including Portugal (1946), Wilkins (1948), Kurbangaleev (1960), Pennybacker (1961), and Sabol'ch & Laslo (1962). The main advantage of the intradural route is that there is probably less bleeding, because there is no need to strip the dura from the floor of the middle fossa, and the reduced risk of exerting traction on the greater superficial petrosal nerve means there is less chance of facial palsy. However, the risk of damage to the hemisphere is inevitably increased; thus, although Henderson (1967) was very concerned about the incidence of facial palsy (10%) and switched to the intradural approach, he found problems with the latter especially relating to the bridging veins between the temporal lobe and the floor of the middle fossa. There is little evidence of much difference in the results of the two approaches except the increased risk of facial palsy in the extradural, and the increased risk of hemisphere dysfunciton in the intradural approach. The other complications and the pain relief are similar for either approach. With regard to facial palsy, in White & Sweet's (1969) and Stookey & Ransohoff's (1959) series the incidence was 7–8% and the former authors stressed the tendency for the palsy gradually to improve with time. This aspect had, in fact, been previously noted by Horrax & Poppen (1935). Overall, in a number of series quoted by White & Sweet (1969), the initial palsy rate varied from 3–18%, it being lower beyond a year. Open root section is not devoid of the complications of root or ganglion injection; eye complications (including diplopia), trigeminal causalgia, and, of course, recurrence of pain all being problems.

The posterior fossa (suboccipital) approach, pioneered by Dandy (1929), might be thought to have advantages, and Dandy himself was so convinced of its efficacy that he was sometimes openly critical of those who did not use it as the definitive treatment but who preferred, for example, alcohol injection (Grant, 1936). Dandy's technical ability in carrying out the operation is legendary and his average time of 30 minutes from skin incision to section of the nerve is unlikely ever to be equalled (White & Sweet, 1969); indeed, Dandy (1932) claimed that sometimes it could be done in 10–15 minutes! The subtleties of the technical aspects can be found in his own original descriptions and drawings. The variations in the anatomy of the petrosal vein are an example of such observations, and certainly dealing with that vein is a very important aspect of a successful operation. It was, of course, Dandy (1929) who believed in the dissociation of light touch and pain fibres, although dispute about this continues (Poulos, 1976). Illingworth (1974), in a small series, agreed with the concept of this dissociation and the results of a larger series using the retrolabyrinthine approach tend to support the theory (Pulec & Hitselberger, 1977). However, even some of Dandy's original comments (1929) may be contradictory (White & Sweet, 1969).

Unfortunately, there are no large series to compare with Dandy's (1932) of 150 operations without any deaths (although there was a 4.5% mortality in his earlier series of 1929). In other series quoted by White & Sweet (1969) the mortality was between 2.5 and 3.5%; these and those of the temporal approach (up to 3.5%) would suggest that experience and a good deal of expertise are needed when carrying out the operation by either approach, and neither of them (especially the temporal one) are operations for the occasional root sectionist. As pointed out by Stookey & Ransohoff (1959),

> 'No region of the skull shows so many minor variations as the area brought into view in the subtemporal approach to foramen spinosum and gasserian ganglion and its divisions. Trivial though these variations appear, their presence may be a source of difficulty to the surgeon'.

I have seen two very experienced neurosurgeons get into very great trouble during an extradural temporal approach and one of the procedures had to be abandoned because of uncontrollable venous haemorrhage. In spite of the technical problems and mortality (the latter being generally greater in the posterior fossa approach — for example, Olivecrona's was 10 times more in this approach than in the temporal approach), it must be acknowledged that some series of the temporal approach have been quite outstanding in terms of low mortality. Rowbotham (1954) had no deaths in 132 operations, Stookey & Ransohoff (1959) 6 deaths in 728 operations (0.8%), and Olivecrona (1961) 2 deaths in 445 operations (0.4%).

There is very little difference between the two procedures (i.e. temporal and posterior fossa) in the expectation of pain relief and, superficially, the effective relief of pain is good. Nevertheless, recurrence of the original pain occurs in as many as 30% (Walker et al, 1956, series which was the posterior fossa approach). White & Sweet (1969) reported seven series of the temporal approach, the incidence of recurrent pain varying from 5-19% with a mean of 13%. Trigeminal causalgia was certainly not unusual in the temporal approach series and occurred at a rate of 30% or more in four of the series where details were given (White & Sweet, 1969); indeed, in one series (Peet & Schneider, 1952) the incidence was 56% and it was noted that, of the original 382 patients, only 29% were completely free of any facial discomfort. It is worth noting that some surgeons, especially Pennybacker (1961), have achieved excellent pain relief together with a low rate of trigeminal causalgia; however, as previously mentioned, Pennybacker (1961) preceded his rhizotomies with a peripheral injection and this may well have accounted for the low rate of the trigeminal causalgia. Nor is the posterior fossa approach devoid of this complication, with Walker et al (1956) having a 27% incidence and Francois et al (1966) a 25% incidence. The ophthalmic complication rate was usually less than 10% in most of the series reported by White & Sweet (1969) although that of Peet & Schneider (1952) was 15%.

Although open root section has had, and no doubt will have, its protagonists, the figures above demonstrate that it does have its problems which need to be taken into account when assessing the severity of the symptoms being treated.

The retrolabyrinthine approach has briefly been referred to and it certainly seems to have impressive qualities. The technical aspects and results have been described by Pulec & Hitselberger (1977) and the operation allows a selective root section to be carried out. Of 28 patients only 3 needed some additional drug therapy to control the pain fully; the complication rate seemed low, although 2 patients sustained hearing loss which was thought to be related to a disturbance of the mastoid cavity. One additional patient had a postoperative c.s.f. leak and this required several operations for it to be cured.

Posterior fossa microvascular decompression of the nerve root
Jannetta (1966, 1979) has been the champion of both this operation and
retrogasserion transtentorial rhizotomy. Because of some postoperative problems
he has abondoned the latter although others (Rand, 1976) have continued to use
it. It has, however, failed to gain great popularity probably because of the
technical difficulties and morbidity. Moreover, a series of such operations has
not been published and it is therefore difficult to judge its attributes.

The microvascular decompression operation is different in that a large number
have been done, the theory being that the neuralgia is due to pulsation of tortuous
branches of the basilar artery pressing on the root of the trigeminal nerve.
Jannetta (1979) has pointed out the great advantage of such a theory and the
operation, namely, relief of pain with no loss of facial sensation. Jannetta (1979)
also claimed a decreased risk of late recurrences in that, of 450 operations, only 2
were followed by recurrent pain beyond a year after surgery. However, closer
analysis of the results does reveal an 11% recurrence of pain after one operation
and 7.4% after two, and such recurrences, when they occurred, did so in less than
6 months. Although postoperative trigeminal causalgia has been very rare, and
success of the procedure has been further reported in small series of patients
(Kelly, 1977; Petty & Southby, 1977; Rhoton, 1978), a more recent series of 46
operations reported by Burchiel et al (1981) was followed by a detailed comment
by Nugent which was as follows:

> 'The results of Burchiel et al would suggest that a patient preparing for
> microvascular decompression would be told that there is a 17% chance of recurrence
> of the pain, a 2% chance of significant morbidity, a 2% chance of death, a 24%
> chance that the nerve will ultimately have to be cut, and a 10-14% chance that a
> second intracranial procedure will be required before the pain is relieved.'

Although Jannetta's (1979) mortality was less than 1% in a much larger group of
patients, he has concluded:

> 'I am in the midst of a dilemma about recommending microvascular decompression
> as a standard procedure, primarily because the procedure, which may be difficult,
> must be carefully learned if the surgeon is to avoid making inaccurate observations
> and causing unnecessary morbidity and mortality.'

Such a comment from the champion of the procedure makes further comment
superfluous.

Decompression and compression operations
The decompression operation of Taarnhoj (1952), the compression procedure of
Shelden et al (1955), plus the variations on these procedures described by White &
Sweet (1969) are now very infrequently used, although they had a brief period of
popularity. The results in terms of pain recurrence have been variable but, on the
whole, would appear to be worse than following other forms of treatment. Thus
Hamby (1960) had an incidence of 54% recurrent pain severe enough to
necessitate reoperation or injection. In addition, there were five series quoted by
White & Sweet (1969) where recurrence rates of 20-30% were documented this
including their own figures of 24%. On the other hand, the mortality was low.
Perhaps one of the more curious aspects, when the results were analysed from

several series, was the lack of correlation between the postoperative sensory disturbance and the recurrence of pain; on the other hand, it might be argued that injury to the pathways rather than elimination of artificial synapses (Shelden et al, 1955) is the object of the operation and such a correlation is hardly relevant. Postoperative trigeminal causalgia has occurred but was reported as being uncommon. In some ways it is, therefore, difficult to see why the procedures have not been more popular. The most likely explanations are probably related to the operations being intradural below the temporal lobe (with ensuing risks of hemisphere dysfunction), and difficulty in understanding how the procedures actually work.

Medullary tractotomy

This operation, originally carried out by Sjöqvist (1938), has had and, in some isolated instances, continues to have its advocates (Hosobuchi & Rutkin, 1971). Sjövist obtained the idea from some earlier findings of Hun (1897). However, both the level and depth of incision into the medulla has remained controversial. Certainly the original level as suggested by Sjöqvist (1938) seems too rostral in that it leaves the patient with a degree of ipsilateral ataxia (Grant & Weinberger, 1941). In addition, recurrent laryngeal nerve paralysis is sometimes a problem. However, with modification of the site of the incision some large series have been reported (Tonnis & Kreissel, 1950; Kunc, 1964). An evaluation of several series was carried out by White & Sweet (1969) and a surprisingly low mortality (1.6%) was reported considering that incisions, albeit small, were being made into the medulla. In addition, trigeminal causalgia and ophthalmic complications were uncommon. However, it was evident that hospitalisation was a good deal longer than for the other forms of surgical treatment, as was the period before the patient could return to a normal life. Tonnis & Kreissel (1950) also felt that the operation might not be suitable for patients with hypertension and vascular disease, and this could be no small drawback in the type of patient who is commonly afflicted by trigeminal neuralgia. Perhaps the main problem is the obvious one, namely, the making of the lesion in the correct place both in terms of pain relief and not leaving a neurological deficit. Hosobuchi & Rutkin (1971), in a small series of patients, attempted to define the correct area by recording from it during stimulation of various areas of the face. Further comments, however, suggested that they thought the operation was unsuitable for idiopathic trigeminal neuralgia although the possibility of using it for other forms of facial pain, including postherpetic neuralgia, was discussed. In spite of the almost unique, and very successful, series of Kunc (1964) widespread enthusiasm for the operation seems to have passed. Detailed analysis of the previous series can be found in White & Sweet (1969). In their monograph Stookey & Ransohoff (1959) were against the operation not least because of sensory deficits remote from the trigeminal area, and because of uncertainty in obtaining analgesia in the division affected by pain, especially the mandibular division. They quote Sjöqvist as saying that tractotomy was inadvisable in patients over 60 years of age or in trigeminal neuralgia involving the mandibular division. As Stookey & Ransohoff (1959) point out, the age of the patients and the site of the pain frequently are in just these categories.

SUMMARY AND CONCLUSIONS

There is no ideal operation for trigeminal neuralgia, the main reason probably being related to lack of knowledge of the aetiology. Depending on how one chooses to interpret the literature, any one of several treatments could appeal. A simple peripheral injection and/or avulsion has the advantage of giving immediate pain relief without any serious morbidity or mortality. When something more permanent is required, the choice probably rests between ganglion or root injection and radiofrequency lesions (or a variation thereof) of the ganglion; both have advantages and disadvantages. Critical reappraisal of the former does reveal a somewhat prejudiced attitude in the literature, whereas the enthusiasm for the latter is inclined to outmatch the realities of its success. It is, however, surely logical to try one of these two procedures before open surgery, whether this be a root section (however selective) or a form of decompression (usually microvascular), since this is the orthodox approach towards any disease. However, it must be admitted that some surgeons will favour open surgery as a first choice.

The main problem today is that, with successful drug treatment, and with radiofrequency gangliolysis gaining in popularity, there are no surgeons who can proudly boast of a series of perhaps several hundred root sections, let alone with very low morbidity and mortality. The days of Dandy (posterior fossa), Grant or Stookey and Ransohoff (temporal) or Olivecrona (both) are past! Moreover, these operations, even in the experts' hands, were not devoid of the complications of the more conservative methods of treatment. Although microvascular decompression seems to be an attractive operation, there are still doubts about the long-term results, and the champion of the operation is himself in some doubt about the indications for the procedure. The other operations are now so infrequently performed that no-one is likely to equal, for example, Kunc's experience with medullary tractotomy. In some ways there is a parallel between the surgery of trigeminal neuralgia and that of Parkinsonism in that effective drug therapy has inevitably reduced the number of patients who require surgical treatment. This must mean that the surgeon of today will not have the same experience as his predecessor.

At the end of the day the referring neurologist or physician will want the surgeon to carry out the operation that he has confidence in and which, in that surgeon's hands, gives good results. I am influenced by my 1977 analysis and lean towards an alcohol injection into the root or ganglion as being the preferred method of treatment if drug therapy has failed. If there is attention to detail with good radiology, and 'clock watching' is resisted, then I am satisfied that the results are very acceptable. They may not be perfect (i.e. 100% success in every case with absolutely no side-effects), but then none of the results of the other procedures are either. It is quite true that patient selection must play a part. It is equally true that there may be too much rigidity in choosing patients for alcohol injeciton in that some with very severe pain may, in spite of the pain, still decline the treatment because of a fear of the numbness. This rigidity reflects the doctor's assumption that the pain is not severe enough. This is surely sometimes wrong and, therefore, the technique of radiofrequency gangliolysis might be a useful alternative. Unfortunately, the recurrence rate following this treatment still seems too high and the often reiterated statement that the procedure can be repeated does not appeal to every patient since some find it an ordeal.

REFERENCES

Burchiel K J, Steege T D, Howe J F, Loeser J D 1981 Comparison of percutaneous radiofrequency gangliolysis and microvascular decompression for the surgical management of tic douloureux. Neurosurgery 9 No.2: 111–119
Cushing H 1920 The role of deep alcohol injection in the treatment of trigeminal neuralgia. Journal of the American Medical Association 75: 441–443
Dandy W E 1929 An operation for the cure of tic douloureux. Partial section of the sensory root at the pons. Archives of Surgery 18: 687–734
Dandy W E 1932 The treatment of trigeminal neuralgia by the cerebellar route. Annals of Surgery 96: 787–795
Ecker A 1974 Tic douloureux eight years after alcohol gasserian injection. New York State Journal of Medicine 74 No.8: 1586–1592
Ecker A 1976 Sensory loss and prolonged remission of tic douloureux after selective alcoholic gasserian injection In: Bonica J J, Albe-Fessard D (eds) Advances in pain research and therapy. Raven, New York, p 895–900
Ferrier D 1890 Removal of the gasserian ganglion for severe neuralgia. Lancet 2: 925–926
Francois J, Hoffman G, Soleme J 1966 La kératite neuroparalytique et sa fréquence après les différentes neurotomies pour néuralgie essentielle du trijumeau. Neurochirurgie 9: 81–98
Garfield J 1972 Trigeminal neuralgia. Update 5 No.7: 643–648
Garfield J 1977 Personal communication
Garfield J 1982 Personal communication
Grant F C 1936 Alcohol injection in the treatment of major trigeminal neuralgia. Journal of the American Medical Association 107: 771–774
Grant F C, Weinberger L M 1941 Experiences with intramedullary tractotomy relief of facial pain and summary of operative results. Archives of Surgery 42: 681–692
Grantham E G, Segeberg L H 1952 An evaluation of palliative surgical procedures in trigeminal neuralgia. Journal of Neurosurgery 9: 390–394
Hamby W B 1960 Effectiveness of various operations for trigeminal neuralgia. Journal of Neurosurgery 17: 1039–1044
Harris W 1912 Alcohol injection of the Gasserian ganglion for trigeminal neuralgia. Lancet 1: 218–221
Harris W 1940 An analysis of 1433 cases of paroxysmal trigeminal neuralgia (trigeminal tic) and the end results of gasserian alcohol injection. Brain 63: 209–224
Härtel F 1912 Die Leitungsanasthesie und injektionsbehundlung des ganglion gasseri und der trigeminusstämme. Archiv für Klinishe Chirurgie 100: 193–292
Härtel F 1914 Uber die intracranielle injektions behundlung der Trigeminusneuralgie. Medizinische Klinik 10: 582–584
Hartley F 1893 Intracranial neurectomy of the fifth nerve. Annals of Surgery 17: 511–526
Henderson W R 1965 The anatomy of the gasserian ganglion and the distribution of pain in relation to injections and operations for trigeminal neuralgia. Annals of the Royal College of Surgeons of England 37: 346–373
Henderson W R 1967 Trigeminal neuralgia: the pain and its treatment. British Medical Journal 1: 7–15
Horrax G, Poppen J L 1935 Trigeminal neuralgia. Experience with, and treatment employed in 468 patients during the past 10 years. Surgery, Gynaecology and Obstetrics 61: 394–402
Horsley V, Taylor J Colman W S 1891 Remarks on the various surgical procedures devised for the relief or cure of trigeminal neuralgia. British Medical Journal 2: 1139–1143, 1191–1193, 1249–1252
Hosobuchi Y, Rutkin B 1971 Descending trigeminal tractotomy. Archives of Neurology 25: 115–125
Hun H 1897 Analgesia, thermic anasthesia and ataxia, resulting from foci of softening in the medulla oblongata and cerebellum, due to occlusion of the left inferior posterior cerebellar artery. A study of the course of the sensory and co-ordinating tracts in the medulla oblongata. New York Journal of Medicine 65: 513–519, 613–620
Illingworth R D 1974 Sensory fibre arrangement in the posterior root of the trigeminal nerve. Journal of Neurology, Neurosurgery and Psychiatry 37: 1279

Jaeger R 1957 Permanent relief of tic douloureux by Gasserian injection of hot water. Archives of Neurology and Psychiatry 77: 1-7

Jannetta P J, Rand R W 1966 Transtentorial retrogasserian rhizotomy in trigeminal neuralgia by microsurgical technique. Bulletin of Los Angeles Neurological Society 31: 93-99

Jannetta P J 1979 Treatment of trigeminal neuralgia. Neurosurgery 4: 93-94

Jefferson A 1963 Trigeminal root and ganglion injections using phenol in glycerine for the relief of trigeminal neuralgia. Journal of Neurology, Neurosurgery and Psychiatry 26: 345-352

Kelly D L 1977 Posterior fossa neurovascular decompression for tic douloureux and hemifacial spasm. North Carolina Medical Journal 38 No.9: 534-536

Kirschner M 1942 Die Behandlung der Trigeminusneuralgie (nach Erfahrungen and 1113 Kranken). Müchener Medizinische Wochenschrift 89: 235-239, 263-269

Krayenbühl H 1969 Idiopathic trigeminal neuralgia. In Acta Clinica No.9. Geigy, Basle

Kulenkampff D 1942 Die Behandlung der Trigeminusneuralgie (zu der Arbeit Kirschners). Münchener Medizinische Wochenschrift 89: 670

Kunc Z 1964 Tractus spinalis nervi trigemini. Fresh anatomic data and their significance for surgery. Publishing House of Czechoslovak Academy of Sciences, Prague

Kurbangaleev S M 1960 Late results of intradural radicotomy of the V-nerve in severe neuralgia. Vestnik Khirurgii imeni I. I. Grekova 85: 8-15

Loeser J D 1978 What to do about tic douloureux. Journal of the American Medical Association 239: 1153-1155

Menzel J, Piotrowski W, Penholz J 1975 Long term results of gasserian ganglion electrocoagulation. Journal of Neurosurgery 42- 140-143

Miles J 1980 Trigeminal neuralgia. In: Lipton S (ed) Persistent pain: modern methods of treatment, vol 2. Academic Press, London, ch 10, p 237

Morgan E J, Cast I P, Wilson P J 1977 Surgical treatment of trigeminal neuralgia (letter to Editor). British Medical Journal 2: 1088

Nugent G R, Berry B 1974 Trigeminal neuralgia treated by differential percutaneous radiofrequency coagulation of the gasserian ganglion. Journal of Neurosurgery 40: 517-523

Olivecrona H 1939 The syndrome of painful anaesthesia following section of the sensory root of the fifth nerve in tic douloureux. Acta Chirurgica Scandinavica 82: 99-106

Olivecrona H 1947 The surgery of pain. Acta Psychiatrica et Neurologica Scandinavica 46: 268-280

Olivecrona H 1961 Trigeminal neuralgia. Triangle 5: 60-69

Onofrio B M 1975 Radiofrequency percutaneous gasserian ganglion lesions. Results in 140 patients with trigeminal pain. Journal of Neurosurgery 42: 132-139

Patrick H T 1912 The technic and results of deep injections of alcohol for trifacial neuralgia. Journal of the American Medical Association 58: 155-163

Peet M M, Schneider R C 1952 Trigeminal neuralgia. A review of six hundred and eighty-nine cases with a follow up study on sixty-five per cent of the group. Journal of Neurosurgery 9: 367-377

Penman J 1968 Trigeminal neuralgia. In: Vinken P J, Bruyn G W (eds) Handbook of clinical neurology. North Holland, Amsterdam, ch 28, p 296

Penman J 1971 Trigeminal sensory root injection. In: Logue V (ed) Operative surgery, neurosurgery, 2nd edn. Butterworth, London, p 191

Pennybacker J 1961 Some observations on trigeminal neuralgia. In: Garland H (ed) Scientific aspects of neurology Livingstone, Edinburgh, p 153

Petty P G, Southby R 1977 Vascular compression of lower cranial nerves: observations using microsurgery, with particular reference to trigeminal neuralgia. Australian and New Zealand Journal of Surgery 47: 314-320

Portugal J R 1946 O tratamento cirurgico da trigeminalgia retrogasseriana por via temporal, intradural. Hospital (Rio) 29: 501-536

Poulos D A 1976 Functional and anatomical localisation in the trigeminal root: in support of Frazier. In: Morley T P (ed) Current controversies in neurosurgery. Saunders, Philadelphia, p 539

Pulec J L, Hitselberger W E 1977 Trigeminal neuralgia: retrolabyrinthine selective posterior root section. The laryngoscope 87: 1861-1868

Putnam T J, Hampton A O 1936 A technic of injection into the gasserian ganglion under roengenographic control. Archives of Neurology and Psychiatry 35: 92-98

Ramb H 1949 Die Alkoholinjektion ins Ganglion Gasseri bei der Trigeminusneuralgie. Deutsche Medizinische Wochenschrift 74: 826-829

Rand R W 1976 Functional and anatomical localisation in the trigeminal root: in support of Dandy. In: Morley T P (ed) Current controversies in neurosurgery. Saunders, Philadelphia, p 533

247

Rhoton A L 1978 Microsurgical neurovascular decompression for trigeminal neuralgia and hemifacial spasm. Journal of Florida Medical Association 65: 425–428

Rowbotham G F 1954 Trigeminal neuralgia: pathology and treatment. Lancet 1: 796–798

Sabol'ch T, Laslo Z 1962 Evaluation of intradural trigeminal radicotomy. Voprosy Neirokhirurgii (Moskva) vol 26: 14–16

Schlösser K 1903 Heilung peripherer Reizzuustände sensibler und motorischer Nerven. Bericht Ophthalmologische Gesellschaft 31: 84–89

Sengupta R P, Stunden R J 1977 Radiofrequency thermocoagulation of gasserian ganglion and its rootlets for trigeminal neuralgia. British Medical Journal 1: 142–143

Sharr M M, Garfield J S 1977 The place of ganglion or root alcohol injection in trigeminal neuralgia. Journal of Neurology, Neurosurgery, and Psychiatry 40: 286–289

Shelden C H, Pudenz R H, Freshwater D B, Crue B L 1955 Compression rather than decompression for trigeminal neuralgia. Journal of Neurosurgery 12: 123–126

Shimizu G 1937 Erfahrungen bei Japanern über Alkoholinjektionbehandlung der Trigeminusneuralgie. Nervenarzt 10: 348–352

Sjöqvist O 1938 Eine neue Operationsmethode bei Trigeminusneuralgie: Durchschneidung des Tractus spinalis trigemini. Zentralblatt fur Neurochirurgie 2: 247–281

Spiller W G, Frazier C H 1901 The division of the sensory root of the trigeminus for relief of tic douloureux: an experimental, pathological and clinical study with a preliminary report of one surgically successful case. Philadelphia Medical Journal 8: 1039–1049

Stookey B, Ransohoff J 1959 Trigeminal neuralgia. Its history and treatment. Thomas, Springfield, Illinois

Sweet W H, Wepsic J G 1974 Controlled thermocoagulation of trigeminal ganglion and rootlets for differential destruction of pain fibres. Part 1. Trigeminal neuralgia. Journal of Neurosurgery 40: 143–157

Taarnhøj P 1952 Decompression of the trigeminal root and the posterior part of the ganglion as a treatment in trigeminal neuralgia. Preliminary communication. Journal of Neurosurgery 9: 288–290

Taptas N 1911 Les injections d'alcohol dans le ganglion de Gasser a travers le trou ovale. Presse Medicale 19: 798–799

Tew J M 1979 Treatment of trigeminal neuralgia. Neurosurgery 4: 93–94

Thiry S 1962 Expérience personelle basée sur 225 cas de neuralgie essentielle du trijumeau traités par électrocoagulation stereotaxique du ganglion de gasser entre 1950 et 1960. Neurochirurgie 8: 86–92

Tonnis W, Kreissel H 1950 Traktotomie nach Sjöqvist in der Behandlung Trigeminusneuralgie. Zentralblatt fur Chirurgie 75: 873–882

Tonnis W, Kreissel H 1951 Die Bedeutung einer sorgfältigen Differentialdiagnose für die chirurgische Behandlung der Trigeminusneuralgie. Deutsche Medizinische Wochenschrift 12: 1202–1205

Von Brücke H 1938 Die Behandlung der Trigeminusneuralgie durch Alkoholinjektion ins Ganglion Gasseri. Archiv für Klinische Chirurgie 192: 328–353

Walker E, Miles F C, Simpson J R 1956 Partial trigeminal rhizotomy using suboccipital approach. Experiences in the treatment of trigeminal neuralgia. Archives of Neurology and Psychiatry 75: 514–521

White J C, Sweet W H 1969 Pain and the neurosurgeon. A forty year experience. Thomas, Springfield, Illinois

Wilkins H 1948 The transdural approach to posterior rhizotomy for trigeminal neuralgia. Paper presented at a meeting of Society of Neurological Surgeons. Omaha, Nebraska June 12

23. Does surgery influence syringomyelia?

P. K Newman, J. B. Foster

'The treatment of syringomyelia . . . should not be neglected, for in some cases it appears to have a considerable influence upon the development of the disease. Hydrotherapeutics, warm baths, tonics, iron, quinine, arsenic, strychnine, iodine and the iodides, and nitrates of silver may prove of service. The remedies which seem to be most commonly employed are warm baths, electricity and counter irritation along the spinal column by means of hot needles, blisters and cauteries. Lastly every form of injury should be particularly guarded against as, even from trivial causes, the consequences are likely to be much more serious than patients would readily realise.'

(Bruhl, 1897).

INTRODUCTION

The above statement illustrates a once common clinical error of attempting to treat a disease without attention to the underlying pathological process, and even now we are often guilty of this. It has been suggested that contemporary surgical techniques can favourably influence the natural history of syringomyelia in some cases, but it is still uncertain which procedure is indicated in which patient. The term syringomyelia implies a cystic cavitation of the spinal cord, and in any individual case pathological classification is usually possible after clinical and radiological assessment. In order to answer the question posed in the title of this chapter, it is first necessary to define the pathogenesis of the major groups of syringomyelia, and then to discuss the available evidence regarding surgery in each category. For the purpose of this discussion, syringomyelia is divided into five groups according to the associated conditions, and the existence is acknowledged of an enigmatic sixth group where no other pathology can be demonstrated and where the cord cavitation is unsatisfactorily termed 'idiopathic'. It is emphasised that by far the most frequently seen type is that associated with an anomaly at the craniovertebral junction.

CLASSIFICATION

1. Syringomyelia and a congenital anomaly at the foramen magnum
2. Syringomyelia and basal arachnoiditis
3. Syringomyelia and spinal arachnoiditis
4. Syringomyelia and spinal cord trauma
5. Syringomyelia and tumour of the nervous system
6. Idiopathic syringomyelia.

SYRINGOMYELIA AND A CONGENITAL ANOMALY AT THE FORAMEN MAGNUM

The literature suggests that 50–90% of cases of syringomyelia are associated with a craniovertebral anomaly, usually the Chiari type 1 malformation. The conflicting hypotheses regarding the pathogenesis of these associated conditions have entertained generations of neurologists and neurosurgeons, and have led to the adoption of a number of surgical approaches, often in an uncritical fashion. The two major opposing views are well known. The first theory, proposed in a series of papers by Gardner and his associates (summarised in the monograph by Gardner, 1973), and modified by Williams (1969), postulates filling of the syrinx from the ventricular system via a patent medullary-cervical communication. The second (Ball & Dayan, 1972; Albouker, 1979) suggests that inflation of the syrinx is caused by the passage across the cord of fluid within the dilated perivascular spaces of Virchow-Robin. Clinical, radiological, pathological, experimental and even mechanical observations are cited for or against either hypothesis, but these two theories are not mutually exclusive and it is very likely that both mechanisms operate. We believe that, in the fetus and in many new-born infants, a patent communication does exist between the fourth ventricle and the central canal of the cervical spinal cord, and that pressure disturbances such as those generated during a traumatic birth may dilate the central canal and even give rise to rupture of the ependymal lining. This will produce a potential syringohydromyelia. In later life a syringomyelic cyst may be further expanded in some patients via a persisting communication with the ventricular system, in others by transfer of fluid from the subarachnoid space across the perivascular channels of the cord, and probably in all cases by destructive fluid shifts within the cavity itself, reflecting physiological pressure changes in the spinal subarachnoid space (Williams, 1978).

Patients with syringomyelia and a Chiari anomaly present most commonly in the fourth or fifth decade when considerable and irrevocable destruction of neural tissue has already occurred. The aims of surgery are therefore to relieve continuing compression at the craniovertebral junction, to restore normal cerebrospinal fluid dynamics, and to drain the syrinx in some cases, thus reducing the risk of further spinal cord damage. Surgery has significantly benefited patients seen at an early stage, those with minimal disability or with rapid progression, and those in whom the major disability is due to compression at the foramen magnum. It must be remembered that the neurological damage is caused by two associated but separate pathological processes: by external compression of the lower medulla and upper cervical cord by the prolapsed cerebellar tonsils, and also by pressure and extension of the syrinx, causing internal destruction of the cord and occasionally of the medullary structures. Thus the ideal surgical approach to this condition should tackle both processes.

Craniovertebral decompression

This procedure was proposed by Gardner (1965), and has subsequently been evaluated by other surgeons. Although, in common with every other surgical approach to syringomyelia, a controlled trial of the technique has never been done, even a sceptical analysis of the crude results from the larger series suggests a significant benefit following craniovertebral decompression, with more than two-thirds of the patients improved, or at least showing no deterioration, several years after the operation (Table 23.1). Since the natural history of this disease is slowly progressive, many more patients would have been expected to deteriorate

Table 23.1 Surgical results in syringomyelia — craniovertebral decompression.

Series	n	Follow-up (years)	Outcome			
			Improved	Same	Worse	Mortality
Gardner (1965)	74	—	52	11	6	5
Hankinson (1978)	69	>5	29	18	19	3
Hurth & Sichez (1979)	58	1–8	32	12	13	1
Logue & Rice Edwards (1981)	68	1–17	21	33	13	1
Total	269		134	74	51	10

during the period of follow-up in the absence of surgical intervention, but as treated and untreated patients have never been satisfactorily compared, it is important to remain critical of the claims for this and any other form of surgery. Unfortunately, most of the tabulated studies deal only superficially with the quality and quantity of improvement, although the assessment of their cases by Logue & Rice Edwards (1981) presented a more detailed and hence more valuable picture.

Figure 23.1 illustrates an attempt to quantify surgical results in a representative sample of our own patients reviewed and examined personally a mean of 9.7 years after craniovertebral decompression. A useful reduction of headache, neck and arm pain, upper-limb sensory symptoms and early long-tract signs may be seen. Little improvement can be expected in amyotrophy, upper-limb sensory signs, trophic changes, neuropathic joints, eye movement disorders (although Thrush & Foster, 1973 recorded decreased nystagmus following decompression in 4 out of 14 cases) or lower cranial nerve palsies, but there may be a worthwhile arrest of the progression of these features of the disease. Steady deterioration uninfluenced by craniovertebral decompression is nevertheless a familiar event.

The precise surgical technique has varied but the general principles have been to remove part of the occipital bone and to combine this with laminectomy at C1 and C2, and frequently at C3. The thickened dura is opened and in many cases

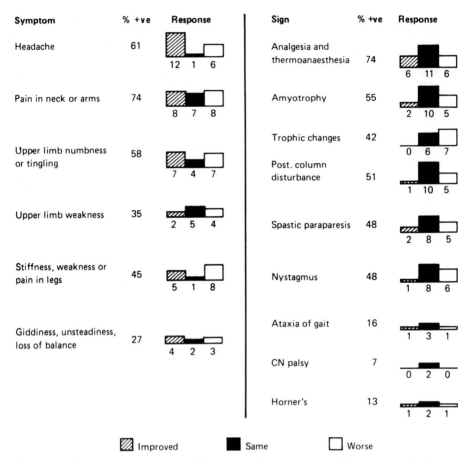

Symptom	% +ve	Response			Sign	% +ve	Response		
Headache	61	12	1	6	Analgesia and thermoanaesthesia	74	6	11	6
Pain in neck or arms	74	8	7	8	Amyotrophy	55	2	10	5
Upper limb numbness or tingling	58	7	4	7	Trophic changes	42	0	6	7
					Post. column disturbance	51	1	10	5
Upper limb weakness	35	2	5	4	Spastic paraparesis	48	2	8	5
Stiffness, weakness or pain in legs	45	5	1	8	Nystagmus	48	1	8	6
Giddiness, unsteadiness, loss of balance	27	4	2	3	Ataxia of gait	16	1	3	1
					CN palsy	7	0	2	0
					Horner's	13	1	2	1

▨ Improved   ■ Same   ☐ Worse

Fig. 23.1 Chiari anomaly and syringomyelia: preoperative symptoms and signs compared with those at mean 9.7 years following craniovertebral decompression (*n* = 35).

the arachnoid is left intact. In others the arachnoid is carefully dissected, the prolapsed cerebellar tonsils are separated, and the opening into the fourth ventricle is re-established. It is difficult to determine which modification is to be favoured as the results appear to be similar, but there is no doubt that the bleeding created by disturbance of the arachnoid results in a stormy postoperative course. The application of microsurgical techniques at this stage of the operation may reduce this complication (Rhoton, 1978). Most patients do not have a significant communication between the fourth ventricle and the syringomyelic cavity by the time thay present to the surgeon: there is therefore nothing to commend the insertion of a piece of muscle or other material in order to 'plug' the obex, as originally described by Gardner. Furthermore, several surgeons have observed disquieting oscillation of vasomotor control when this procedure has been adopted, and it now appears that this elaboration of the basic operation of decompression is futile.

In summary, surgical decompression of the cerebellar tonsils is indicated in most cases of syringomyelia associated with the Chiari anomaly and appears to help the majority of patients; however, the extent of the benefit may be disappointing. Severely disabled patients are not helped by craniovertebral decompression, and gross syringobulbic disturbance is associated with a high postoperative morbidity and mortality. Exclusion of such cases may improve surgical figures. It is logical to operate on early cases and those who present with minimal disability, since the arrest of the natural history of deterioration must be the main aim of surgery.

Syringostomy

The results of primary syringostomy are superficially similar to those of craniovertebral decompression, although some further comment is necessary. Table 23.2 summarises the more important documented series. Pitts & Groff (1964) found that two-thirds of their patients were improved or stable at least 2

Table 23.2 Surgical results in syringomyelia — syringostomy.

Series	n	Follow-up (years)	Outcome		
			Improved	Same	Worse
Syringostomy					
Pitts & Groff (1964)	37	>2		25	12 (1†)
Love & Olafson (1966)	33	1–10	10	12	11
Tator et al (1982)	20	5	11	4	5
Terminal ventriculostomy					
Gardner et al (1977)	12	12–20 months	8	2	2
Williams & Fahy (1983)	34	–	21 (?)	13	?

years after surgery, but did not observe any additional benefit when gutta percha drainage of the syrinx was compared with simple myelotomy. It is difficult to draw conclusions from the data of Love & Olafsen (1966), as a variety of syringostomy techniques were used (predominantly a syringo-subarachnoid fistula) in patients who had sometimes previously undergone posterior fossa decompression. Moreover, the length of follow-up is not clear, the description of the underlying pathology is difficult to interpret, and details regarding the extent of the improvement are sparse. The report by Tator et al (1982) is of more value; each patient was treated by a syringo-subarachnoid shunt, and a mean follow-up period of 5 years is stated. Although cerebellar tonsillar prolapse was minimal or absent in the majority of these patients and this was therefore an unusual group, the findings do suggest that a syringostomy may be indicated in some cases, particularly where a Chiari anomaly is not present.

Gardner and his colleagues (1977) have recently enthusiastically published the results following 'terminal ventriculostomy'. In this procedure a syringostomy is attempted by excision of the filum terminale, theoretically permitting drainage from the syrinx into the subarachnoid space. However, radiological and pathological studies usually demonstrate termination of the syrinx cavity at a higher level than the conus, and hence this technique cannot be expected to help many patients. Furthermore, it is not possible to accept the figures given by

Gardner et al (Table 23.2) as the length of follow-up of their cases is much too short. The more critical evaluation of this technique by Williams & Fahy (1983) will have dampened the ardour of its proponents. Twenty-one of 34 patients were reported to have shown some improvement, but when the authors analysed these results this improvement was insignificant in the majority of cases. Williams (1980) has also made the point that there are theoretical disadvantages in the existence of a free communication between the syrinx cavity and the subarachnoid space, because physiological pressure changes within the latter compartment could actually inflate the syrinx. Despite these objections, terminal ventriculostomy may have a place in the management of syringomyelia and further experience should be sought in the selected group of patients in whom extension of the syrinx into the conus can be demonstrated preoperatively. Computerised tomography may be useful in identifying such cases.

Syringostomy has not been evaluated adequately, partly because of Gardner's assertions regarding craniovertebral decompression, but also because many surgeons have had problems with patency of the shunt. The adoption of valved syringo-peritoneal shunts may reduce the failure rate, provide a more effective and theoretically satisfying means of syrinx drainage, and permit further assessment of this relatively simple form of treatment.

Ventricular drainage
A small proportion of patients have significant hydrocephalus at the time of presentation, or at an interval following craniovertebral decompression. These patients are best treated by means of a ventriculo-peritoneal or ventriculo-atrial shunt. In addition to the expected improvement due to the relief of symptoms of raised intracranial pressure, there may often be a worthwhile functional improvement with reduction of ataxia and long-tract signs. It has been suggested that this therapeutic approach should be used in all cases regardless of ventricular size (Krayenbuhl & Benini, 1971), and anecdotal reports have been cited in support. No evidence can be found to justify this recommendation, which is further invalidated when the underlying mechanisms are considered. Drainage of the fourth ventricle through a Silastic tube leading to the cervical subarachnoid space also has its advocates, this procedure being performed during craniovertebral decompression. However, it does not appear that this technique further improves the outcome after decompression alone (Cahan & Bentson, 1982).

Craniovertebral decompression and syringostomy
In many cases a craniovertebral decompression has been followed by continued deterioration over months or years, and in this situation a secondary syringostomy has sometimes been performed. The results have often been unimpressive and this is hardly surprising, for the surgeon has remained one step behind the advancing disease process. In patients who have both syringomyelia and its associated Chiari anomaly (and unlike those with an uncomplicated Chiari malformation who tend to fare better after decompression), there are two separate sites of neurological damage, with distinct but associated pathological processes operating. It is not common for a significant communication between

the fourth ventricle and the syringomyelic cavity to be demonstrated: thus, decompression of the craniovertebral anomaly cannot usually be expected to have any useful influence on the behaviour of the fluid in the isolated syrinx, with the possible exception of the effect of restoration of normal craniospinal-cerebrospinal fluid dynamics. Hence, a rational approach to treatment will involve a dual procedure, with attention to both the craniovertebral obstruction and to the cord cavity itself. In those patients in whom a high cervical syringomyelia is found at laminectomy during craniovertebral decompression, a combined operation may be possible, but in others syringostomy should follow shortly after craniovertebral decompression as a comparatively straightforward secondary procedure. A systematic trial of such a combined approach in early and minimally disabled patients has much to commend it, and might produce better results than present surgical methods.

SYRINGOMYELIA AND BASAL ARACHNOIDITIS

A chronic meningeal reaction in the region of the foramen magnum and occluding the basal cisternae is found in a significant proportion of cases of syringomyelia. The hydrodynamic mechanisms producing the syrinx cavity are probably similar to those occurring in patients with cerebellar tonsillar prolapse and, indeed, a Chiari malformation and a basal arachnoiditis may be found in the same patient. Birth trauma may be an important aetiological factor in these cases, both in production of the arachnoiditis and in promoting the potential for syrinx formation (Newman et al, 1981). In other cases the arachnoiditis may be acquired in later life, and factors such as tuberculous meningitis have been implicated (Appleby et al, 1969).

To attempt posterior fossa and upper cervical decompression is particularly hazardous in this group of patients and cannot be recommended, as little improvement can be expected and an advancing deficit as a result of surgery is well recognised (Williams, 1978). For this reason it is important to establish the diagnosis radiologically: in this situation, myelography with oil-based contrast is more useful than with water-soluble media. Where significant hydrocephalus is present, a ventriculo-peritoneal or ventriculo-atrial shunt may lessen the disability associated with the dilatation of the ventricles. Drainage of the syringomyelic cavity, preferably via a syringo-peritoneal catheter, is theoretically justified, but in practice the results are often disappointing. It is, nevertheless, reasonable to attempt to drain the syrinx cavity in most cases, and certainly in those patients in whom clinical progression is observed.

SYRINGOMYELIA AND SPINAL ARACHNOIDITIS

In cases of spinal arachnoiditis, as distinct from those with basal arachnoiditis, an association with syringomyelia is very rare. Barnett (1973) discovered only seven cases reported in the literature of the previous 40 years, and added seven more. An underlying cause of the arachnoiditis is usually evident in the form of a preceding meningitis, haemorrhage into the subarachnoid space, spinal trauma, or as a result of intrathecal injections. Unfortunately, the progressive neurological deficit in these cases is not usually produced by the syrinx, but by the inexorable constrictive process of the arachnoiditis which strangles the cord and its nutrient vessels. Little can be done to alleviate this progression. However, should an ascending deficit occur above the level of the arachnoiditis, then this may suggest extension of a syringomyelic cyst, and the insertion of a syringo-thecal (or better, syringo-peritoneal) shunt may be worthwhile. Barnett has stated that improved long-term results followed the insertion of a shunt in four of his patients.

SYRINGOMYELIA AND SPINAL CORD TRAUMA

It is well recognised that syringomyelia may arise in a small proportion of patients as a late complication of spinal cord trauma. An ascending myelopathy, with pain as a prominent feature, will alert the clinician to this possibility and radiological confirmation will usually follow. Although the cavity may be extensive, communication with the ventricular system cannot be demonstrated and it has been concluded that these cavities develop as a sequel to the coalescence of microcysts formed as a result of the initial cord trauma. Enlargement of these lesions is presumably a consequence of destructive fluid shifts within the cavities reflecting pressure changes in the subarachnoid space. In most instances where cavity fluid has been analysed, it has been shown to have a composition similar to that of cerebrospinal fluid, and this suggests that transudation of fluid across the cord into the cavity may also have an important role.

Surgical treatment of post-traumatic syringomyelia may alleviate pain, and in some cases is followed by relief of motor or sensory disability. Barnett & Jousse (1973) described favourable results in all 7 patients treated and, of the 13 cases reported by Shannon et al (1981), improvement followed surgery in 11. If the disability below the level of the cord trauma is only partial, then syringostomy is indicated. However, where no function exists caudal to the traumatic lesion, then either a syringo-subarachnoid shunt just above this site, or amputation of the cord at the traumatic level, appear to be equally acceptable techniques. A formal comparison of these two related approaches has not been made. It should be emphasised that the results of surgery are not always dramatic, and that spontaneous improvements have occurred in conservatively managed cases. Nevertheless, early surgery is likely to prove beneficial and should not be withheld unless a strong contraindication exists.

SYRINGOMYELIA AND TUMOUR OF THE NERVOUS SYSTEM

A tumour of the spinal cord may mimic syringomyelia and true cord cavitation has been demonstrated at autopsy in less than one-third of such cases (Barnett &

Rewcastle, 1973). Moreover, the frequency of intramedullary tumour found at autopsy in cases of syringomyelia is low: the review by Poser (1956) of a number of published series gave a frequency of 16.4%. It has been suggested that this form of cord cavitation arises by liquefaction within the tumour, by secretion of fluid from the tumour into a cyst, and by means of secondary vascular factors, and it is likely that all three factors play their part. Where primary excision is not possible, as is the case in many intramedullary tumours of glial origin, then aspiration of an associated syringomyelic cyst may help in diagnosis, and drainage of the cavity by means of a longitudinal myelotomy incision may materially improve the condition of the patient (Guidetti et al, 1982).

Intraspinal extramedullary tumours associated with syringomyelia are exceptional, and secondary vascular factors have been implicated in the pathogenesis of the cord cavitation. The treatment is that of the obstructing tumour.

Posterior fossa tumours have occasionally been reported in association with syringomyelia, and in these cases the syringomyelic cavity may have been produced by obstruction of cerebrospinal fluid egress from the fourth ventricle, together with the persistence of a communication between the ventricle and the central canal of the cord. An arachnoid cyst in the posterior fossa may have the same effect. The treatment of these lesions is usually by means of a direct surgical approach to the tumour or cyst.

IDIOPATHIC SYRINGOMYELIA

A proportion of cases of syringomyelia are extensively investigated by modern radiological methods and yet none of the above associated factors can be demonstrated. The precise pathogenesis in this group remains mysterious, and it is possible that in some cases this is an acquired lesion attributable to vascular disturbances within the cord or to an unrecognised intramedullary tumour. In others, perhaps the majority of this group, the lesion is likely to be congenital and related to the persistence of a dilated central canal of the cord. A surgical approach to the foramen magnum is not indicated, and the experience of Tator and his colleagues (1982) suggests that syringostomy should be carefully considered.

CONCLUSION

In some patients the surgical treatment of syringomyelia remains a frustrating and disappointing exercise, yet in others some amelioration may be expected and the progressive nature of the condition may be stabilised in many more. Thoughtful assessment of each case with due regard to the underlying pathogenesis will allow the clinician to select the appropriate technique for each individual. In those cases with an associated Chiari anomaly, the combination of craniovertebral decompression and primary syringostomy offers the best hope for a successful outcome from surgery, but sadly we remain therapeutically impotent in those patients who continue to deteriorate despite these procedures.

The authors wish to acknowledge the contribution made to our studies of syringomyelia by the neurosurgeons of the Regional Neurological Centre, Newcastle. In particular, our colleague Professor John Hankinson has been responsible for the surgical treatment of the majority of our patients and we thank him especially for his continuing interest and encouragement.

REFERENCES

Albouker J 1979 La syringomyélie et les liquides intra-rachidiens. Neurochirurgie 25 Suppl. 1: 1–144
Appleby A, Bradley W G, Foster J B, Hankinson J, Hudgson P 1969 Syringomyelia due to chronic arachnoiditis at the foramen magnum. Journal of the Neurological Sciences 8: 451–464
Ball M J, Dayan A D 1972 Pathogenesis of syringomyelia. Lancet 2: 799–801
Barnett H J M 1973 Syringomyelia associated with spinal arachnoiditis. In: Barnett H J M, Foster J B, Hudgson P Syringomyelia. Saunders, London ch 15, p 220–244
Barnett H J M, Rewcastle N B 1973 Syringomyelia and tumours of the nervous system. In: Barnett H J M, Foster J B, Hudgson P Syringomyelia. Saunders, London, ch 17, p 261–301
Barnett H J M, Jousse A T 1973 Nature, prognosis and management of post-traumatic syringomyelia. In: Barnett H J M, Foster J B, Hudgson P Syringomyelia. Saunders, London, ch 11, p 154–164
Bruhl I 1897 A contribution to the study of syringomyelia. Translated with notes and additions by Galloway J, Scott L. New Sydenham Society, London p 105
Cahan L D, Bentson J R 1982 Considerations in the diagnosis and treatment of syringomyelia and the Chiari malformation. Journal of Neurosurgery 57: 24–31
Gardner W J 1965 Hydrodynamic mechanism of syringomyelia: its relationship to myelocele. Journal of Neurology, Neurosurgery and Psychiatry 28: 247–259
Gardner W J 1973 The dysraphic states from syringomyelia to anencephaly. Amsterdam, Excerpta Medica
Gardner W J, Bell H S, Poolos P N, Dohn D F, Steinbery M 1977 Terminal ventriculostomy for syringomyelia. Journal of Neurosurgery 46: 609–617
Guidetti B, Mercuri S, Vagnozzi R 1982 Long-term results of the surgical treatment of 125 intramedullary spinal gliomas. Journal of Neurosurgery 54: 323–330
Hankinson J 1978 The surgical treatment of syringomyelia. In: Krayenbuhl, H (ed) Advances and technical standards in neurosurgery, vol 5. Springer Verlag, Vienna, p 127–151
Hurth M, Sichez J P 1979 La chirurgie de la charnière craniocervicale: étude critique à propos de 63 cas d'hydrosyringomyélie opérés. Neurochirurgie 25 Suppl. 1: 114–131
Krayenbuhl H, Benini A 1971 A new surgical approach in the treatment of hydromyelia and syringomyelia. The embryological basis and the first results. Journal of the Royal College of Surgeons of Edinburgh 16: 147–161
Logue V, Rice Edwards M 1981 Syringomyelia and its surgical treatment — an analysis of 75 patients. Journal of Neurology, Neurosurgery and Psychiatry 44: 273–284
Love J, Olafson R 1966 Syringomyelia: a look at surgical therapy. Journal of Neurosurgery 24: 714–718
Newman P K, Terenty T R, Foster J B 1981 Some observations on the pathogenesis of syringomyelia. Journal of Neurology, Neurosurgery and Psychiatry 44: 964–969
Pitts F W, Groff R A 1964 Syringomyelia: status of surgical therapy. Surgery 56: 806–809
Poser C M 1956 The relationship between syringomyelia and neoplasm. Thomas, Springfield, Illinois
Shannon N, Symon L, Logue V, Cull D, Kang J, Kendall B 1981 Clinical features, investigation and treatment of post-traumatic syringomyelia. Journal of Neurology, Neurosurgery and Psychiatry 44: 35–42
Rhoton A L 1978 Microsurgery of Arnold-Chiari malformation and hydromyelia in adults. In: Rand R W (ed) Microneurosurgery, 2nd edn. Mosby, St Louis, p 265–277
Tator C H, Meguro K, Rowed D W 1982 Favourable results with syringosubarachnoid shunts for treatment of syringomyelia. Journal of Neurosurgery 56: 517–523
Thrush D C, Foster J B 1973 An analysis of nystagmus in 100 consecutive patients with communicating syringomyelia. Journal of the Neurological Sciences 20: 381–386

258

Williams B 1969 The distending force in the production of communicating syringomyelia. Lancet 2: 189–193

Williams B 1978 A critical appraisal of posterior fossa surgery for communicating syringomyelia. Brain 101: 223–250

Williams B 1980 On the pathogenesis of syringomyelia: a review. Journal of the Royal Society of Medicine 73: 798–806

Williams B, Fahy G 1983 A critical appraisal of 'terminal ventriculostomy' for syringomyelia. Journal of Neurosurgery 58: 188–197

24. In infantile hydrocephalus how much brain mantle is needed for normal development?

A. P. Lonton

INTRODUCTION

Deeply embedded in the folklore of many cultures is the belief that highly gifted individuals are endowed with disproportionately large brains. Morley Fletcher in 1900 referred to 'the large brains . . . of great weight found in certain individuals characterised by their intellectual power'. Although this simplistic faith may have waned, a corollary of this assumption is widely held. Until very recent years, the vast majority of clinicians and neuroscientists would have considered it axiomatic that significant thinning of the brain mantle would inevitably be associated with profound loss of intellectual, sensory and physical powers. Scarff (1952) reflected the current opinion when he proposed that hydrocephalic infants with less than 1 cm of cortex were of subnormal intelligence and should not be offered any treatment. However, doubt was cast on this unproven assumption when Macnab (1961) reported several cases of hydrocephalic infants who had mantles of 0.5 cm but with subsequent IQs in the 85–100 range. Hadenius et al (1962) also found examples of mantles less than 1 cm compatible with normal intellect. They proposed that the long-term prognosis was more related to the nature of the underlying lesion and not the degree of hydrocephalus. In these studies measurements were made by air ventriculography which was not particularly accurate, nor without risk to the patient.

The first clinically useful and commercially viable CT scanner was invented by Hounsfield in 1971. This superior imaging technique has been used extensively for brain scanning from the mid 1970s. Therefore, for those conditions in which both CT scanning and psychometric assessment are routine procedures, there is now a vastly improved capacity to explore the relationship between brain anatomy and quantifiable intellectual skills.

REVIEW OF STUDIES CORRELATING INTELLIGENCE WITH CT SCAN FEATURES

There have been remarkably few attempts to correlate IQ test scores with appropriately measured CT scan features. Furthermore, since the majority of published studies are on less than 40 patients, many significant correlations must inevitably have been missed because of the relatively small numbers in the various sub-groups examined. Levin et al (1981) showed a tendency for lower IQs to be associated with severe ventricular dilatation in cases of closed head injury, normally after motor vehicle accidents. Cala et al (1978), in a facinating study of 26 Australian heavy drinkers, demonstrated a good correlation between the degree of cerebral atrophy and the patient's drinking history as well as his intellectual and motor deficits. Large ventricles were commonly found in children with minimal brain damage (Bergstrom & Billie, 1978), in dementia in the elderly (Roberts et al, 1977), in schizophrenic patients (Golden et al, 1979), and in adult metachromatic leukodystrophy (Manowitz et al, 1978). There have been a number of small studies of hydrocephalics (Mueller et al, 1977; Jansen et al, 1982), and Hammock & Milhorat (1981) give many illustrations of the diverse pathology of hydrocephalus as well as psychometric details of many patients. The findings of a large scale survey of the relationship between CT scan features and the intellectual skills of hydrocephalics (Lonton, 1979) are expanded in this chapter.

PATIENTS AND METHODS

The information in the 1979 study, and the additional up-dated analyses, were derived from a computerised data bank on 1234 patients with spina bifida. A second data bank of several hundred children with other neural tube malformations provided patients principally with congenital or acquired hydrocephalus. All had been treated at birth or subsequently at the Sheffield Children's Hospital. Of these patients, 467 had cranial CT scans 449 of which were sufficently well defined to be measurable. Their ages ranged from 2–22 years with a mean of 9.3 and a standard deviation of 3.7 years. Two hundred and fifty-nine had myelomeningocele, 98 congenital hydrocephalus, 23 post-meningitic and 19 post-haemorrhagic hydrocephalus, 22 meningoceles, 14 encephaloceles, and the remaining 32 had a variety of related disorders, including a few with macrocephaly. Three hundred and two were tested on the Wechsler Intelligence Scale for Children (WISC); 98 on the Stanford Binet, usually because they were too young for the WISC; and 11 on other tests, giving a total of 411 patients with psychometric assessments. Unless stated otherwise, the statistical technique used was analysis of variance, performed by computer using version 6.5 of the statistical package for the social sciences (SPSS) by Nie et al (1975).

Measuring the degree of hydrocephalus
A number of researchers have had difficulty in deciding the best way to measure the ventriculo-cephalic ratio on CT scans. Ideally volumes should be measured, but this would be impossibly laborious. A popular one dimensional method which needs nothing more elaborate than a ruler is fully described by Hahn & Rim (1976). Their most important measure is the ratio of the distance between the

frontal horns of the lateral ventricles, and the total brain width at that level. This is perfectly adequate for symmetrical scans but totally inappropriate for the abnormal scans which may account for up to 10% of those of hydrocephalic patients. Synek & Reuben (1976) measured the ventricle brain ratio just above the third ventricle.

Manual planimetry can be used to find the area of ventricle and brain on the slice which shows the greatest degree of ventricular dilatation (Lonton, 1979). The ventricle brain percentage ratio (VBR) is then used as a two dimensional index of the degree of hydrocephalus. Others have also used VBR type measurements (Golden et al, 1979; Levin et al, 1981; Jansen et al, 1982). Rapid evaluations of VBRs can now be obtained with digital planimeters and many pathology laboratories have one of these costly but useful microelectronic devices for measuring areas. All of these ratios are approximations, but all are infinitely better than purely subjective assessments of 'mild', 'moderate', 'severe', and 'gross' hydrocephalus. It is quite astonishing that some researchers fail to realise that such judgments can not be replicated with reliability either by other researchers or even themselves.

RESULTS

The variation in severity of hydrocephalus

Table 24.1 shows the distribution of the VBRs, and the groupings adopted. Group 1 comprised all scans with VBRs from 0-10%. Groups 2, 3, 4 and 5 contain successive intervals of 10%. All scans with VBRs above 50% were in group 6. The mean VBR for all groups was 30.9%. There was a 12-fold difference between the mean VBRs for groups 1 and 6. However, there was at least a hundred-fold difference between the volume of the very smallest compared with the largest ventricles.

Table 24.1 The distribution of degrees of hydrocephalus ($n = 449$). The right hand column relates to the 259 spina bifida (SB) patients only.

Group	VBR range (%)	VBR mean (%)	n	%	% of SB scans
1	0–10	5.5	81	18	13
2	11–20	15.4	76	17	19
3	21–30	25.6	76	17	19
4	31–40	35.2	84	19	24
5	41–50	45.7	56	12	12
6	51–100	62.9	76	17	13
Mean/total		30.9	449	100	100

At this time it is impossible to evaluate the distributions of VBRs in the non-handicapped population. There have been attempts to establish norms for one dimensional measures (Hahn & Rim, 1976; Goodwin et al, 1981), but none of the existing studies have been based on sufficiently large numbers of obviously normal patients. Indeed, it would be difficult to see how such a study could be ethically justifiable in view of the dosage of radiation involved. Because patients tend to be selected for cranial CT scans for suspected abnormalities, this reported series can not be considered to give distributions of VBRs for all patients with neural tube malformations. One group that is probably under-represented is spina bifida without obvious signs of hydrocephalus. It is important to bear this in mind when interpreting the last column of Table 24.1, which shows the percentages of the 259 spina bifida children in each VBR grouping. As will be mentioned later, there is also a slight under-representation of children with CSF shunts who were also of low intelligence.

Degree of hydrocephalus and IQ

In crude terms, Table 24.2 indicates that even grossly enlarged ventricles are not associated with dramatically lowered IQ for patients with or without valves. Analysis of variance did, however, show a statistically significant lowering of performance scale IQ with increasing VBR (but in absolute terms, a mean difference of 14–16 points is small, and only likely to be of statistical significance in large scale studies).

Table 24.2 The relationship between degree of hydrocephalus and mean IQ scores ($n = 302$ for the WISC verbal and performance scales; $n = 411$ for the full scale IQs which include 109 scores on other tests).

Group	Verbal Scale IQ			Performance scale IQ			Full scale IQ		
	No valve	Valve	Both	No valve	Valve	Both	No valve	Valve	All
1	111	101	104	96	86	90	100	93	95
2	104	107	106	94	87	90	95	94	94
3	99	102	100	87	85	86	92	95	94
4	99	104	101	86	86	86	91	94	92
5	95	109	101	82	82	82	85	96	91
6	102	90	96	80	72	76	90	81	86
Mean	101	102	101	87	84	85	92	92	92
$P =$	NS	NS	NS	0.001	0.001	0.001	NS	NS	NS

The extraordinary findings of the 1979 study advanced the previous observations of Macnab (1961) and Hadenius (1962) that some thin brains could have normal functions, to the much more extreme conclusion that most thin hydrocephalic brains are minimally different in intellectual power from normal sized brains. Subsequently, there have been a number of small scale studies which have upheld this conclusion, but unfortunately the majority do not use any of the recognised measures of degree of hydrocephalus. However, two recent papers are particularly noteworthy. Hammock et al (1981), after considerable expereience of preoperative assessment of hydrocephalus by cranial CT scan, concluded that there was no direct correlation between intellectual capabilities and CT findings. It must be emphasised that most of the CT research so far, including my own, is predominantly postoperative, in the sense that although there are patients without valves included in the research, few of these patients subsequently needed shunting operations. The work of Jansen et al (1982) is particularly interesting because it concentrates on adult hydrocephalics. This well documented study also found no correlation between VBR and full scale IQ.

One further conclusion that can be drawn from Table 24.2 is that valves only seem to be associated with lower IQ when the ventricles are very large or very small, i.e. under and over-corrected conditions, respectively. However, this very study also highlights the fact that the spina bifida patients were not randomly selected for CT scanning. An analysis of 966 patients (Lonton, 1982), which included the patients in the 1979 study, showed mean IQs of 81 and 93 for spina bifida patients with and without valves, respectively. The corresponding IQs for the spina bifida patients in the 1979 study were 92 and 93. Hence, by accident or otherwise, patients with valves and of lower intelligence were less likely to have a postoperative scan, and are consequently under-represented here.

Which skills are most affected by increases in severity of hydrocephalus?
The Wechsler series of tests can be used to give a profile of skills. In conditions such as hydrocephalus, where patients are known to have very unevenly developed abilities, skill profiles are of greater diagnostic and prescriptive utility than global IQs. The published means for the non-handicapped population on each of the 11 sub-scales is in the region of 10 (Wechsler, 1949). Previous research has shown that patients with hydrocephalus are particularly deficient in motor and perceptuo-motor tasks (Lonton, 1977). Table 24.3 shows that the WISC sub-scales that involve these skills (picture arrangement, block design, object assembly and coding) are clearly the ones which are most affected by increasing severity of hydrocephalus. Some skills, particularly short-term memory (digit span sub-scale) and comprehension, are minimally changed by massive increases in VBR.

Table 24.3 Degree of hydrocephalus and sub-scale scores on the Wechsler Intelligence Scale for Children ($n = 302$).

VBR Group	Infor-ma-tion	Comp-rehen-sion	Arith-metic	Similar-ities	Voca-bul-ary	Digit span	Pict. comp.	Pict. arrgt.	Block design	Object assembly	Coding
1	8.7	10.5	9.6	12.0	12.0	9.4	8.7	9.0	9.1	7.1	7.9
2	9.2	10.7	9.5	13.3	11.9	9.5	8.8	8.7	9.3	7.9	8.3
3	8.4	9.9	9.2	11.7	11.6	8.7	9.3	8.0	8.5	7.0	7.4
4	8.7	10.7	9.2	11.9	11.2	9.9	8.8	8.0	8.6	7.5	7.1
5	8.7	9.7	9.4	11.2	11.4	9.2	8.5	7.3	8.2	6.5	6.2
6	7.4	9.7	7.8	10.5	9.8	9.0	7.3	6.1	6.5	5.5	5.7
Mean	8.5	10.3	9.1	11.8	11.3	9.4	8.6	7.9	8.4	7.0	7.1
$P =$	NS	NS	NS	0.05	NS	NS	0.05	0.001	0.001	0.05	0.005

Reading involves the harmonius interaction of many psychological skills including visual and auditory memory, visual perception, and varied linguistic and semantic processes. In spite of the complexity of the task, reading quotients, obtained from Schonell Graded Word Reading Tests, are not significantly affected by increasing VBR (Table 24.4). It is again noticeable that patients with valves have lower scores than untreated patients, only in groups 1 and 6.

Table 24.4 Degree of hydrocephalus and reading ability.

VBR Group	No valve	Reading quotients Valve	All	n
1	98	91	93	47
2	91	99	95	42
3	85	93	88	49
4	88	97	92	70
5	85	99	92	34
6	93	78	85	45
Mean/total	89	92	91	287
$P =$	NS	NS	NS	
n	144	143	287	

Asymmetrical and other abnormal scans

Although the numbers of abnormal scans in Table 24.5 have been slightly augmented since 1979, there are still too few of them to warrant detailed analysis. However, as a group, the abnormal scans are associated with lower full scale IQs than the symmetrical scans ($P = 0.005$). The location of greatest brain loss seems to bear little relation to skill deficits. Most patients with unilateral hydrocephalus show reasonable development of skills attributable to the affected hemisphere,

Table 24.5 Type of scan related to IQ and degree of hydrocephalus.

Type of scan	Verbal IQ	Performance IQ	Full IQ	Mean VBR %	n
Symmetrical	102	86	93	29	413
Asymmetrical (R>L)	75	66	68	51	5
Asymmetrical (L>R)	96	80	87	44	12
Porencephalic cyst (R)	85	76	80	48	12
Porencephalic cyst (L)	98	74	80	41	7
Porencephalic cyst (R + L)	119	98	106	42	3
Dandy Walker syndrome	100	82	87	51	6
Mean	101	85	92	31	458

and several patients have their best skills located in the most severely affected side! One of the patients with Dandy Walker syndrome and a VBR of 61% (Fig. 24.1) has verbal, performance and full scale IQs of 140, 88 and 117 respectively, in spite of the generally poor intellectual prognosis for this condition (Sawaya & McLaurin, 1981). This patient obtained average scores on some of the WISC sub-scales involving perceptuo-motor skills and visual perception and has normal vision, but also has massive deficits in the relevant parts of the brain.

Viewing CT scans from the perspective of IQ

It is interesting to see in Table 24.6 that the whole range of VBRs are represented among the 28 patients with IQs of 120 or above. The most extraordinary patient

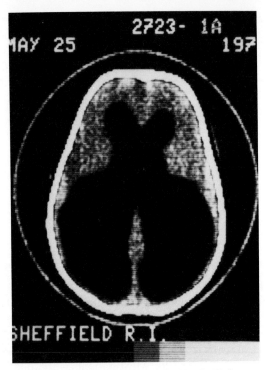

Fig. 24.1 CT scan of a 4-year-old hydrocephalic boy with Dandy Walker syndrome, and VBR of 61%. His full scale IQ is 117 (reproduced by kind permission of Sheffield Health Authority).

Table 24.6 The CT scan features of groups with extreme or abnormal IQ scores.

IQ range	Mean VBR (%)	Range of VBRs (%)	Abnormal scans (%)[a]	n
IQ $\geqslant$ 120	25	2–95	0	28
IQ $\leqslant$ 50	51	21–84	38	24
(VIQ–PIQ) > 45	32	2–71	11	10
(VIQ–PIQ) < 10	21	6–44	0	10
Total population	31	1–95	9	467

a Asymmetrical, Dandy Walker syndrome, porencephalic cysts etc.

(Fig. 24.2) has a VBR of 95% and verbal, performance and full scale IQs of 143, 99 and 126 respectively. He has a first class degree in mathematics, and thus represents the incredible combination of the thinnest brain, but highest academic attainment in this group. This young man was seen at the age of 21 years because, in addition to an endocrine disorder, he had a very large head. Another patient has a VBR of 90% and an IQ of 118.

The percentage of abnormal scans and the mean value of the VBRs is higher in the group with IQs of 50 or below, but quite a number of these children have normal CT scans. Another interesting group in Table 24.6 is the 10 children where the verbal IQ is more than 45 points higher than the performance scale IQ. The mean VBR for this group is similar to that of the whole group. A right-handed boy had a massive discrepancy of 84 points between his verbal IQ of 144, and his performance IQ of 60. If anything, his scan (Fig. 24.3) shows that his left

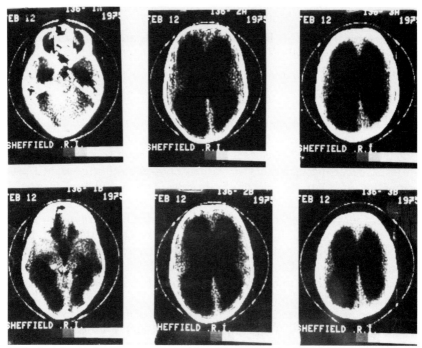

Fig. 24.2 Set of scans from a young man with an IQ of 126 and a first class degree in mathematics (reproduced by kind permission of Sheffield Health Authority).

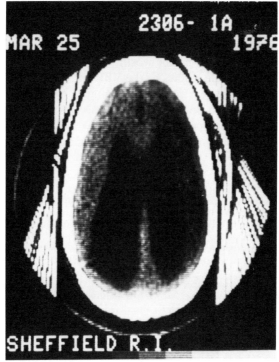

Fig. 24.3 CT scan of a right-handed boy with a verbal IQ of 144, and performance IQ of 60. His left ventricle is slightly more distended than the right, and thus his best skills are located in the most affected side! (reproduced by kind permission of Sheffield Health Authority).

ventricle is more dilated, i.e. his most powerful skills are probably located in his most affected hemisphere.

CONCLUSIONS

The most important issue arising from this research is that under certain limited circumstances there seems to be no gross correlation between quality of intellect and quantity of brain. The relevant circumstances seem to be a relatively slow brain insult occurring in infancy or earlier, coupled with a presumed massive overprovision of relatively 'plastic' brain cells. This would explain why some hydrocephalics are brilliant but brainless, and it also accommodates the possibility of massive intellectual losses due to sudden brain trauma at any time, or slow deterioration after the period of relative plasticity of the brain. Research fails to explain why performance skills are more adversely affected by increasing VBR than verbal skills. One possible reason could be that language skills are more readily transferred to other brain locations than are non-verbal skills, i.e. the latter may be more firmly localised.

Another point arising from this study is that valves only seem to be associated with skill deficits when ventricles are abnormally small or grossly enlarged. The explanation for this seems to be that the former condition is one of overcorrection, the so-called 'slit ventricle', and the latter one of undercorrection. Presumably, in both cases, the chronic valve malfunctioning results in intellectual deficits.

A most important consequence of this research is that thickness of cortex should never be used as the sole, or even as a highly significant factor in deciding when surgery would or would not be worthwhile. An interesting area of further research could be large scale studies of the VBRs of the normal population. The recent development of nuclear magnetic resonance imaging techniques, which produce better pictures with no damaging radiation (Husband & Hobday, 1981), should make this an exciting possibility. Perhaps we will find that brainlessness is quite a common phenomenon in the supposedly normal population.

REFERENCES

Bergstrom K, Billie B 1978 Computed tomography of the brain in children with minimal brain damage. Neuropaediatrie 9: 378–384
Cala L A, Jones B, Mastaglia F L, Wiley B 1978 Brain atrophy and intellectual impairment in heavy drinkers. Australian and New Zealand Journal of Medicine 8: 147–153
Golden C J, Graber B, Moses J A, Zatz L M 1979 Relationships of neuropsychological test scores to ventricular enlargement in schizophrenic patients. Journal of Computed Axial Tomography 3: 563
Goodwin L S, Hellmann J, Vannucci R C, Maisels M J 1981 Ventricular dimensions of the brain in premature and full term infants. Archives of Neurology 38: 447–449
Hadenius A M, Hagberg B, Hyttnes-Bensh K, Jorgen S 1962 The natural prognosis of infantile hydrocephalus. Acta Paediatrica Scandinavica 51: 117–123
Hahn F J Y, Rim K 1976 Frontal ventricular dimensions on normal computed tomography. American Journal of Roentgenology 126: 593–596
Hammock M K, Milhorat T H 1981 Cranial computed tomography in infancy and childhood. Williams and Williams, Baltimore
Hammock M K, Milhorat T H, Brailler D R 1981b Computed tomography in the evaluation of patients with spina bifida. Zeitschrift fur Kinderchirurgie 34: 334–345

Husband J E, Hobday P A 1981 Computerised axial tomography in oncology. Churchill Livingstone, Edinburgh

Jansen J, Gloerfelt-Tarp B, Pedersen H, Zilstorff K 1982 Prognosis in infantile hydrocephalus. Acta Neurologica Scandinavica 65: 81–93

Levin H S, Meyers C A, Grossman R G, Sarwar M 1981 Ventricular enlargement after closed head injury. Archives of Neurology 38: 623–629

Lonton A P 1977 Location of the myelomeningocele and its relationship to subsequent physical and intellectual abilities in children with myelomeningocele associated with hydrocephalus. Zeitschrift fur Kinderchirurgie 22: 510–519

Lonton A P 1979 The relationship between intellectual skills and the computerised axial tomograms of children with spina bifida and hydrocephalus. Zeitschrift fur Kinderchirurgie 28: 368–374

Lonton A P 1982 Predicition of intelligence in spina bifida neonates. Zeitschrift fur Kinderchirurgie December 1982

Macnab G H 1961 Hydrocephalus in infancy. In: Carling E R, Ross J P (eds) Surgical progress. Butterworth, London

Manowitz P, Kling A, Kohn H 1978 Clinical course of adult metachromatic leukodystrophy presenting as schizophrenia. Journal of Nervous and Mental Disorders 166: 500–506

Morley Fletcher H 1900 A case of megalencephaly. Transactions of the Pathological Society of London 51: 230

Mueller S M, Bell W, Cornell S, de S Hamsher K, Dolan K 1977 Achondroplasia and hydrocephalus. Neurology 27: 430–434

Nie N H, Hull C H, Jenkins J G, Steinbrenner K, Brent D H 1975 Statistical package for the social sciences. McGraw Hill, New York

Roberts M A, Caird F I, Steven J L, Grossart K W 1977 Computerised axial tomography and dementia in the elderly. In: du Boulay G H, Mosely I F (eds) Computerised axial tomography in clinical practice. Springer Verlag, Berlin

Sawaya R, McLaurin R L 1981 Dandy Walker syndrome. Journal of Neurosurgery 55: 89–98

Scarff J E 1952 Non-obstructive hydrocephalus. Journal of Neurosurgery 9: 164–176

Synek V, Reuben J R 1976 The ventricular-brain ratio using planimetric measurement of EMI scans. British Journal of Radiology 49: 233–237

25. Febrile convulsions in children: are prophylactic anticonvulsants needed?

Neil Gordon

Attitudes to the treatment of epilepsy are changing and not before time. It is no longer accepted that fits must be stopped at all costs and the possible long-term effects of anti-epileptic drugs are being increasingly questioned. There is much yet to learn about the adverse effects of seizures on the one hand and the toxic effects of treatment on the other. It is against this background that the treatment of febrile convulsions has to be judged.

EPIDEMIOLOGY AND NATURAL HISTORY

There is no doubt that there are a number of children, about 3% of those aged between 3 months and 5 years of age, who appear to be liable to convulsions when their temperatures rise rapidly above a certain level unassociated with infections of the nervous system. A rectal temperature of 38°C or more is usually accepted in the definition of this type of epilepsy. There is evidence that the liability is inherited as a dominant trait (Ounsted et al, 1966). The pyrexia is most often due to an upper respiratory infection of viral origin, but an association with a specific virus is unproven.

The first febrile convulsion is often the severest but there is a high risk of recurrence. This is over 50% for girls under the age of 13 months at the time of the first attack, and about 30% for boys of the same age. Among older children the presence of a family history is of more importance, increasing the chances of further febrile fits from 25 to 50% (O'Donohoe, 1979).

Opinions vary on the risks of subsequent epilepsy, probably due to the varying criteria used in different series. Frantzen (1971) found an incidence of later epilepsy of less than 2%, but in Wallace's series at least one spontaneous seizure occurred in 17% (Wallace, 1977). The chance of a child developing epilepsy after febrile convulsions will depend on such factors as the duration of the initial seizure, particularly if this is over 30 minutes, whether the febrile fits are of a focal type or are recurrent, evidence of antecedent brain damage, and an early age of onset. In one of the most reliable follow-up studies Nelson & Ellenberg

(1976) have shown that 2% had recurrent afebrile seizures by the age of 7, but if the febrile seizures were complex with prolonged duration, recurrence within 24 hours and focal features, the risk of developing epilespy rose to over 4%. If development had been abnormal before the first febrile fit the child was eight times more likely to develop epilepsy. This study also showed that the majority of afebrile fits occurred within 3 years of the first febrile seizure.

This research does confirm that parents of the vast majority of children who develop convulsions with fever can be reassured that their child can lead a perfectly healthy life. However this does not mean that a febrile fit is ever a trivial affair. The majority of parents when directly asked about the experience of their child's first attack of this kind said that they thought the child was dying (Baumer et al, 1981). Parents must therefore be reassured that the majority of children with febrile convulsions do progress normally into adult life.

There can be no doubt that the liability to febrile convulsions does place the child at risk from brain damage from severe convulsions. Anyone who is involved in the care of physically and mentally handicapped children hears the story too often to ignore it of a child who developed normally for the first few years of life, contracted an infection with a high temperature associated with severe convulsions and has remained handicapped ever since. Ounsted and his colleagues (1966) found that a third of the hundred children they were studying with hyperkinesis, catastrophic rage and mental defect gave a history of severe febrile convulsions earlier in life. Aicardi & Chevrie (1970) reviewed 239 patients who were under the age of 15 years at the time of their first attack of status epilepticus and just under a third of them were febrile at the onset of the fits. They confirmed that the possibility of permanent brain damage occurring as a consequence of the status was considerable, especially if this happened before the age of 18 months.

The major risk run by children liable to develop severe seizures with fever is undoubtedly brain damage. Animal studies suggest that removal of factors such as arterial hypotension and hyperpyrexia protect against cerebellar damage but only to a slight extent against neocortical and hippocampal lesions. Sustained neuronal discharge with elevated metabolic rate may cause ischaemic changes in neurones by an accumulation of metabolites. One consequence of this is swelling of astrocytic end-feet, resulting in impaired transport of substrates and metabolites to and from active neurones (Meldrum, 1978). Evidence has been found in children which strongly suggests brain damage as the result of cerebral hypoxia after convulsions lasting more than 30 minutes or after rapidly recurring short convulsions. This is based on studies of cerebrospinal fluid, acid-base status and lactate and pyruvate concentrations after convulsions of varied duration and aetiology (Simpson et al, 1977). It has been shown that intracranial pressure rises during and after fits of any kind, even with minor seizures. These changes may often be related to increased cerebral blood flow, but when repeated major convulsions occur cerebral oedema may complicate the picture so that cerebral blood flow is impaired and brain damage likely. Then treatment to reduce the pressure, with mannitol for example, may be of vital importance and is a strong argument for intracranial pressure monitoring in status epilepticus (Minns & Brown, 1978).

TREATMENT AND PROPHYLAXIS AT TIMES OF FEVER

Should treatment be given to prevent convulsions associated with fever? Generalisations are to be avoided but surely guide lines are needed to help make this decision for each individual child. Few if any would attempt to justify treating every child who has such fits. Equally to never treat them as a matter of principle seems equally unreasonable. It is most likely that the right decision lies somewhere between these two extremes and that first of all an effort must be made to identify those at particular risk. Lennox-Buchthal (1973) maintained that the children at greatest risk were those whose fits started before the age of 13 months, or between 13 and 36 months if there was a family history, or if two or more such episodes occurred. Wallace (1974) also found an increased risk of recurrence of febrile convulsions if there were repeated seizures in the initial illness, persistent neurological abnormalities, or if the initial fit was a prolonged and unilateral one and lasted more than 30 minutes. Girls with an early age of onset and boys with a family history seem to be in particular need of protection.

Boys experience more febrile convulsions than girls and over a longer period of time, but girls are more liable to serious complications as they have more frequent fits at a younger age. A possible explanation for these findings and for the fact that a generalised insult may result in focal lesions is the increased liability to damage of immature brains or parts of the brain (Taylor, 1969). Ounsted (1971) has suggested that the message of the Y chromosome is to delay the maturation of the male from about mid-pregnancy onwards and there is no doubt that girls are in advance of boys in early childhood, especially in certain aspects of language development. This means that boys are exposed to the risks of brain damage for a longer period than girls. For the majority of people in the early months of life the right side of the brain is more active developing perceptual functions, and then the left cerebral hemisphere predominates as language is acquired. As a result the likelihood of right hemisphere lesions gradually rise over the first 3 years of life while left hemisphere lesions fall sharply through the first 2 years.

The persistence of grand mal after febrile convulsions is largely determined by events preceding the initial fit, such as complications during pregnancy and birth, while temporal lobe seizures are related to prolonged, repeated and unilateral febrile convulsions and may therefore be prevented by adequate treatment (Wallace, 1977). Chevrie & Aicardi (1975) also emphasise that the expression of the first febrile convulsion depends upon multiple factors such as age, sex, genetic predisposition, previous brain damage and the nature of the febrile illness. The EEG is of little practical value in the assessment of children with febrile seizures (O'Donohoe, 1979).

Severe febrile convulsions are often unilateral and the association of hemi-convulsions, hemiplegia and later epilepsy has been designated the HHE syndrome (Gastaut et al, 1960). Severe, prolonged and mainly unilateral convulsions occurred with fever among children under the age of 2. They were frequently followed by permanent hemiplegia, often by mental handicap, and by epilepsy. The pathological findings included venous congestion, vascular thrombosis and cerebral oedema. This was followed by cortical atrophy which can now be easily confirmed by the CT scan.

It seems reasonable to consider prophylactic treatment for selected children using the above criteria to identify those at particular risk, as children with high risk factors do have a significantly greater chance of developing epilepsy in later life with an incidence around 13% as opposed to 2-3% of those with no risk factors. The high risk group constitutes about a third of children with febrile fits (N.I.H. Consensus statement, 1980; Table 25.1). The reasons for this must be explained to parents and the wishes of parents to accept such treatment or not has

Table 25.1 Risk factors in children liable to febrile convulsions.

1. Febrile convulsions which occur under the age of 13 months especially in girls
2. Febrile convulsions which occur between the ages of 14 and 38 months with a family history of epilepsy, especially in boys
3. The history of significant complications during pregnancy and birth
4. The presence of neurological abnormalities prior to the first febrile convulsion
5. A prolonged (over 15 minutes) or unilateral febrile convulsion (complex) or repeated fits at the time of the first attack
6. The persistence of neurological abnormalities after a febrile convulsion, temporary or permanent
7. Two or more febrile convulsions associated with separate illnesses.

to be taken into account. One factor is the ability of parents to cope with the management of the prolonged and severe febrile fit, and the nearness of medical aid if this is needed. The importance of treatment of the infection and associated temperature will have been stressed and one of the options which is increasingly favoured is to confine anti-epileptic treatment to the occurrence of a febrile fit if and when it occurs. When the doctor cannot be contacted as a matter of urgency if the child has a severe fit, the parents can be instructed in the use of emergency treatment and most parents are able to cope with this. In view of the dangers from seizures lasting for more than 30 minutes the treatment must be effective within this period. Diazepam given rectally is the drug of choice, rectal paraldehyde being a much more complicated procedure. It is doubtful if diazepam is absorbed quickly enough by suppository, and the use of the i.v. preparation is preferable. The dose is 0.5 mg per kg body weight and a preparation is now available in which 5 mg and 10 mg of the liquid are prepared in rectal tubes which can be administered without difficulty. Rectal Valium can also be used for prophylaxis, the appropriate dose being given when a child at risk is found to have a rectal temperature greater than 38.5°C (Knudsen, 1979). It may then be reasonable to use suppositories rather than the i.v. liquid as obtaining a quick therapeutic level in the body is not so important.

LONGTERM PROPHYLAXIS

The alternative is prophylaxis with long-term drug treatment and has to be considered if the risk factors are particularly high, or for one reason or another it is not possible to consider rectal diazepam. Another factor in favour of such a course of action is that repeated febrile fits may impair intellectual development (Aldridge-Smith & Wallace, 1982). It is claimed that treatment with phenytoin sodium does not prevent febrile convulsions, although it may modify their severity (Melchoir et al, 1971). Another study from Denmark (Faero et al, 1972) suggests that phenobarbitone is effective if a constant serum level of 16 μg/ml is obtained. The sedative effects of phenobarbitone can be counteracted by giving the drug in the evening and gradually increasing the dose up to 5 mg/kg body weight. However, in a number of children the phenobarbitone has to be stopped due to side-effects such as irritability, hyperactivity, sleeplessness and aggression although the possibility of toxic side-effects can be reduced by careful monitoring of serum levels. In a carefully controlled trial of infants on long-term treatment with phenobarbitone Camfield & Camfield (1981) found evidence of impaired memory and poor comprehension, and also increased fussiness and irritability and a tendency to wake in the middle of the night, but no overactivity. Also the effective role of phenobarbitone in the treatment of febrile fits has been questioned (Heckmatt et al, 1976).

Sodium valproate is an alternative drug. It is responsible for a number of side-effects, some of them severe, but these may be less troublesome than those of phenobarbitone. If the sodium valproate is given in a dose of 20–40 mg/kg/day to obtain a serum concentration of 60 μg/ml or more it can be as effective as phenobarbitone (Ngwane & Bower, 1980; Wallace & Smith, 1980).

There is one suggestion that should be considered and that is the possibility that a significant number of children with febrile seizures are suffering from anoxic rather than epileptic attacks, the fever precipitating reflex cardiac arrest. This conclusion is based on the type of seizure, the family history, clinical and EEG findings and the response to the oculovagal or oculocardiac reflex. If this possibility can be confirmed the management of these children will obviously be different (Stephenson, 1978). The suspicion is that such a mechanism is unlikely to account for the severer or prolonged febrile fits.

If continuous anti-epileptic treatment is started for how long should it be continued? There are no definite criteria except that the liability to febrile seizures becomes progressively less as the child grows older, so that even if the risk factors are high it seems reasonable to consider gradually stopping the treatment after a fit-free period of 18 to 24 months (Gordon, 1982). Three-quarters of second convulsions occur within a year (Addy, 1981).

CONCLUSIONS

Prophylactic treatment for febrile convulsions in addition to antipyrexial measures should be considered for children when high risk factors are identified. Among these children the chance of brain damage from severe or prolonged seizures outweigh the known risks of long-term treatment and 30 to 40% of children who have had one febrile fit will have another if not given such treatment. Rectal diazepam used prophylactically and for the emergency treatment of such fits is to be preferred. When this is not a practical proposition long-term treatment for 18 to 24 months with sodium valproate, with phenobarbitone as an alternative, is the drug of choice. However the situation is still unsatisfactory and more research is needed into the management of febrile convulsions (Fishman, 1979). The first of such seizures is often the most severe so that more education of the general public is needed, especially among affected families. It must be emphasised that there is much more to the management of epilepsy than prescribing pills. There are understandable risks of overprotection on the part of the parents and the children leading a restricted life to an unjustifiable degree. If the parents do know something about the subject, realise that their children can be helped if this is necessary and that the vast majority of children with febrile convulsions develop normally, this is much less likely to occur. One of the most important factors in the prophylaxis of these fits is the ability of parents to carry out preventive measures such as steps to stop the child rapidly developing a high temperature, contacting medical aid if a severe attack occurs and giving rectal diazepam as indicated. Another important aspect of prevention is to ensure an accurate diagnosis, especially of the first seizure in very young infants. It may well be difficult to exclude meningitis in infancy without examining the cerebrospinal fluid, and Ounsted (1978) considers that whatever the type of meningitis the risk of convulsions resulting in brain damage is sufficiently great to warrant the use of prophylactic anticonvulsant treatment as soon as such an infection is suspected.

REFERENCES

Addy D P 1981 Prophylaxis and febrile convulsions. Archives of Diseases of Childhood 56: 81–83
Aicardi J, Chevrie J J 1970 Convulsive status epilepticus in infants and children. A study of 239 cases. Epilepsia 11: 187–197
Aldridge-Smith J, Wallace S J 1982 Febrile convulsions: intellectual progress in relation to anticonvulsant therapy and to recurrence of fits. Archives of Diseases in Childhood 57: 104–107
Baumer J H, David T J, Valentine S J, Roberts J E, Hughes B R 1981 Many parents think their child is dying when having a first febrile convulsion. Developmental and Medical Child Neurology 23: 462–464
Camfield C S, Camfield P R 1981 Behavioural and co-operative effects of phenobarbitol in toddlers. In: Nelson K B, Ellenberg J H (eds) Febrile seizures. Raven, New York, p 203–210
Chevrie J J Aicardi J 1975 Duration and lateralisation of febrile convulsions. Etiological factors. Epilepsia 16: 781–789
Faero O, Kastrup K W, Lykkegard Nielsen E, Melchior J C, Thorn I 1972 Successful prophylaxis of febrile convulsions with phenobarbitol. Epilepsia 13: 279–285
Fishman M A 1979 Febrile seizures: the treatment controversy. Journal of Pediatrics 94: 177–184
Frantzen E 1971 The prognosis of febrile convulsions. Epilepsia 12: 192
Gastaut H, Poirier F, Payan H, Salaman G, Toga A, Vigouroux M 1960 HHE syndrome Hemiconvulsions, epilepsy. Epilepsia 1: 418–447
Gordon N 1982 Duration of treatment for childhood epilepsy. Developmental and Medical Child Neurology 24: 84–88
Heckmatt J Z, Houston A B, Clow D J, Stephenson J B P, Dodd K L, Lealman G T, Logan R W 1976 Failure of phenobarbitone to prevent febrile convulsions. British Medical Journal 1: 559–561
Knudsen F U 1979 Rectal administration of diazepam in solution in the acute treatment of convulsions in infants and children. Archives of Diseases of Childhood 54: 855–857
Lennox-Buchthal M A 1973 Febrile convulsions. A reappraisal. Electroencephalography and Clinical Neurophysiology, Suppl. 32
Melchior J C, Buchthal F, Lennox-Buchthall M 1971 The ineffectiveness of diphenylhydantoin in preventing febrile convulsions in the age of greatest risk under three years. Epilepsia 12: 55–62
Meldrum B 1978 Physiological changes during prolonged seizures, and epileptic brain damage. Neuropadiatrie 9: 203–212
Minns R A, Brown J K 1978 Intracranial pressure changes associated with childhood seizures. Developmental and Medical Child Neurology 20: 561–569
Nelson K B, Ellenberg J H 1976 Predictors of epilepsy in children who have experienced febrile convulsions. New England Journal of Medicine 1029–1032

Ngwane E, Bower B 1980 Continuous sodium valproate or phenobarbitone in the prevention of 'simple' febrile convulsions. Archives of Diseases of Childhood 55: 171–174

NIH Consensus Statement 1980 Febrile seizures: long-term management of children with fever-associated seizures. Summary of an NIH Consensus statement. British Medical Journal ii: 277–279

O'Donohoe N V 1979 Epilepsies of childhood. Butterworth, London

Ounsted C 1971 Some aspect of seizure disorders. In: Gardner D, Hull D (eds) Recent advances in paediatrics. Churchill Livingstone, Edinburgh, p 363–400

Ounsted C 1978 Preventing febrile convulsions. Developmental and Medical Child Neurology 20: 799–800

Ounsted C, Lindsay J, Norman R 1966 Biological factors in temporal lobe epilepsy. Clinics in development Medicine, No. 22. S.I.M.P./Heinemann

Simpson H, Habel A H, George E L 1977 Cerebrospinal fluid acid-base status and lactate and pyruvate concentrations after convulsions of varied duration and aetiology in children. Archives of Diseases of Childhood 52: 844–849

Stephenson J B P 1978 Two types of febrile seizure: anoxic (syncopal) and epileptic mechanisms differentiated by oculocardiac reflex. British Medical Journal ii: 726–728

Taylor D C 1969 Differential rates of cerebral maturation between sexes and between hemispheres: Evidence from epilepsy. Lancet 2: 140

Wallace S J 1974 Recurrence of febrile convulsions. Archives of Diseases of Childhood 49: 763–770

Wallace S J 1977 Spontaneous fits after convulsions with fever. Archives of Diseases of Childhood 52: 192–196

Wallace S J, Aldridge Smith J 1980 Successful prophylaxis against febrile convulsions with valproic acid or phenobarbitone. British Medical Journal i: 353–354

26. The evaluation of treatment

Klim McPherson

'As we learn from our mistakes our knowledge grows, even though we may never know — that is, know for certain. Since our knowledge can grow, there can be no reason here for despair of reason. And since we can never know for certain, there can be no authority here for any claim to authority, for conceit over our knowledge, or for smugness.'

Karl R. Popper,
Conjectures and Refutations

In the evaluation of the relative merits of different treatments for the same condition, it has become very clear that several explanations for an apparent treatment difference which are independent of their intrinsic merits can, and do, have dramatic and unexpected effects. Thus the casual, or indeed careful, observation that patients treated in one way appear to fare better than patients treated in another can have nothing to do with the actual relative efficacy of the two treatments. There are three plausible alternative explanations:

1. *Chance.* In so far as the response to any treatment is variable between patients, then the chance element which determines that response, or the choice of responsive patients, can result in the observation of an aggregated difference which appears to favour one treatment. Statistics have become a basic part of the evaluation of therapy to answer the first question that comes to mind when faced with any apparent treatment difference, that is, the extent to which that difference could have arisen by chance. Now that statistical methods have become commonplace, the control and quantification of some chance effects is routine and one has to be more wary of other explanation, especially when chance is an unlikely one (e.g. $P < 0.05$).

2. *Patient selection.* The choice of therapy for a particular patient is generally the result of complex processes of selection. In those processes there are many opportunities for systematic bias in the selection of patients as well as in their treatment. Moreover, patients with different prognoses may systematically differ in their degree of compliance with prescribed therapy.

3. *Ancilliary treatment.* Clearly patients who receive one kind of therapy may necessarily or habitually have particular ancilliary treatments associated with it which might make sufficient difference to the outcome to mislead an observer.

This is perhaps more likely if the ancilliary treatment is not expected to have an important effect.

The recognition of these errors in the interpretation of clinical evidence has lead to the development of the randomised controlled trial so that the real effects of treatment can be established. Thus, to quantify the likely extent of chance, one always calculates the probability of observing an effect which is more extreme than the one actually observed. Patients are allocated randomly to treatments to ensure that any differences between patients on different treatments are a matter solely of chance, and not systematic selection. It is worth pointing out that this is more than a convenient device — it is essential.

It is often argued that any measurable attributes of patients which might affect prognosis can be adjusted for in the analysis which compares methods of treatment, so that patient selection will have less influence upon results. However, the great merit of random allocation is that characteristics not thought to affect prognosis, or which are not measurable, are also balanced. It then becomes a matter of straightforward logic that the extent of systematic differences in all characteristics between randomly allocated groups has probable limits, defined by the chance nature of the randomisation process. Indeed, it is this that puts the statistical calculations in context because, in the absence of randomisation, systematic selection biasses are not known to be absent. For example, if an observed difference has a P-value associated with it of 0.01, it means that this particular outcome could be a consequence of random imbalance betweem the treatment groups, but the chance of that occurring is only 1%. If the groups are not randomised such an argument becomes very much less pertinent, particularly if there is a chance of systematic selection at any stage in the therapeutic decision.

Lastly, if we are worried about ancillary treatment muddying the treatment comparison, double-blind procedures become necessary if possible. Then not only will supposedly unimportant aspects of treatment be comparable between groups, but also the designation of important end-points will not be influenced by knowledge of, and preferences for, particular treatments.

If we consider other possible sources of deception, then, apart from deliberate fraud, it is difficult to think of any that do not come under these three headings. So much, therefore, for the theory and the formal justification for randomised clinical trials as opposed to uncontrolled non-random comparisons. However, in essence the persuasiveness of the theory rests on the kind of effect that these alternative explanations can actually have in real comparisons.

The first example I shall cite comes from a comparison of several clinical trials in the treatment of lung cancer at the National Institute of Health (Pocock, 1977). In each trial with strict protocols and well defined eligibility criteria, two treatments were compared. Patients were randomly allocated to the treatments and at the end of each trial the better treatment was then compared, in a subsequent trial, with another treatment. Thus it was possible to compare the outcome in patients on the same treatment, but in consecutive rather than concurrent trials. In all, 19 such comparisons were made. Clearly, because the treatments were the same and tightly controlled by protocol, any differences which occurred had to be the consequence of one of the three alternative explanations (see above) for an observed treatment effect and could not be anything to do with the real effect of that treatment. For chance to be the explanation of any differences we would expect to see only 1 of the 19 comparisons different at less than the 5% level of significance. In fact 4 of the comparisons were significant indicating that some other factor was the explanation for these observed differences. Indeed, the probability of observing 4 significant comparisons out of 19 is less than 2%. So the number of significant differences is significantly higher than expected if chance were the only explanation. Moreover, because therapeutic efficacy cannot be the explanation, the only plausible alternatives are either patient selection or ancillary treatment.

Clearly patient selection is the most likely because the treatment schedules were themselves tightly defined even though the patients who were eligible were also well defined, by protocol (which is not true in general). In other words, here we have a set of comparisons for which we know a priori that treatment efficacy cannot be the cause of any differences, and for which conventional statistical calculations indicate a significant effect. Indeed, quite apart from the statistics, the differences were qualitatively quite marked; the death rate in one comparison was half the death rate in a consecutive series on the same treatment. If this can occur with unambiguous end-points like death in carefully controlled historical comparisons then comparing two non-randomised groups of patients who are treated differently becomes a very hazardous procedure. Moreover, the degree of hazard is unknown. If one believes that a new treatment is better because one is desperately seeking therapeutic advances it is all too easy to persuade oneself that in a particular case a non-random comparison is valid. Often it is not possible to identify a strong reason why such a comparison is invalid, and general principles may not be enough to control one's enthusiasm. Thus, in the example above, it is impossible to identify explanations although the general conclusion is unequivocal. In the general way in which we evaluate therapies, using significance tests and so on, we would have been unequivocally misled if we had deduced from a significant difference that one treatment was better than another.

The principle illustrated by this particular example is, of course, extremely important in the evaluation of all medical and surgical therapy. It is important because, as we shall come to later, clinical trials are difficult and expensive and can easily be seen to be unnecessary. This leads some (e.g. Kranberg, 1979 and Gehan & Freineich, 1974) to advocate the use of historical controls to evaluate new therapies. An interesting example of the lesson that can be learned from uncritical reliance on such comparisons can be obtained from the response to Kranberg by Doll & Peto (1980). These latter workers cite a review of anticoagulant therapy for myocardial infarction by Chalmers et al (1977). The British Medical Journal (1979) had recently pronounced firmly in favour of such therapy while the New England Journal of Medicine (1979) firmly against, presumably on the basis of the same literature. How one interprets the literature depends, among many other considerations, on the value one places on historical comparisons. Chalmers et al used the information from 16 000 patients in 32 studies; 18 historically controlled, 8 concurrently controlled, and 6 randomised. The pooled evidence from the historically controlled comparisons suggested that the reduction in mortality attributable to anticoagulant therapy was 53% while for the randomised series the pooled reduction in mortality was only 20%. Clearly the difference could easily be explained by the selection of particularly favourable patients for anticoagulant therapy in some of the non-randomised comparisons. We know already that, even when there is no reason to suspect that selection occurred a priori, mortality rates can be halved in consecutive series of similar patients on the same treatment.

Therefore, the case for randomised clinical trials is obvious. However, in avoiding biases that exaggerate the efficacy of treatments, over-compensation which could create the opposite bias must be avoided. Unfortunately this can only be done in trials with large numbers of patients when random errors become relatively small. Of course this is only true when therapeutic differences are slight. When major differences are expected then they easily overwhelm sampling variation in even quite a small number of patients. Where there are uncertainties about an optimal treatment then the actual efficacy is bound to be small. However, detecting small treatment effects is important in common conditions.

In statistical terms, a clinical trial is designed so that the chance of being deceived in two quite separate ways is made as small as possible. The first deception is to believe there is a treatment difference when in fact there is none. This is avoided in a randomised study by accepting a difference only when the correctly calculated P-value is low. This is what the P-value means; when it is low, the observed treatment difference is likely to be real.

On the other hand, if there really is a difference, we would like the chance of obtaining a non-significant result to be small. This is where the formal requirement for large numbers in clinical trials comes from. Given a certain level of significance and a given real treatment difference, the only way of ensuring that the chance of a non-significant result is low, is to increase the number of patients in the trial. In practice there is a strong tendency to organise a clinical trial recruiting as many patients as possible in a reasonable period of time and, at the end, analyse the results for a significant difference. Under these circumstances the chance of believing there to be a real effect when there is not (called a Type I error) is controlled by only believing significant effects. However, the chance of obtaining a non-significant difference when in fact the therapies are importantly different (called Type II error) is not necessarily well controlled.

In Figure 26.1 these two kinds of errors are illustrated. If there is no real treatment difference we would prefer a non-significant result; the calculation of statistical significance is precisely the calculation of the chance that, in the absence of a treatment difference, any given trial yields a significant result and this probability is denoted by 2α. Because we always calculate significance levels the probability of being misled in this way is always low. This means that clinicians who interpret clinical trials are unlikely to claim an effect for a treatment when it does not in fact exist. On the other hand, we can control the probability of claiming a non-significant difference if the treatments really are different (which is denoted by β) by statistical calculation of the sample size of trial before it is started. These calculations are done by reference to a particular size of expected treatment difference.

280

	REAL TREATMENT DIFFERENCE	
	NONE	NEW TREATMENT BETTER
CLINICAL TRIAL RESULT — NOT SIGNIFICANT	**NOT MISLEADING** PROBABILITY $= 1 - 2\alpha$	**TYPE II ERROR** PROBABILITY $= \beta$
SIGNIFICANT	**TYPE I ERROR** PROBABILITY $= 2\alpha$ $=$ LEVEL OF SIGNIFICANCE	**NOT MISLEADING** PROBABILITY $= 1 - \beta$ $=$ POWER

Fig. 26.1 The two probabilities of certain results in any clinical trial when either the two treatments are equivalent or the new treatment is better. 2α: Probability of claiming a significant effect when there is no treatment difference. β: Probability of claiming a non-significant effect when there is a treatment difference of a certain magnitude.

As an example, let us suppose that an investigator is testing a new treatment against traditional therapy. A clinical trial is started randomising patients between the two treatments until 200 patients are recruited into each arm (i.e. 400 in all). By contemporary standards this is a large trial and will have involved an enormous amount of care, work and money. Let us say that the old treatment cures 50% of patients and the remainder relapsed or had to undergo a second line of therapy. If we now imagine that the new treatment actually cures 60% of patients, then there is a worse than even chance that this trial will finish with a difference that is significant at 5%. In other words, in most trials of this size a therapeutic difference of this magnitude will be missed. It is true that most such trials will show a tendency in favour of the new treatment, but only a minority will be statistically significant ($P < 0.05$). This is a necessary and sufficient basis for controversy and yet these calculations are performed assuming an important therapeutic effect. If, however, the real cure rate with the new treatment is 70%, then only 3% of such trials will end up with a non-significant difference and 97% will be significant at 5%. But in a trial with 60 patients in each arm, even this quite large treatment difference will result in non-significant differences more often than not.

The sad truth is that to resolve therapeutic controversies one always requires large or very large trials. The formal requirement is to specify in advance the chance of achieving a significant difference if a specified difference in treatment efficacy actually exists. This chance is called the power of a trial. For example, if we thought, on the basis of existing knowledge, that an improvement from 50% to 60% was plausible and worth knowing about, then we might say that we wanted a clinical trial to have a chance of 90% of detecting such an effect. (Power equals 90%.) We then could calculate (see for example Lachin, 1981) that the minimum number of patients required in each arm is 550, or more than 1000 patients altogether. We could also look this up in tables (e.g. Fleiss, 1973) and discover that an 80% power would only require 420 in each arm and so on. There is a great advantage in this exercise compared to running a clinical trial with 200 patients in each group which has a less than even chance of achieving a significant result. Moreover, it is no help to anticipate and plan for a real therapeutic difference greater than 10% if, in reality, that is desirable rather than plausible. Such a strategy is extremely tempting because the sample size requirement for a reasonable power of detecting an important but small difference is often so large.

An example of the kind of problems that can arise from over-estimating the expected therapeutic effect can be obtained from one enormous multi-centre trial of the secondary prevention of myocardial infarction. The Anturane reinfarction trial (1978) was designed to include enough patients to have a 90% power of detecting a halving of the cardiac mortality rate in the first year after infarction. That is, it was hoped that Anturane would reduce the mortality from 10% to 5% at 1 year. It was not explained why this was the expectation but these constraints required at least 1200 patients altogether and, in 24 centres throughout North America, 1500 patients were recruited in 2 years. This is no mean undertaking and required great expense and organisation. However, according to the published findings, the reduction in cardiac mortality in the Anturane group compared to placebo was 32% at 2 years which, as it happens, is not quite significant at 5%. Needless to say this presents a terrible dilemma for the organisers because results which are not significant are not convincing and one cannot change all the rules simply because the trial is expensive and complicated.

Therefore, the organisers of the trial did what must be overwhelmingly tempting in such circumstances; they looked closely at the results to see if they could discover any patterns which might provide further insights into the nature of the effect. They discovered that the reduction in cardiac mortality was largely attributable to a reduction in the rate of sudden deaths, particularly in the first 6 months postinfarction. However, Anturane derived its plausible therapeutic effect in the first place because of its antithrombotic properties. This was why a halving of cardiac deaths was expected, not because anyone supposed that the rate of *sudden* deaths (presumably due to arrhythmia) would be changed. The results were finally reported as a beneficial effect on sudden death rate, in spite of the fact that the trial was designed to detect another effect, for which at least the mechanism would have been understood.

Of course there was much controversy surrounding this trial, particularly when the FDA refused to license the drug for the secondary prevention of myocardial infarction. Ultimately it appeared that Anturane had about the same effect as aspirin on the reduction of total mortality after myocardial infarction — about 20%. Therefore, it would be reasonable to conclude that, had the sample size been determined on the basis of a plausible reduction in cardiac mortality then, firstly, the drug would have been licensed and secondly we would now know considerably more than we do about the treatment of patients with myocardial infarction.

It is also worth emphasising that searching for sub-groups of patients, or end-points, or time periods in which or during which the test treatment appears to work particularly well is a very hazardous procedure (Lee et al, 1980). Unless such sub-groups are strongly indicated before the data are examined, by reference to information quite separate from the trial, then such sub-groups are almost bound to be misleading. This is because chance has peculiar manifestations and dredging the data will always produce some combination of circumstances (because there are usually so many possible) in which apparently interesting effects are seen. Therefore, restricting the search to only those sub-groups for which there is a prior suggestion at least provides some control over the unhappy chance of being misled in a framework which is logically coherent. In the Anturane example no one would have suggested looking at arrhythmic deaths but now everyone is trying to work out a plausible biological explanation; the most likely one is merely the play of chance and inadequate prior definition of what is a sudden death.

Of course it is essential when trying to keep the sample size as small as possible (consistent with a reasonable power of detecting a plausible treatment difference) to utilise as much information as possible in the comparison of treatments. The point of doing this is to be in a position to compare an index of response which does not ignore useful information and thus require more patients for a given power. In general, if the outcome of a trial is death or serious event like a stroke of myocardial infarction, it is inefficient merely to compare the proportion of patients in each group with such an event. In the example we discussed earlier to illustrate the meaning of power we simply used an illustrative cure rate, but in fact if we had incorporated the time to an event we could often achieve a greater power for a given number of patients. If it is the case that one treatment is better than another then not only will fewer people die (or whatever), but the average length of time between treatment and death may be longer. Thus, to compare only numbers of deaths may miss an important advantage of therapy. Efficient and easy methods for utilising time to an untoward event in clinical trials have been described by Peto et al (1976, 1977).

We have spent much time discussing the role of chance and of selection in misleading clinical opinion and it is as well to end with an example which illustrates the extent of the possible influence of undefined aspects of compliance or simply poorly understood biological mechanisms. The Coronary Drug Project (1973) experience is an example of the hazards associated with selecting sub-groups of patients according to their compliance with therapy (Coronary Drug Project Research Group, 1980). In fact it raises a number of very perplexing questions of a general nature. It was a double-blind, randomised, placebo controlled trial of five different drugs in the secondary prevention of coronary heart disease. More than 5500 patients were randomised to each of the five drug groups and nearly 3000 to the placebo group. The patients were men aged 30-64 with a history of myocardial infarction in the previous 3 months. In one drug group, Clofibrate, the 5 year mortality was 20% which was no different from the 5 year mortality in the placebo group. The investigators thought that if they looked only at the patients who took more than 80% of the prescribed dose they might observe a difference in overall mortality between adherers and non-adherers. Indeed they did — it was 15% at 5 years among the former and 25% among the latter. In normal circumstances this would constitute quite convincing evidence in favour of a therapeutic effect for Clofibrate because the difference is highly significant ($P<0.0001$) and cannot be easily attributable to any of three alternative explanations outlined earlier.

Fortunately, however, these investigators also examined the placebo group for a possible effect of adherence and discovered that the 5 year mortality was respectively 15% and 28%. Clearly this is not a therapeutic effect and this piece of evidence immediately contradicts the most obvious inference from the Clofibrate group. It must be said, of course, that the possibility that good placebo adherers are measurably different in terms of known risk factors from non-adherers was investigated. Adjusting for 40 baseline risk factors made little difference to the mortality comparison — it narrowed to 16% versus 26% but remained significant at $P<0.000\,000\,01$. The explanation is not at all clear.

Epilogue

> 'For the simple truth is that truth is often hard to come by, and that once found it may easily be lost again. Erroneous beliefs may have an astonishing power to survive, for thousands of years, in defiance of experience, with or without the aid of conspiracy. The history of science, and especially of medicine, could furnish us with a number of examples.'
>
> Karl R. Popper,
> Conjectures and Refutations

REFERENCES

Anturane Reinfarction Trial Research Group 1978 Sulfinpyrazone in the prevention of cardiac death after myocardial infarction. New England Journal of Medicine 298: 289-295

British Medical Journal 1979 2: 1244-1245

Chalmers T C, Matta R J, Smith H, Kinzher A M 1977 Evidence favouring the use of anticoagulants in the hospital phase of acute myocardial infarction. New England Journal of Medicine 297: 1091

Coronary Drug Project Research Group 1973 The coronary drug project: design methods and baseline results. Circulation Suppl. 1:I. 47-48

Coronary Drug Project Research Group 1980 Influences of adherence to treatment and response of cholesterol on mortality in the coronary drug project. New England Journal of Medicine 303: 1038-1041

Doll R, Peto R 1980 Randomised controlled trials and retrospective controls. British Medical Journal 1: 44

Fleiss J 1973 Statistical methods for rates and proportions. Wiley, Interscience

Gehan E A, Freineich E J 1974 Non-randomised controls in cancer clinical trials. New England Journal of Medicine 290: 198-203

Kolata G B 1980 FDA says no to Anturane. Science 208: 1130-1132

Kranberg L 1977 Do retrospective controls make clinical trials 'inheritantly' fallacious. British Medical Journal 2: 1265-1266

Lachin J M 1981 An introduction to sample size determination and power analysis for clinical trials. Controlled Clinical Trials 2: 93-113

Lee K L, McNeer J F, Stanmer C F et al 1980 Clinical judgement and statistics: Lessons from a simulation randomised trial in coronary artery disease. Circulation 61: 508-515

New England Journal of Medicine 1979 301: 836-837

Peto R, Pike M C, Breslow N E et al 1976 Design and analysis of randomised clinical trials requiring prolonged observation of each patient. 1 Introduction and design. British Journal of Cancer 34: 585–612

Peto R, Pike M C, Breslow N E et al 1977 Design and analysis of randomised clinical trials requiring prolonged observation of each patient. 2 Analysis and Examples. British Journal of Cancer 35: 1–32

Pocock S J 1977 Randomised clinical trials. British Medical Journal i: 1661

Temple R, Pledger G W 1980 The FDA's critique of the Anturane reinfarction trial. New England Journal of Medicine 303: 1488–1492